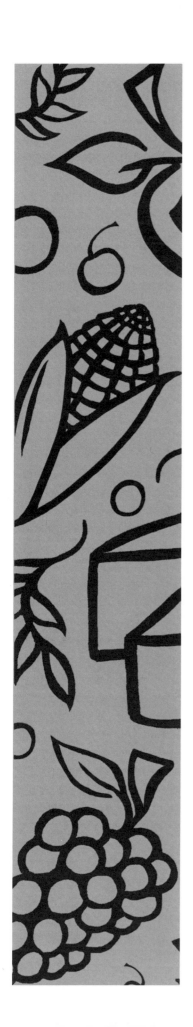

"I am truly impressed after finishing my review of the excellently written book, 'The Executive Chef's Arthritis Cookbook and Health Guide' by Chef Prentiss Carl Haupt and Dr. James McKoy. As a rheumatologist, I was most delighted with the review of those medical conditions which are so common in medical practice these days (fibromyalgia, chronic fatigue syndrome, etc.). Dr. McKoy's comprehensive overview of these conditions, along with modern management principles, adds tremendous depth to the book. Chef Haupt and Dr. McKoy are to be commended for an outstanding job covering a subject which is timely and so poorly understood by many.

"Finally, plaudits to the authors of 'The Executive Chef's Arthritis Cookbook and Health Guide.' I have no doubt that it will become a new and unique reference source for patients and physicians alike."
Peter T. Singleton, MD
Clinical Professor
Stanford University Medical Center

"A comprehensive book that addresses the many facets of food preparation for sufferers of arthritis, from nutritional concerns to cooking methods. A practical guide for those who want to improve their health through the food they consume."
Ferdinand E. Metz, Certified Master Chef
President, The Culinary Institute of America

"'The Executive Chef's Arthritis Cookbook and Health Guide' is a wonderful example of how appropriate changes in diet and nutrition can have profound effects on alleviating the causes and symptoms of arthritis. Executive Chef Prentiss Carl Haupt and nationally known rheumatologist Dr. James McKoy have created a 'delicious' guide to naturally treating arthritis. So often we forget that what we eat has a direct biochemical effect on key 'modulator molecules' (enzymes, cytokines, eicosanoids, and hormones) that can either lessen the symptoms of arthritis or aggravate them. By combining healthy dietary habits with the appropriate use of nutritional supplements, the authors have given arthritis patients an enjoyable guide to alleviating their pain and suffering."
Joseph Pepping, PharmD
Co-Director, Integrative Medicine Service
Kaiser Permanente Medical Center, Hawaii

"Prentiss Carl Haupt, CEC has created a resource for those suffering from arthritis that offers an approach to combining wellness and eating well. 'The Executive Chef's Arthritis Cookbook and Health Guide' will benefit those looking to learn about the nutritional effects of food and how to incorporate these recipes into everyday living."
L. Tim Ryan, Certified Master Chef
Executive Vice President, The Culinary Institute of America

"I was fortunate to receive training in rheumatology from Dr. McKoy earlier in my career. I appreciated his enthusiasm and desire to share his knowledge in rheumatology. He has put some of that wisdom into this book, which I found both educational and easy to read. The content is clinically focused and provides the appropriate level of information for the average patient. Dr. McKoy also gives useful perspectives on his integrative approach to treating patients with complementary medicine. The book contains charts, tips, and resources which patients as well as professionals will find helpful."
Dr. David Finger, M.D., Chief, Rheumatology Service
Tripler Army Medical Center, ` Honolulu, Hawaii

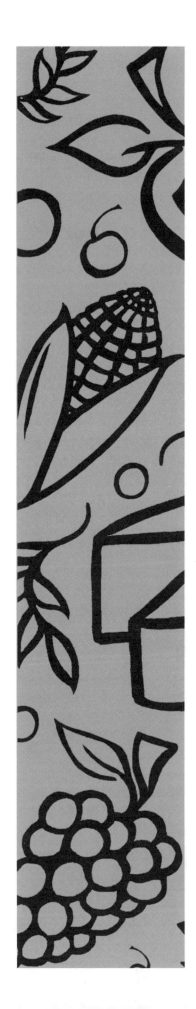

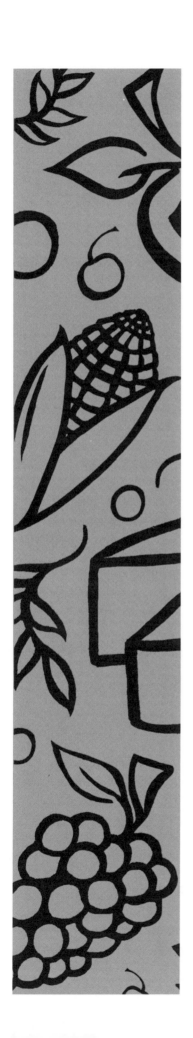

THE EXECUTIVE CHEF'S
ARTHRITIS COOKBOOK
AND
HEALTH GUIDE

by
Certified Executive Chef
Prentiss Carl Haupt
and
James McKoy, M.D.

The Executive Chef's Arthritis Cookbook and Health Guide
by Executive Chef Prentiss Carl Haupt and James McKoy, M.D.

Published by:
Arthritis Cookbook Corporation
P. O. Box 880130
Pukalani, HI 96768

All rights reserved. No part of this book may be reproduced or transmitted in any form or by any means, electronic or mechanical, including photocopying, recording, or by any information storage and retrieval system without written permission from the authors, except for the inclusion of brief quotations in a review.

Copyright © 2001 by Arthritis Cookbook Corporation
Printed in the United States of America

Publisher's Cataloging-in-Publication

Haupt, Prentiss Carl.
    The executive chef's arthritis cookbook and health guide / by Prentiss Carl Haupt and James McKoy. -- 1st ed.
    p. cm.
    Includes bibliographical references and index.
    LCCN: 00-110239
    ISBN: 0-9700833-1-9 (hrdbk.)
    ISBN: 0-9700833-2-7 (pbk.)

    1. Arthritis--Nutritional aspects. 2. Arthritis--Diet therapy. I. McKoy, James. II. Title.
III. Title: Arthritis cookbook and health guide

RC933.H38 2001   616.7'220654
                           QBI01-200877

DISCLAIMER

This book is not intended as a substitute for the advice of a physician. Readers who suspect they may have specific medical problems should consult a physician about any suggestions that are made in this book.

The term *diet* in this book does not refer to a typical calorie-counting diet. Diet in this book refers to good, fresh, healthy, wholesome food. It also refers to health food store products not related to animal products.

Remember, before trying anything new which involves your health, always consult your physician.

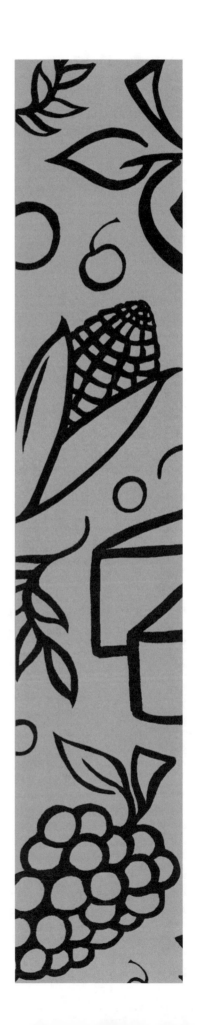

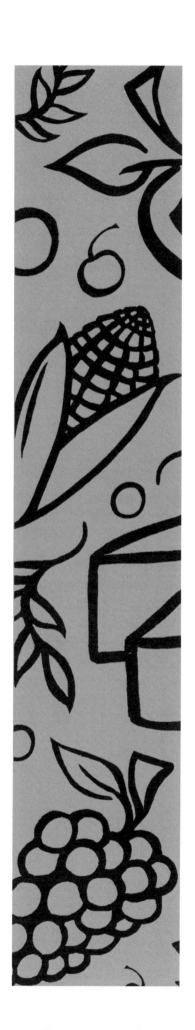

Table Of Contents

Chapter 1	The Facts About Arthritis	19
Chapter 2	Innovative Treatments for the 21st Century	39
Chapter 3	Alternative & Complementary Approaches to Treating Arthritis	49
Chapter 4	Arthritis And Nutrition	67
Chapter 5	The **NO Foods**	85
Chapter 6	Apples And Honey	97
Chapter 7	Facts About Water	105
Chapter 8	Facts About Fats & Roux	117
Chapter 9	Kitchen Tools	125
Chapter 10	Herbs And Spices	135
Chapter 11	Cooking Methods	145
Chapter 12	Stocks and Broths	151
Chapter 13	Sauces, Marinades, and Butters	159
Chapter 14	Appetizers	179
Chapter 15	Soups	187
Chapter 16	Salads and Dressings	205
Chapter 17	Rice and Grains	227
Chapter 18	Potatoes	237
Chapter 19	Facts About Veggies and Garlic	249
Chapter 20	The Beak Recipes	275
Chapter 21	Fin and Seafood Recipes	289
Chapter 22	Desserts	311
Chapter 23	Health Foods	321

Appendices

Table of Equivalents	335
Suggested Weights for Men and Women	336
Bibliography	337
Arthritis Resources	338
Glossary of Arthritis Terms	345
Nutritional Analysis	347
Contact Pages	348
Index	355

ABOUT THE AUTHORS

Prentiss Carl Haupt, Certified Executive Chef

Chef Haupt was born and raised in Pennsylvania. He graduated from Pennsylvania State University, Berks Campus, in 1975. While at Penn State he studied Food Service and Hotel Administration. Soon after graduation he was accepted into the prestigious Culinary Institute of America in Hyde Park, New York. He graduated with the highest honors in 1978.

Upon graduation, Chef Haupt was offered a fellowship at the Culinary Institute. As a fellow he was an Instructional Assistant in the schools Escoffier Room. The Escoffier Room is a four star Mobil Guide restaurant, and is also an Ivy Award winner. The restaurant was named after Auguste Escoffier, the King of Chefs. While Chef Haupt was a fellow, the Escoffier Room was directed by French Master Chef Eugene Bernard, who won numerous gold medals in international cooking competitions. While a student and fellow at the Culinary Institute, Chef Haupt became a protégé of Certified Executive Chef Anthony Gillette, who is a Gold Medal winner in the Culinary Olympics and other international competitions.

Chef Haupt moved to Hawaii in 1979 and has worked in several outstanding restaurants, mainly on Maui. At Chez Paul French Restaurant, he worked as sous chef. He and his fellow Culinary Institute graduate Executive Chef Drew Previti made Chez Paul the talk of Maui and recognized by gourmet eaters as a top restaurant for world travelers.

Chefs Haupt and Previti then helped open and design Erik's Seafood Grotto. Their menu was a silver medal winner in two categories in the Gourmet Guide of Hawaii, for best special and best seafood. From Erik's, Chef Haupt became the Executive Chef at Napili Kai Beach Club's Sea House Restaurant, where he made the restaurant one of the Top 500 Restaurants in America three years in a row in Restaurant Holiday Magazine. Chef Haupt, with his tasty, innovative, and beautifully presented recipes, was one of the true pioneers of Hawaiian Regional Cuisine.

In 1986, Chef Haupt wrote his first cookbook, *Heavenly Hawaiian Recipes: A Glorious Collection of Recipes*. This successful book contains 101 of Chef Haupt's favorite recipes, designed for the home cook, with most products available nationwide.

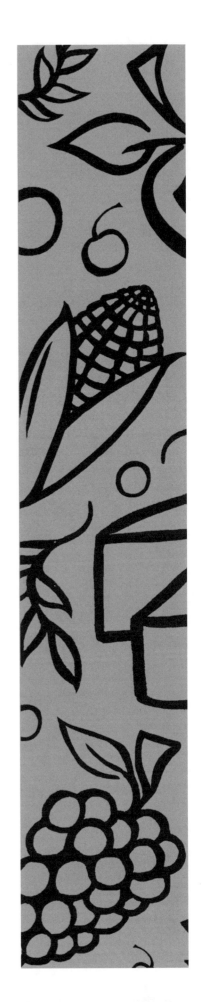

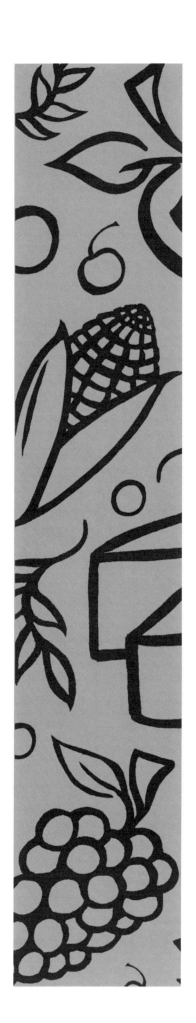

Chef Haupt was asked to teach for the University of Hawaii at Maui Community College, where he suggested the school try for national accreditation through the American Culinary Federation's Educational Institute. In 1990, Maui Community College became the 33rd accredited school in the United States, and the first in Hawaii. A Governor's Recognition award was given to all six instructors who participated in this extremely demanding accomplishment, including Chef Haupt.

In 1991, Chef Haupt's good friend Chef Ron Smith and his family bought the beautiful seaside Waterfront Restaurant in Maalaea Village on Maui. Chefs Haupt and Smith were in the same group at the Culinary Institute of America, and for five years Chef Haupt worked for his friend Chef Ron. Together they made Waterfront Restaurant one of Hawaii's most award winning restaurants.

In 1997, at the tender age of forty-eight, Chef Haupt retired from active cooking to write a cookbook and health guide about arthritis and the correlation between food and arthritis, *The Executive Chef's Arthritis Cookbook and Health Guide.*

At present, Chef Haupt lives on the slopes of Haleakala volcano on Maui, where he continues to write and consult for the food service industry.

James McKoy, M.D.

Dr. James McKoy is a board certified internist and rheumatologist who has been practicing clinical rheumatology since 1981. He served for twenty-two years in the United States Army, sixteen of which were spent primarily teaching residents and students how to optimally manage patients with arthritis. He retired from military service on February 1, 1996, as a full colonel. Since that time he has been in clinical practice at Kaiser Permanente, Hawaii. He is presently Chief of Rheumatology, Chief of the Chronic Pain/Integrative Medicine Program, and Assistant Chief of the Department of Neuroscience.

Dr. McKoy has served as an Associate Clinical Professor of Medicine at John Burns School of Medicine, University of Hawaii. He is on the medical advisory board of *Arthritis Today* magazine and reviews the alternative medicine articles submitted for publication. He also answers the write-in questions from patients on alternative medicine.

Dr. McKoy is a frequent guest on local TV talk and news shows. He often speaks at national medical meetings. His opinion on complementary/alternative care for arthritis is sought after by reporters and health writers around the country. Dr. McKoy has an arthritis holistic practice that includes complementary medicine (vitamins/herbal therapy, aromatherapy, guided visual imagery, massage therapy, thought field therapy, mind-body medicine, and prayer).

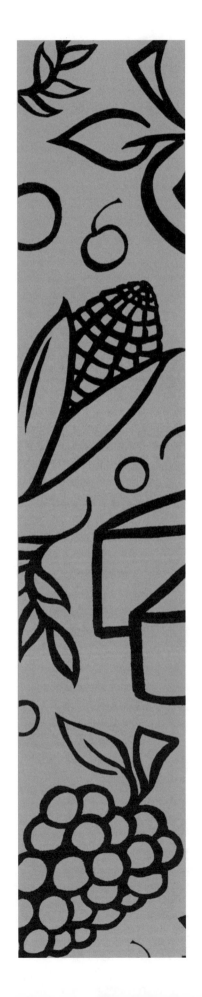

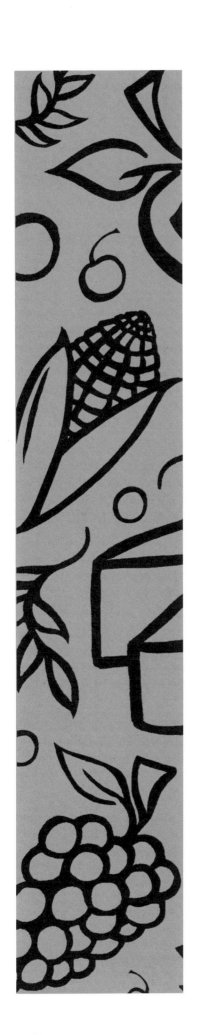

DEDICATION
by Executive Chef Prentiss Carl Haupt

To my mother, Juanita Jameson, who has always stood behind me in whatever I have done.

To my sister, Holly Jacobs, and my brother, Curt Haupt.

To Francine, my other half–without her there would not be a book.

To Master Chef Eugene Bernard and Certified Executive Chef Anthony Gillette, my mentors.

To Kahle Innes, my Pennsylvania State University professor who taught me so much about the industry.

To Thomas E. Walk, CRC, Department of Veterans Affairs Vocational Rehabilitation Specialist, whose support and guidance from the beginning made this project possible.

DEDICATION
By James McKoy, M.D.

To my wonderful wife Gwendolyn and five children Rachel, Rebekah, Joshua, Jonathan, and Abigail who offered suggestions and constantly encouraged me and gave me the time to devote to completing this project. Without their help and encouragement, this book would not have been possible.

To all the patients who have given me the opportunity to be a channel for change in their mental, spiritual, and physical transformations. Most of the knowledge, tips, and cases needed to make this an informative and interesting book have come from those who have touched me in a special way.

ACKNOWLEDGEMENTS
by Executive Chef Prentiss Carl Haupt

I would like to take this time to say a big mahalo or, as I always say, Thank You Very Much! for all the time and effort of all the fine professional people who helped us with our book.

Thomas E. Walk, CRC, Vocational Rehabilitation Specialist, Department of Veterans Affairs
Thomas fully believed in our project and was instrumental in getting us funding through the Vocational Rehabilitation for Disabled Veterans program. Thomas' favorite banana bread recipe is included in this book. Thank You Very Much!

Ed Gavigan, VRC Officer, Department of Veterans Affairs
Ed is Thomas Walk's boss. He also believed in our project and gave the OK for all the monies involved. Thank You Very Much!

David Fisher, MBA, Center Director, Hawaii SBDC Network
David was our first contact. He led Carl to the Maui Writers Conference and to Keith Gilchrist of The Mindworks, who has been his consultant for the project. Thank You Very Much!

Terry Conlon, Librarian, Kahului Public Library
Terry was a great asset in helping getting information needed for this book. Thank You Very Much!

Carla Mauri, Librarian, Makawao Public Library
Carla was of great assistance with locating material necessary for this book. Thank You Very Much!

Ferdinand Metz, Certified Master Chef, President, The Culinary Institute of America
I want to personally thank Ferdinand once again for his wonderful professional support and comments on the book. Thank You Very Much!

Mary Gilchrist, Shakti Creations
Mary did many of the wonderful drawings you see in the book. Thank You Very Much!

Tim Ryan, Certified Master Chef, Vice President, The Culinary Institute of America
Tim, again Thank You Very Much! for your great professional support and comments on the book.

Donnie McGean and Michele Heick, Hawaiian Moons Natural Foods
Thank you for all the help with the health food chapter.

Jethro Kloss, Back to Eden Books® Publishing Company
The information provided in *Back to Eden* is a valuable part of this book. Jethro Kloss was a true hero for his devotion to the betterment of mankind. Thank You Very Much! to the Kloss Family.

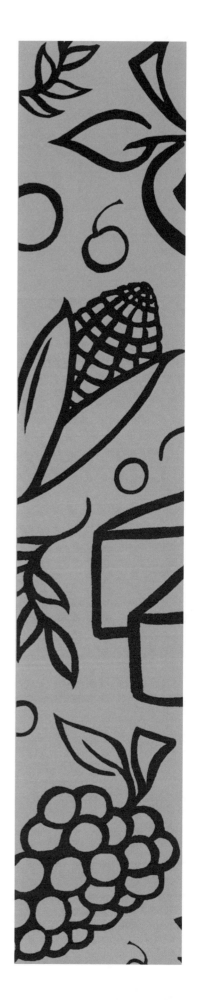

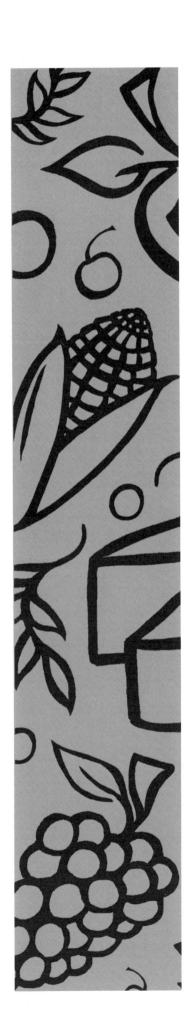

Phyllis A. Balch, CNC, and James F. Balch, MD, PAB Books, Inc.
What a great wealth of information and help these authors of *Prescription for Dietary Wellness* have provided to people looking to better their own health in today's world. Thank You Very Much! for allowing me to use your work.

Mary Hermann, Marketing Director, National Honey Board
A great big mahalo to Mary for all the information she provided about honey for Chapter 6. What a great resource! Thank You Very Much!

Jan Lisa Goo Potratz and Ruth Goodfellow, Agape Design
The wonderful people at Agape Design, Jan Lisa the owner and Ruth the artist, are responsible for the beautiful front and back covers of the book and all the chapter cover pages as well. The time and dedication they gave to our project is very valuable to us. Thank You Very Much!

Siobhan Halsted, Manager, Down to Earth Natural Foods
Siobhan is truly dedicated, with a great knowledge of her field which she is always willing to share with others. Thank You Very Much! for all your help writing the product descriptions and brand names for the health food chapter.

Keith Gilchrist, The Mindworks
Keith has worked on this project with us since we first got the grant to do the book. He was such a very valuable part of this book from start to finish that 1,000 Thank You Very Muches! would only begin to thank him.

**Karen Tanaka, MEd Educational Administration,
Certified Culinary Educator, Food Service Program Director,
University of Hawaii, Maui Community College**
Thank You Very Much! to my great friend and former boss for the wonderful professional comments and support she gave us for the book.

**Robert Santos, Certified Culinary Educator, Chef Instructor,
University of Hawaii, Maui Community College**
My lifelong true friend and fellow student at the Culinary Institute of America took the time to read the book page by page and offer his valuable insights to the betterment of our project. Thank You Very Much, Bobby!

The Culinary Institute of America, Hyde Park, NY
The recipes I learned in my first class with Chef White at The Culinary Institute of America gave me the foundation for my cooking career and some of the recipes in this book. Thank You Very Much!

**Leigh Delozier, Director, Consumer Publications,
Arthritis Foundation**
Thank You Very Much! for permission to use information from the Arthritis Foundation.

ACKNOWLEDGEMENTS
by James McKoy, M.D.

**Dr. Peter T. Singleton, M.D., Clinical Professor,
Stanford University Medical Center**
I am grateful to Dr. Peter T. Singleton, my mentor and inspiration to become an arthritis specialist.

**Dr. Joseph Pepping, PharmD, Nutritional Pharmacologist,
Co-Director Integrative Medicine Service, Kaiser Hawaii,
and Founder of the Wellness Institute International**
I thank my good friend Dr. Joe Pepping who over the years has shared his stories, knowledge of herbs, vitamins, nutrition, and principles of wellness.

**Susan Milton, Program Director,
Arthritis Foundation, Hawaii Branch**
I thank Susan for reviewing this book and sharing her knowledge and insight, and for being a valuable resource to me in planning conferences for patients and physicians so I can share my integrative approach to treating arthritis

**Valerie Matsunaga, PharmD, Manager, Pharmaceutical Services,
Kaiser Permanente Medical Center, Hawaii**
Valerie is the hardest working and most disciplined woman that I know. I thank her for her professional and personal support. I really appreciate the time she took out of her busy schedule to devote to this book.

**Dr. David Finger. M.D., Chief, Rheumatology Service,
Tripler Army Medical Center, Hawaii**
Dr. Finger was one of my most outstanding trainees. I would like to thank him for his professional support and comments on this book.

**Karen Lee, Attorney at Law,
Board of Directors of the Arthritis Foundation, Hawaii Branch**
Karen is a delightful woman whose counsel and great wisdom I appreciate.

**Dr. Bernard Robinson, M.D., Chief, Department of Neuroscience,
Kaiser Permanente Medical Center, Hawaii**
Dr. Robinson is a skilled neurosurgeon, administrator, and leader who is very creative and knows how to bring together the necessary resources to do the impossible. I thank him for all his support and encouragement over the many years that I have known him.

Alicia Rivero
Alicia is a friend of many talents. She assists me with computer graphics for the many lectures that I do around the country. She did the computer graphic for the cornucopia on the front cover and the traditional and alternative treatment charts. I can never thank her enough for all that she does for me.

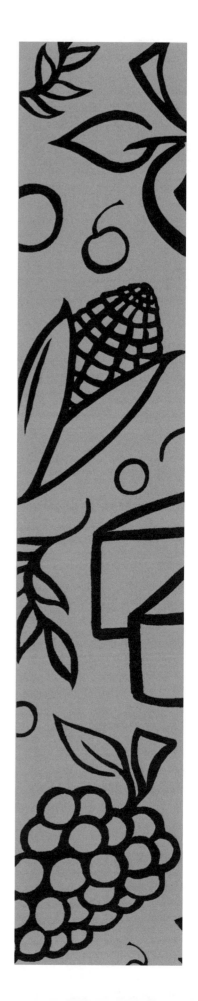

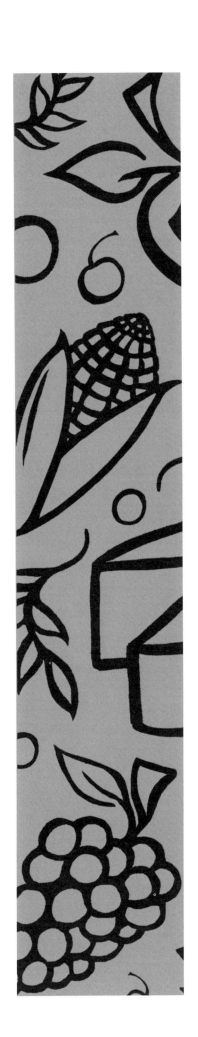

Dr. Wayne E. Anderson, Pastor of the City of Refuge Christian Church, Hawaii

I thank Dr. Anderson, who is my Pastor and my friend for his prayers and encouragement over the years. Through his anointed teaching and preaching, I have come to believe that all things are possible. About ten years ago, by way of prophecy, he planted a seed that I would begin to put what I do in writing. This book is the first fruits of that seed.

FOREWARD
by James McKoy, M.D.

This book is part of our commitment to provide useful information that will help you develop a healthier lifestyle. We want to give you the tools that will enable you to live well with arthritis. Long-term good health requires a commitment to take care of yourself and a willingness to improve in every way. Simple changes can have a profound impact on your arthritis.

By focusing on nutrition, you can join the people around the world that are already reaching increasing levels of success as they work to alleviate/minimize the effects of arthritis and improve their overall health. Through nutrition we can help you look better, feel better, and live better. Modern medicine ignores the fact that many of our common degenerative diseases could be prevented or cured by lifestyle changes, nutrition, and the appropriate use of nutritional supplements. Research shows that fruits and vegetables can enhance the immune system and protect against arthritis. Hippocrates said, "Let thy food be thy medicine and let thy medicine be thy food."

This book is designed to assist you in taking charge of your life as you become knowledgeable about the need for and role of optimal nutrition and supplements for arthritis. Knowledge and lifestyle changes are essentially today's medicine for a healthier tomorrow, for what you do today will determine your tomorrow.

FOREWARD
by Executive Chef Prentiss Carl Haupt

In life, you have to look for an idea that excites you–something that will help mankind, while it keeps on exciting you for years to come.

I was brought up with good Christian values. We went to church quite a bit. When I was fifteen I only went to church on special occasions such as Easter and Christmas. I used to ask a lot of questions, especially about belief. I never believed that God whispered in anyone's ear. I used to think people who claimed He did were crazy, or braggarts who wanted to show normal people that they were better than we were. Little did I know...

After I returned home from Vietnam with the Marine Corps, I didn't have time for church. Being a college student, paying my own way, plus working fifty or more hours a week (especially Sundays!) didn't allow me much time for church.

I had always noticed how happy my beloved sister Holly was. She told me I was missing something special. Boy, she was right. About 12 years ago I returned to church. I have never looked back. I really enjoy everything about it, but I still didn't believe God talked to anyone.

On Christmas Eve, 1996, God whispered in my ear. I was crying and didn't know why. He told me to do the project I had in mind–a book about how food affects people with arthritis. He told me that He would help me in any way I needed help. Francine asked me why I was crying, but I was speechless and couldn't answer. Later, I told her what had happened.

Since then I received a grant from the Veterans Administration to fund this project. Everyone I asked has helped me and given me permission to use their materials. Thank you, everyone. God was right!! And He does whisper in people's ears. With God on our side, how can we go wrong? *The Executive Chef's Arthritis Cookbook and Health Guide* is the project that enables me to keep experimenting with foods that seem to help arthritis sufferers, and the subject continues to excite me.

We have many things in the works:

- A web page (www.arthritiscookbook.com)
- Salt substitute you can buy at the grocery store
- A video of people with arthritis who cook, and their hints and tips

Plus much more as time passes. We've only just begun!

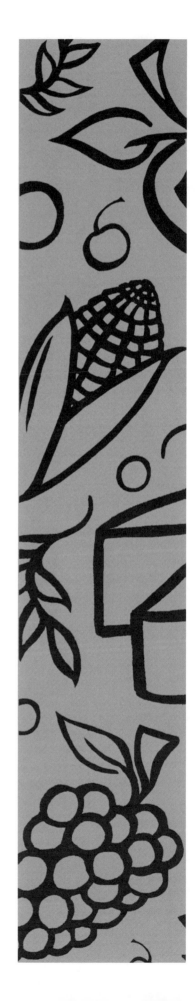

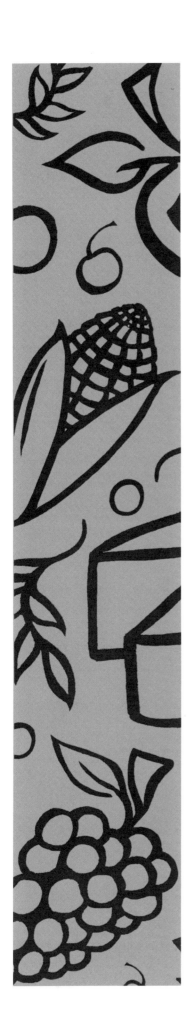

PREFACE
by Pastor Vernon Tom

Aloha Pumehana,

In the gracious Hawaiian language, that means "warm-hearted affection." Isn't that what happens when people gather around food, especially in Hawaii? Eating in an atmosphere of warmth nurtures the soul as well as the body. In Hawaii getting together to eat is a fine art that specializes in making people feel welcomed and loved. The phrase *E komo mai* means "come on in, kick back, and feel at home." Native Hawaiians were the host nation that welcomed all other ethnic groups to Hawaii many years ago, and today local people have learned to do the same to anyone else. So that is why I write in loving support of Carl Haupt's cookbook. It is in affirmation of a wonderful ministry of gathering people in the love and mercy of God.

The Bible tells in the book of Genesis of how God created foods of all kinds, for human beings' sustenance and total enjoyment. Human beings from Adam and Eve on are given the mandate to take care of the earth. That does not mean to subjugate in exploitation, but to truly care for all of creation as a gift from God. It is such a splendor to see the varieties of plant and animal life God created for our enjoyment, living together in harmony. Out of that system we carefully take only what we need for physical sustenance.

In Hawaii we are able to enjoy such a wide variety of dishes, because so many ethnic groups have learned to live together in harmony. Some of us crave "local food" when we are away from the islands. The best metaphor to describe our ethnic mix of peoples is stew: each ingredient adding flavor to the total dish but retaining individual identity. In Hawaii stew can include meat, potatoes, celery, and carrots, but also kim chee, kamaboko, Portuguese sausage, eggplant, and anything else local people enjoy. Praise God for creating such *ono* ("delicious") foods for our enjoyment.

The Bible also talks about taking care of our health. That includes the body, soul, and spirit according to I Thessalonians 5:23, "May your whole spirit, soul, and body be kept blameless at the coming of our Lord Jesus Christ." For the spirit, that means being reconciled to God the Father through Jesus Christ's death on our behalf for the forgiveness of sins. For the soul, that means good mental health and nurturing of human emotions that enrich all of life. For the body, that means proper exercise and a complete diet of food that takes care of all the body's nutritional needs. St. Ireneus put it all together when he said, "The glory of God is the human being fully alive!"

Speaking personally, that also means I spend time in prayer and reflection of the Word of God, loving my wife and children and caring for their needs, a well-balanced diet, and regular disciplined exercise. That includes an hour on the treadmill three to four times a week, and tennis and golf once a week. I have never felt healthier in my life, and I give all of this high priority because God calls me to a careful stewardship of a whole and healthy life on earth. How blessed we are with all the resources God provides so we can live an abundant life on earth. When we go on to the fullness of heaven we can hear our dear God welcome us with the words, "Well done, thou good and faithful servant."

So read on, and enjoy all the recipes in my friend Carl's good book!

Pastor Vernon Tom
Po'okela Church
September 18, 2000

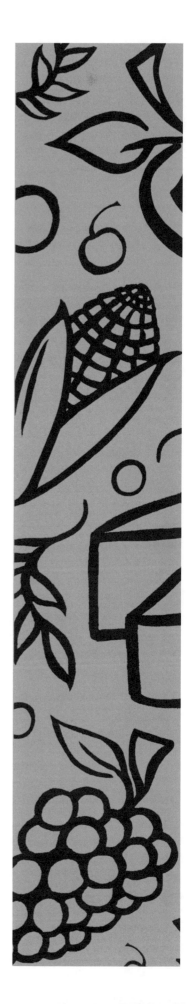

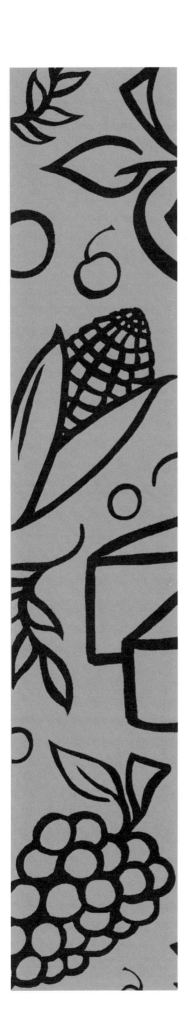

KITCHEN PRAYER

Bless my little kitchen, Lord
I love its every nook.
And bless me as I do my work,
Wash pots and pans and cook.
May the meals that I prepare,
Be seasoned from above,
With Thy blessings and Thy grace,
But most of all Thy love.
As we partake of earthly food,
The table Thou has spread,
We'll not forget to thank Thee, Lord,
For all our daily bread.
So bless my little kitchen, Lord,
And those who enter in;
May they find naught but joy and peace,
And happiness therein.

              Amen.

                    Anonymous

18

THE FACTS ABOUT Arthritis

CHAPTER 1

20

THE FACTS ABOUT ARTHRITIS
by James McKoy, M.D.

Arthritis is among the most chronic medical conditions in the United States. It is a leading cause of activity limitation, and has a substantial impact on healthcare resources. Arthritis affects approximately forty million people in the United States. By the year 2020, over sixty million people will be affected by arthritis. Twenty-one million people are presently suffering from the clinical signs and symptoms of osteoarthritis (OA) or degenerative joint disease (DJD). Approximately 2.1 million people are suffering from rheumatoid arthritis (RA).

Each year 31.5 million patients visit their doctor for arthritis related symptoms, eight million are hospitalized. More than seventeen million people, 42% of those with arthritis, are limited in their daily activities. The prevalence of activity limitation increases with aging. The total annual cost for caring for patients with arthritis is approximately $150 billion a year. That's approximately 2.5% of the yearly gross national product (GNP). The following is a brief overview of four of the most common disorders affecting bones, joints, and surrounding tissues.

Osteoarthritis

Osteoarthritis (OA) is the most common form of joint disorder and leading cause of disability in the United States. Osteoarthritis is usually described as joint "wear and tear" but can be more complex. Biomechanical stress to the joint can lead to a chain of chemical events that cause destruction of the joint cartilage and the appearance of the clinical signs and symptoms of OA. Risk factors for the development of osteoarthritis include advancing age, obesity, quadriceps muscle weakness, joint overuse or injury, athletic activity, developmental abnormalities, and a small percentage occur from genetic predisposition. Twelve percent of the adults over the age of twenty-five have symptomatic OA and this percentage increases sharply with advancing age. Osteoarthritis is more common in women but osteoarthritis of the knee is more common in men. Women are generally affected at a younger age than men are. Osteoarthritis more often affects older people (85% of the population will be affected by OA by age seventy). Osteoarthritis can co-exist with other forms of arthritis.

Signs and Symptoms of Osteoarthritis

Osteoarthritis predominantly affects the hands (base of thumb and distal fingers), spine, hips, and knees. It is characterized by the progressive deterioration of the joint cartilage. As the arthritis progresses, the joint cartilage thins and softens and begins to break down. Inadequate attempts to repair the deteriorating cartilage causes thickened, irregular bony formation and osteophytes (bone spurs). The degenerative changes produce a variety of signs and symptoms. Patients may complain of pain, swelling, crepitus (grinding), deformity, and limitation of motion of various joints.

Pain is the most pronounced symptom of OA. Pain is increased by joint use and relieved by rest. Pain may become more persistent as the arthritis progresses. Stiffness may be experienced after periods of inactivity, especially on awakening in the morning which might last for approximately thirty minutes. On examination, the doctor might find crepitus, which reflects the rubbing of adjacent bones when the joint is moved. Localized tenderness, bony enlargement, and soft-tissue swelling also may be present. In advanced disease, there is deformity, bony enlargement, and malalignment of the joint and marked loss of joint motion. These effects contribute to the disability, pain, and suffering associated with osteoarthritis. Sometimes, your doctor may order certain tests to help confirm the diagnosis, to determine how much joint damage exists, or to distinguish between different types of arthritis. These tests may include x-rays, blood tests, or joint fluid tests.

Treatment

The goals of arthritis therapy are to relieve pain and inflammation, minimize risks of therapy, retard disease progression, provide patient education, prevent work disability, and enhance the quality of life and functional independence. Drug therapy for osteoarthritis ranges from simple analgesics to investigational agents such as minocycline. The drug of choice widely used for pain in OA is Extra Strength Tylenol (two tablets by mouth three to four times a day). For inflammatory phases of OA, non steroidal anti-inflammatory drugs (Motrin, Naprosyn, Voltaren, etc.) are generally used. Topical agents such as capsaicin and Penetran Plus can be rubbed on the joints for pain relief. Heat or cold can provide temporary relief of symptoms. Heat helps relax aching muscles and relieve joint pain and soreness, and cold helps by decreasing pain and swelling. An ice pack should be applied if there is swelling because it helps constrict blood vessels and reduce swelling.

For severe pain and inflammation, a powerful anti-inflammatory drug, called corticosteroid, can be injected directly into the affected joint. An injection can provide almost immediate relief for a tender, swollen, and inflamed joint. However, this treatment can only be used safely about three times in the same joint over a one-year period. Too frequent injection of corticosteroids can

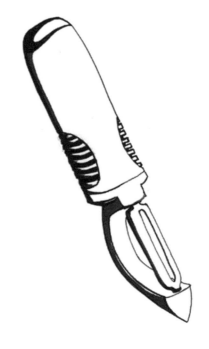

Large-Handled Vegetable Peeler
You can buy a large-handled vegetable peeler or build up the handles on yours and take a lot of pain and strain out of this chore.

Chapter 1 The Facts About Arthritis 23

weaken the cartilage and de-mineralize (and weaken) the bone, resulting in further joint weakness. Physical therapy for muscle strengthening and range of motion exercises with appropriate mechanical devices can be very beneficial in relieving pain and improving use of involved joints. Some people with severe, advanced OA may require surgery. The benefits of surgery can include less pain and better movement and function. Arthroscopic surgery can be used to clean cartilage debris from the joint or remove osteophytes. Surgery can be used to fuse joints, rebuild part of a joint, or completely replace the joint.

Rheumatoid Arthritis

Rheumatoid arthritis (RA) is an autoimmune disease in which the body's immune system attacks healthy joint linings and other body tissues causing inflammation and damage. Rheumatoid arthritis is a chronic, progressive disease affecting more than 2.1 million Americans. It is most common between ages twenty to fifty years of age. There are genes such as HLA-DR antigens, which play a role in some people being more susceptible to the arthritis. Women are two to three times as likely as men to have rheumatoid arthritis. Over the age of seventy, men and women develop rheumatoid arthritis at about the same frequency.

Rheumatoid arthritis is one of the most serious, disabling, and common forms of arthritis. It is characterized by the inflammation of the membrane lining the joint, which causes pain, stiffness, warmth, redness, and swelling. Some patients describe it as "a firestorm in my body." The inflamed joint lining, the synovium, can invade and damage bone and cartilage. Inflammatory cells release enzymes that may digest or eat away bone and cartilage. The involved joint will eventually lose its shape and alignment resulting in deformities, loss of motion, decreased strength, mechanical pain, and loss of useful function of the involved joint.

Research suggests that rheumatoid arthritis occurs because of a genetic predisposition coupled with an as yet unknown environmental trigger. Viruses and bacterial infections have been considered as possible trigger agents for rheumatoid arthritis. I truly believe that stress, poor nutrition, food allergies, sleep deprivation, toxins, and chemicals play a major role in causing or aggravating rheumatoid arthritis.

Symptoms

Patients complain of pain and stiffness and of having difficulty in making a fist and walking upon first getting up in the morning. Rheumatoid arthritis is predominantly a symmetric small joint arthritis, involving the hands, wrists, and small joints of the feet.

Even the small bones of the ear and temporal mandibular joint can be involved. RA can also involve large joints such as shoulders, knees, and hips.

The signs and symptoms of rheumatoid arthritis occur in the joints and throughout the body. The joint manifestations of RA consist of reversible signs and symptoms related to inflammation of the joint lining that can lead to irreversible structural damage. Pain, stiffness, and soft tissue swelling around the joint are early findings of RA. The second and third fingers of the hands are most commonly involved. Some patients might have associated low-grade fevers, weight loss, fatigue, and bone thinning (osteoporosis). Patients who have had arthritis for ten to fifteen years may suffer from dry eyes, dry mouth, enlargement of the salivary glands, scar tissue (fibrosis) of the lungs, inflammation around the heart, and inflammation of blood vessels.

Evaluation

Accurate history, physical exam, laboratory tests, and x-rays will help to make the diagnosis. Early referral to a rheumatologist is recommended. X-rays can be helpful in making a diagnosis of rheumatoid arthritis. X-rays can show increased joint space secondary to effusion and later show joint space narrowing secondary to cartilage destruction, malalignment, bone thinning, and erosions. Destructive joint changes can be seen as early as four months from the beginning of the disease.

Laboratory tests such as rheumatoid factor (RF), erythrocyte sedimentation rate (ESR), and complete blood count (CBC) can be very helpful. Rheumatoid factor can be present in 70 to 80% of patients. High titers correlate with a poorer prognosis. ESR is a measurement of inflammation in the body. Prolonged elevation of ESR also correlates with a poorer prognosis. Most patients with chronic inflammation will develop an anemia that is seen on the CBC. The anemia correlates with severity and chronicity of the inflammation.

Poor prognosis in rheumatoid arthritis is suggested by earlier age at onset, female patient, high titer rheumatoid factor, elevated erythrocyte sedimentation rate, swelling of more than twenty joints, early appearance of erosions, early involvement of large joints, and extra-articular manifestations of RA. These manifestations include rheumatoid nodules on places like the elbows, dry eyes, dry mouth, inflammation of eyes, lung involvement, inflammation of the heart, inflammation of blood vessels and involvement of various organs like spleen and bone marrow (Felty's Syndrome).

Diagnosis of the Disease

The diagnosis is generally made by a set of criteria established by the American College of Rheumatology (ACR). These criteria are as follows: 1) morning stiffness in and around joints lasting at least one hour before maximal improvement; 2) at least 3 joint areas simultaneously have had soft tissue swelling or fluid; 3) soft-tissue swelling (arthritis) of the finger or wrist joints; 4) symmetric joint swelling (arthritis); 5) radiographic erosions and/or thinning of the bone around the small joints; 6) rheumatoid nodules (lumps consisting of inflammatory scar-like tissue on surfaces like the elbow); and, 7) the presence of an abnormal amount of rheumatoid factor in the blood. Criteria 1 through 4 must have been present for at least six weeks. In order to have a definitive diagnosis of rheumatoid arthritis (RA), you must have four or more of the seven criteria.

Management of Rheumatoid Arthritis

The goals of therapy of rheumatoid arthritis focus on reducing swelling, relieving pain and stiffness, maintaining normal joint function in daily activities, and improving the quality of life. Current management strategies include early diagnosis, rapid assessment of likely prognosis and initiation of appropriate therapy, early use of effective disease modifying anti-inflammatory rheumatic drugs (DMARDs), and appropriate use of physical therapy and occupational therapy.

In the past, drug management of RA has been based on treatment with non-steroidal anti-inflammatory drugs (NSAIDs), with DMARDs administered to most patients only in the later phases of the disease. Now a more aggressive approach is being recommended, with the introduction of DMARDs early in the course of the arthritis. The first line of drug therapy is usually a non-steroidal anti-inflammatory drug (NSAID) such as Motrin, Naprosyn, Relafen, Voltaren or a COX-2 (celebrex,vioxx). The NSAIDs have a rapid suppressive effect through blocking several enzymes (cyclo-oxygenase and prostaglandins), thereby reducing pain, stiffness, and inflammation. A new class of drugs similar to these called the Cyclo-oxygenase pathway #2 inhibitors will be discussed later. Corticosteroids (prednisone) can be used to decrease pain, stiffness, and swelling while waiting for effective DMARD therapy to be established. Corticosteroids are often given by mouth or within the joint or muscle. In patients with RA, early use of disease-modifying drugs may allow control of the disease.

Disease modifying drugs include methotrexate (MTX), Plaquenil (hydroxychloroquine), Azulfidine, cyclosporine, Arava (lefluno-

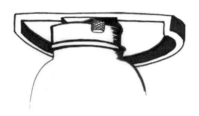

Under-Cabinet Jar Opener
This easy to use jar opener mounts under your cabinet and will open jars from 3/8˜ to 3˜ with hardly a twist of the wrist.

mide), Enbrel, Remicade, and Anakinra. These drugs may be used in combination, i.e., MTX and Plaquenil; or MTX, Plaquenil, and Azulfidine; or MTX and Enbrel. Single dose therapy should be titrated to maximum dose before adding another drug. DMARDs act by a variety of means, with the common mechanism of inhibiting proinflammatory cytokines, the most inflammatory and destructive cells.

While some patients have been able to alleviate the pain of arthritis through medications, exercise, proper diet, and physical therapy, it's sometimes necessary to seek a more permanent solution to the problem Corrective surgery is available for joints that are damaged and painful. Joints can be replaced and in some cases deformities can be corrected. Most often hip or knee replacement is a possible way for arthritis patients to resume their normal activity and eliminate pain.

Nonpharmacologic Therapy

For the patient, arthritis is a multifaceted problem, so its management must focus on many aspects of life. Drug therapy is essential for reducing chronic pain. Also important are diet and nutrition, physical and vocational therapy, education, patient motivation, and psychosocial counseling. Having a strong support structure from a social worker, a nurse, pastor, and family members is vital to improving quality of life. A variety of treatments that are considered alternative are integrated in my overall treatment plan, including acupuncture, massage, dietary changes, vitamins, herbal supplements, aromatherapy, and mind/body exercises. All are aimed at enhancing the patient's quality of life.

A physician needs to know what type of person is receiving these newer therapies. Each treatment plan is individualized, based on the personality and lifestyle of the patient. My treatment plan includes a structured day of balanced activity and rest, with a given number of hours dedicated to sleep. A therapeutic program that includes low-impact or aquatic exercise is invaluable in maintaining muscle strength and tone. A balance of rest and exercise can help conserve energy and maintain range of motion and use of joints. The stronger the muscle, tendons, and ligaments around joints, the less pain and deformities.

A health care provider must know who a person is before the person is poked with a needle. Effective communication among the patient and members of the healthcare team is an essential part of any treatment program. A cooperative relationship must exist between the physician and the patient so the patient adheres to a mutually agreed upon regimen.

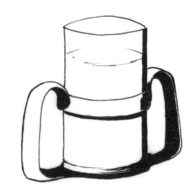

Two-Handled Glass Holder
For people who have a little tremor, this two-handled glass holder makes drinking completely secure.

Nutrition and Arthritis

The relationship between nutrition and arthritis remains elusive because the disease may be caused by many factors, including genetic, environmental, hormonal, viral, bacterial infections, and physical and emotional stress. There is no known specific diet for arthritis. In general, the diet that is right for arthritis is pretty much the diet that is right for everybody with and without arthritis. And most often that means that you have to eat a wide variety of foods in moderation. The more variety you get in your diet, the more chance you will get everything you need for a healthy body and immune system.

For years people have suspected that foods are an important factor in the development of rheumatoid arthritis. There is no question that certain substances in the diet may aggravate or alleviate arthritis symptoms. Many people notice an improvement in their condition when they avoid high protein diets (red meats), high salt intake, preservatives, alcoholic beverages, caffeine, high fat diets, refined sugars, gluten (wheat products), high caloric diets, white flour, citrus fruits, and nightshade plants (tomatoes, eggplant, bellpeppers, etc.). Foods that appear to be helpful in preventing and, in some cases, ameliorating arthritis include more of a vegetarian diet, cold water fish (salmon, mackerel, tuna, herring, etc.), increased water intake, beans, and non-citrus fruits.

Vegetables are rich in antioxidants that can neutralize free radicals. Oxygen free radicals attack many parts of the body and contribute not only to arthritis but heart disease, cancer, and the aging process. High consumption of red meats contributes to arthritis because of the high content of iron and preservatives. Preservatives and iron act as catalysts and encourage the production of dangerous molecules harmful to the joints and tissues.

So-called food allergies or sensitivities have been linked to increased joint pain by evoking an immune response. It has been estimated that such immunologic sensitivities cause joint symptoms in approximately 5 to 10% of patients. Use of an elimination diet can minimize such reactions. An allergy elimination diet might help to identify hidden food allergens that may be causing some or all of your symptoms. During the elimination period, possible common food allergens are eliminated from the diet for two to three weeks. After symptoms improve, foods are added back one at a time to determine which foods provoke symptoms.

There seems to be little doubt that fasting alleviates inflammation. Fasting induces rapid changes in the endocrine and central nervous systems and in the lipids and proteins, all of which are intimately involved in inflammatory reactions. Fasting can modulate the sensation of pain and swelling.

We know that it's often difficult for people with arthritis to prepare meals on a daily basis. This *Executive Chef's Arthritis Cookbook and Health Guide* is an excellent resource for easy to prepare recipes and it's filled with nutritional information. Through the delicious recipes in this book people can be helped to manage their weight and the symptoms of arthritis by eating healthy foods.

Exercise and Arthritis

Regular physical exercise is effective in slowing the age-related, progressive deterioration of biological functions. It is difficult to get people to see the benefit of a regular exercise program when they are suffering from stiffness, pain, weakness, and have retired to a rocking chair. Exercise is a vital part of the overall treatment program for patients with arthritis. Exercise relieves muscle tension, stress, and anxiety. Exercise improves muscle and bone strength, joint mobility and function, posture, balance, and coordination. Exercise also helps to control weight, improve sleep, increase mental alertness, and develop a positive attitude and a better self-image.

Flexibility exercises, strengthening exercises, and aerobic or endurance exercises are the three types of exercises the body needs. Flexibility exercises help to remove morning stiffness and increase the range of motion of the joints. Strengthening exercises help to improve the tone and strength of muscles around joints which helps to reduce pain. Aerobic or endurance exercises contribute to overall fitness, improve energy, and help in weight reduction. Walking is the most common weight-bearing activity and can produce an increase in related bone strength in people of all ages. For those who find walking too painful, exercising in a pool is an excellent alternative. Before starting any exercise program, consult with your doctor. Physical therapists and occupational therapists are trained to examine you and design an exercise program tailored to your needs.

Stress and Arthritis

Stress is the cumulative effects of all the psychological and emotional hits we take daily. The body actually has a physical reaction when it is under pressure and produces the "stress hormones" epinephrine and cortisol, which can cause serious damage to the body. People usually experience the most stress when they're in situations in which they feel they have little or no control. With daily burdens and stresses, too many of us do not take the time and care to eat well, relax, and practice good health habits. Under these conditions, the onslaught of physical disease is inevitable and so the stress continues. Medical science has shown that stress can decrease T-lymphocytes which can contribute to the onset and flares of inflammatory arthritis. None of the possible causes of rheumatoid arthritis rules out the important role that stress may play in its onset and aggravation.

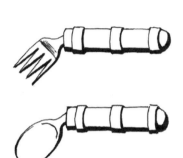

Large-Handled Bent Utensils
The built-up handle and the angle on this spoon and fork remove the strain on your wrist and make eating a pleasure again.

Since 1936, researchers have shown how personality and behavior could affect certain disease syndromes, and how emotional and psychological factors affected various body functions and health. Arthritis or a flare-up may occur because an individual cannot cope with some particularly stressful event, or because their coping response is inappropriate or exaggerated. Socially isolated individuals have higher stress levels and many more illnesses. The mind/body relationship is a two-way street that can strongly influence the course of many illnesses, particularly arthritis. Arthritis itself can be a significant source of stress. There are financial concerns because of doctor bills and medical expenses, possible adverse side effects from medications, and deformities, which have a negative impact on quality of life.

Top 10 Stressors in Arthritis Patients

1. Decreased quality of life by living with chronic pain and suffering
2. Strained male-female relationships caused by decreased sexual enjoyment and not being able to continue doing the customary household chores or attending functions
3. Concern for children's well-being and not being able to be involved in their activities
4. Financial burdens
5. Job pressure because of not being able to perform at the same pace as before
6. Job discrimination
7. Erosion of social values and the impact on families and community
8. Loss of independence, mobility, and function
9. Living with decreased energy
10. Caretaking responsibilities

Many interrelationships exist between stress and arthritis. Chronic stress can make individuals much more sensitive to pain, causing additional stress that intensifies the discomfort. The relief of pain and/or the reduction of stress can relax tense muscles and break the vicious, self-perpetuating cycle.

Evidence suggests that the onset of arthritis flare-ups is often preceded by stressful events. Current research has shown that stress can also have a significant effect on the functioning of the immune system influencing arthritic signs and symptoms, as well as the course of the disease. Several studies suggest that stress is involved in the onset of rheumatoid arthritis and in causing a flare-up of symptoms in people who had been relatively stable and pain free. In one British survey, almost all the women studied reported an emotionally stressful event before the onset of symptoms. The stress was usually some disruptive personal relationship or business problem, the breakup of a love affair, the death of a close friend, or an unpleasant job.

Research has shown that there seems to be more joint destruction in people with sustained high stress versus those with low stress or no stress. People who believe that they have greater control over their health have fewer problems. Relieving pain, developing a sense of control, and improving social support are three of the most effective stress busters for rheumatoid arthritis.

Little research has been devoted to emotional and psychological factors in causing osteoarthritis. Emotional stress does not seem to be as important in osteoarthritis as in rheumatoid arthritis. The stress of loss or separation from a spouse is mentioned most often as a factor in the pain of osteoarthritis. Pain is an important source of stress. In turn, stress intensifies concern about arthritis and causes even more pain.

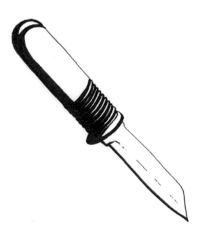

Built-Up Handle Knife
You can build up the handles on your knives with plastic tape or buy one already made, making peeling and cutting much easier.

Stress plays a major role in fibromyalgia/chronic fatigue. There seems to be no clear line that separates the biological versus psychological factors in the manifestations of fibromyalgia. Any form of stress, whether psychological or physical, triggers chemical changes in the body. These changes can lead to the symptoms or exacerbation of pain and the symptoms of fibromyalgia or chronic fatigue.

Reducing stress is one of our best weapons against disease.

Fibromyalgia Syndrome

Fibromyalgia syndrome (FMS) is a relatively common condition with generalized muscular pain and tender points. According to unpublished data from the National Arthritis Data Workgroup, some six million Americans have fibromyalgia, making it one of the most common types of pain syndromes. Over four million of them are women and fewer than two million are men. The name *fibromyalgia* means pain in the muscles and the fibrous connective tissues (the ligaments and tendons). The condition is called a syndrome because it is a set of signs and symptoms that occur together. Although it may feel like a joint disease, it is not a true form of arthritis and does not cause deformities of the joints.

The first indication that fibromyalgia pain had a biologic basis came in 1975 when a pair of Canadian researches described distinct sleep abnormalities in patients with chronic diffuse musculoskeletal pain. In 1990, the American College of Rheumatology (ACR) published a set of criteria for the diagnosis of fibromyalgia. This recognition, coupled with the lobbying efforts of affected patients and their advocates and spurred by a tremendous amount of research, made fibromyalgia a household word. Research has shown that fibromyalgia affects approximately four million Americans and 87% of these are women.

The central feature of fibromyalgia is pain. Recent research points to a central cause of fibromyalgia rather than a primary muscular cause. Pain is believed to be originating from altered central nervous system processing. Biochemical investigations, histochemical, immunologic, and electrophysiologic studies support this claim. There appears to be upregulation for the hypothalamic/pituitary-adrenal axis that causes a stress-like response. Patients with fibromyalgia have been found to have a low level of growth hormone and abnormalities of the thyroid and gonadal axes. Researchers have found elevated levels of substance P, low serotonins, elevated nerve growth factor, and other chemicals that generate pain. There is a correlation between decreased blood flow in the brain and symptoms of fibromyalgia. Small cervical canals have been associated with chronic widespread pain, particularly following whiplash injuries.

The criteria for diagnosis as established by ACR in 1990 are as follows: 1) widespread pain defined as pain above and below the waist, right and left side of the body, and along the midline, of at least three months' duration and, 2) pain upon palpation of at least eleven of eighteen specific tenderpoints. In addition to the ACR criteria, people with fibromyalgia are likely to experience a number of other manifestations such as severe fatigue, difficulty sleeping, joint pain, headaches, weakness, numbness/ tingling, mood swings, memory lapses, and pain in the chest, abdominal, pelvic or rectal area.

Fibromyalgia is not a discrete or unique disease, so the ACR criteria should not be rigidly used. Fibromyalgia may represent the end of a continuum where chronic fatigue is to the far left and decreased pain threshold and generalized pain (fibromyalgia) to the far right. Fibromyalgia frequently coexists with other autoimmune disorders such as rheumatoid arthritis, osteoarthritis, and lupus.

Chronic Fatigue Syndrome

Chronic fatigue syndrome (CFS) was defined in 1994 by specific requirements of severe fatigue lasting for at least six months which impairs daily activity and is not resolved by rest, and exclusion of fatigue associated with malignancy, auto-immune disease, infections, neuropsychiatric disease, endocrine disease, and side effects of medication or other toxic agents. There are nonspecific requirements that must have begun at or after the time of onset of increased fatigue. Symptoms include fever, sore throat, painful lymph nodes, muscle weakness, muscle pain, headaches, migratory joint pains, forgetfulness, inability to concentrate, depression. As you can see there is a lot of overlap between chronic fatigue and fibromyalgia. Fibromyalgia and chronic fatigue syndrome are diagnoses of exclusion where no other diagnosis fits well. I don't try to separate them. On one end of the spectrum, you have chronic fatigue and on the other end you have predominantly a chronic pain syndrome.

Various ideas about the cause of FMS and CFS have been developed in recent years. These include genetic predisposition triggered by another illness, stress, organ injury, neurohumoral deregulation, viral infection, pain amplification disorder, deficiency of sleep, organ system dysfunction, and a psychological or psychiatric disorder. Recent research has not indicated that FMS or CFS is a psychological or psychiatric disorder.

A more recent theory to explain the reason why people get CFS and FMS is dysfunction of coagulation (blood clotting). These patients might have a genetic deficiency for elements which control the clotting system in our blood causing a hypercoagulable state. This hypercoagulable state may not cause clotting but leads to decreased oxygen, nutrient, and cellular passage to tissues causing systemic compromises and symptoms characteristic of CFS/FMS complex. Once this hypercoagulable state is detected, appropriate anticoagulant therapies may be given to relieve patients' symptoms.

Another new theory is that certain bacteria induce the immune system to generate elements causing an abnormal clotting system. Abnormal gut bacteria, staph A bacteria found in the nose, and mycoplasma infections have been associated with the symptoms of fibromyalgia and chronic fatigue. There is clinical evidence now to support an association between various forms of hypotension and chronic fatigue. Research has suggested that patients with CFS have an increased incidence of neurally mediated hypotension and open treatment of this autonomic dsyfunction has been associated with improvement of CFS symptoms.

Within a group of patients who have been diagnosed with fibromyalgia/chronic fatigue, there will be those who, with the proper MRI and neurological exams, prove to have what is called "posterior fossa compression" (Chiari malformation) or a narrowing of the spinal canal called cervical spinal stenosis. Patients with these conditions complain of pain, numbness, and difficulty with concentration and that is why some end up with the diagnosis fibromyalgia. This does not mean that everyone with fibromyalgia/chronic fatigue has this structural defect and not all patients with fatigue and chronic muscle pain should be labeled fibromyalgia/chronic fatigue syndrome.

Although this structural defect is being reported in media as the cause of fibromyalgia/chronic fatigue, that is not the case. Yes, there are patients with constriction of the brain or spinal cord with some symptoms consistent with fibromyalgia, but the numbers of fibromyalgia patients are very low for those who fit the neurological criteria for this structural defect. The treatment for this problem is major brain surgery and some of the operations may be unnecessary and not beneficial. Patients who have had the surgery have touted it a success in relieving some of their symptoms, which has been publicized—creating a lot of interest in desperate patients looking for a miracle cure. This has become a topic of hot debate. More research is needed in this area.

Many patients with fibromyalgia/chronic fatigue are often misdiagnosed and have seen numerous doctors over several years before a correct diagnosis is made. Common conditions that may mimic fibromyalgia include hypothyroidism, lupus, rheumatoid arthritis, and infections. These can usually be excluded by a good history, physical examination, and laboratory tests. Because the diagnosis is often not made and the search continues for a diagnosis and treatment, many patients undergo numerous unnecessary tests and procedures, and some are placed on inadequate and dangerous treatments. Although fibromyalgia does not produce obvious physical impairment, patients perceive themselves as being equally or more incapacitated than are patients with RA.

For the very first time there are unique testing and treatment protocols for FMS/CFS based on the newer theories. Abnormalities of the clotting system can be measured through a company called Hemex, and a company called Bioscreen can test for infections, abnormal fat metabolism, and abnormal amino acid metabolism. If there are abnormalities with the clotting system, anti-clotting agents such as low dose heparin can be used. Antibiotics and other agents can be used to treat infections and to restore normal bacteria flora.

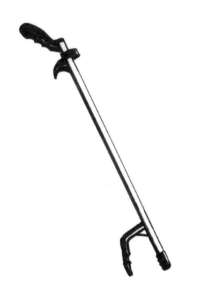

Reacher
A lightweight aluminum reacher takes the strain out of getting objects that are difficult to get to. This one has a magnet for picking up small metal objects.

To effectively treat fibromyalgia and chronic fatigue, the pathogenesis (causative pathways) must be understood. Treatment should be directed to each abnormal pathway. The most important principle of treatment is education that empowers the patient to self-care. Other principles of management include treating background pain, treating pain generators, managing sleep, treating associated syndromes (headaches, restless leg syndrome, premenstrual syndrome, sleep disorders-sleep apnea, muscle cramps, dizziness, and neurally mediated hypotension), managing psychological distress, initiating a physical conditioning program, and cognitive behavior therapy.

Firstline treatment for pain is an NSAID and/or Extra Strength Tylenol. This may not be adequate as a single therapy or even in combination with other drugs like Elavil. Elavil (tricyclic medication) is the most commonly used medication and shows benefits in one month. Not only does it reduce pain by decreasing a pain generator, substance P, but helps you to get into deep restorative sleep. Uses of other antidepressants called serotonin inhibitors (Prozac, Zoloft, Effexor, and Paxil) have been helpful in treating the symptoms of fibromyalgia. If there are a few very severe tender points, injection with procaine (anesthetic) is very helpful. If there is gonadal dysfunction, DHEA and testosterone may be helpful.

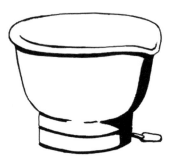

Mixing Bowl with Suction Base
A molded polypropylene bowl mounted on a lever-operated suction base makes mixing a one handed job. The bowl twists off the base for cleaning or serving.

Neurontin (gabapentin) and related compounds have been helpful in treatment of other centrally mediated painful processes and have shown to be beneficial in some patients with fibromyalgia. Growth hormone can be very beneficial in the minority of patients who are deficient in this hormone. It takes six months for growth hormone to have an effect on muscles and to see any improvement. The long wait in improvement and cost of growth hormone prohibit its use. Some doctors use low dose narcotics to manage the pain of fibromyalgia that fails the more conservative pain medications. The concerns about physical dependence, abuse, and addiction prevent many physicians from writing for these agents on a continuous basis. Most well educated and motivated patients will do well with a wholistic approach which is discussed in the alternative section instead of a drug approach.

Osteoporosis

Osteoporosis is the most common human bone disease affecting approximately ten million people in this country, with eighteen million more at increased risk due to low bone mass. One in two postmenopausal white women will experience an osteoporotic fracture in her remaining lifetime. The lifetime risk of hip fracture for a 50-year-old woman today is about 15%. More than 700,000 spine fractures, 200,000 wrist fractures, and 300,000 hip fractures occur each year in the United States, predominantly in postmenopausal women. Osteoporosis is a silent disease process that takes an enormous medical and economic toll on an aging population.

Although osteoporosis is preventable and treatable, its first clinical manifestation is usually a fracture, sometimes a major and disabling one. Osteoporotic fractures create a heavy economic burden. In 1995, 432,000 hospital admissions, almost 2.5 million physician visits, and about 180,000 nursing home admissions in the United States were caused by osteoporotic fractures. Direct medical costs alone for osteoporotic fractures in 1995 were estimated at $13.8 billion. The cost, disability, and deaths associated with osteoporotic fractures will increase with the aging population if this disease is not taken more seriously by patients and physicians. A Gallup survey in 1991 found that three fourths of all women aged 45 to 75—the group at highest risk—had never even discussed osteoporosis with their doctors.

Osteoporosis, once acknowledged as a natural part of aging, does not need to be a consequence of aging any longer. It is largely a preventable disease due to the remarkable progress that has been made in the scientific understanding of its causes, diagnosis, and treatment. Prevention, detection, and treatment of osteoporosis should be a mandate of primary care. There is no longer any reason for a physician or patient to feel that osteoporosis is a hopeless situation.

Osteoporosis is no longer just a disease of elderly women with fractures. Osteoporosis is a disorder of low bone mass which results in thinning of the bone and increased fracture risk. At menopause, lowered estrogen levels cause loss of bone faster than it can be replaced, so there's a drop in bone density or bone thickness. The once healthy bone material is now considerably thinner, pitted, and brittle. Fractures are the complication of osteoporosis that can lead to decreased quality of life and death. As stated before, this is a silent disease without any signs or symptoms until there is a fracture, loss of height, or marked curvature of upper back causing a bent over posture. The most common fractures are those near the hip joint, spine, and distal forearm (wrist). Less than full recovery, severe pain, disability, chronic suffering, and even death can follow these fractures.

There are more deaths associated with the complications of osteoporosis than breast cancer. The most serious outcome of osteoporosis is hip fracture, 10-20% of which can result in death within one year. Up to 25% of hip fracture patients may require long term nursing home care, and only a third fully regain their pre-fracture level of independence. It is possible that the patient

36 The Executive Chef's Arthritis Cookbook and Health Guide

who is at risk for the complications of osteoporosis can be identified early and, with appropriate interventions, these complications can be prevented. If you have no symptoms and are in the age group for osteoporosis, you can ask your doctor to assess your risk factors. If you have any risk factors for osteoporosis, you can ask your doctor if a bone density test is right for you.

Risk Factors

Several risk factors have been associated with the development of osteoporosis, including old age, being female, Caucasian race, being postmenopausal, having a small build, having had late menarche (after 14 years of age) and/or early menopause (before 40 years of age), having had surgical removal of ovaries, poor health, current cigarette smoking, alcoholism, inadequate weight bearing exercise, high protein diet, and soft drinks (phosphate binds calcium). There are secondary causes of osteoporosis, which include a broad range of disease states (i.e., arthritis, removal of stomach, liver disease, diabetes, cancer, poor functioning of the adrenal glands and hyperfunctioning of the thyroid gland), and therapeutic drugs (i.e., corticosteroids, heparin, Dilantin, cancer drugs, excessive thyroxine). Impaired eyesight, dizziness, lack of house safety (throw rugs, floor cords, and slippery bathtubs with no handrail), and muscle weakness cause falls resulting in fractures in the elderly. All patients being considered for drug treatment of osteoporosis should also be counseled on risk factor reduction.

Monitoring, Prevention, and Treatment

Bone mineral density (BMD) testing is a necessary component in evaluating patients with several risk factors for osteoporosis, patients on drugs that contribute to bone loss, and those with medical disorders that contribute to bone loss. The best single predictor of a woman's risk of future fracture is bone density, which can be easily and non-invasively measured through a variety of tests, including dual-energy X-ray absorptiometry (DEXA).

Everyone does not need a bone density study. Generalized screening for osteoporosis is not indicated at menopause. If you are a healthy postmenopausal woman without medical risk factors for osteoporosis who is undecided about, unwilling, or unable to take estrogen, a BMD test would be very useful in the decision to consider preventive measures or alternatives. In most cases, the diagnosis of established osteoporosis (fractures and X-ray evidence of bone thinning) can be made without bone density testing. In these patients, the main reason for BMD testing is to establish a baseline with which therapeutic response can be measured.

Calcium supplementation inhibits bone reabsorption and decreases bone loss. Therefore, patients who are post-menopausal should maintain an adequate calcium intake of approximately 1500mg of calcium a day. Pre-menopausal women should take 1000mg of calcium a day. There are many different brands of calcium. Calcium citrate appears to be better absorbed.

Vitamin D is of benefit especially in patients who are taking corticosteroids. Corticosteroids can cause rapid bone loss and Vitamin D may be of benefit in preventing or reducing this bone loss. Vitamin D, 400-800 IU found in one to two multivitamins is usually adequate. A blood test called 25-Hydroxy D can be done in patients who are on corticosteroids to make sure they are taking adequate amounts of Vitamin D.

Drug Treatment

Federal Drug Administration (FDA) approved drug options for osteoporosis prevention and/or treatment are hormone replacement therapy (HRT), bisphosphonates (alendronate/fosamax, risedronate/actonel), raloxifene, and calcitonin.

Estrogen deficiency must be corrected to prevent bone loss. Studies of HRT indicate an 80% decrease in vertebral fractures and a 25% decrease in hip fractures with five years of use and an anticipated 50-75% decrease in all fractures with ten or more years of use. Based on its effectiveness in preventing and treating osteoporosis, along with other potential benefits for post-menopausal health, HRT provides the greatest benefit relative to cost. Men with low testosterone levels may benefit from testosterone replacement. Medroxyprogesterone, 200mg IM every six weeks can be used to treat men with bone loss.

Bisphosphonates are potent drugs that inhibit bone remodeling by decreasing the function of the cells causing absorption of bone while allowing bone formation to continue at a normal rate. Bisphosphonates increase bone mass in the spine and hip and reduce new vertebral and hip fractures. Alendronate has been available for several years. with Risedronate or actonel may have less stomach irritation such as heartburn or nausea.

Raloxifene is a selective estrogen-receptor modulator (SERM) that maintains bone mass in the spine and reduces the risk of vertebral fractures. Unlike estrogen, raloxifene does not stimulate proliferation of the uterine lining and has no known adverse effects on breast tissue. Some studies have suggested that raloxifene might reduce a woman's risk of breast cancer. Unlike HRT, it does not treat the symptoms of menopause, such as hot flashes.

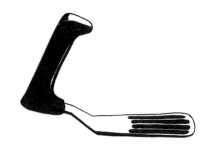

Angle Handle Spatula
The light weight, angled handle on this spatula is designed for those with reduced grip strength. It is comfortable to use and helps provide balance to prevent strained joints and muscles.

Researchers are investigating factors beyond effects on bone mass to explain effects of anti-resorptive therapies. It appears that these therapies have effects on bone mass, bone turnover, and bone quality that contribute to their efficacy in preventing new fractures. The available therapies have different effects on bone mass, but all of them reduce the risk of fracture.

Calcitonin (a nasal spray, also available as an injection) is a mild anti-resorptive agent that inhibits the activity of cells responsible for bone loss. It is somewhat less effective than the above mentioned drugs. It has been shown to maintain bone mineral density in the spine and to reduce the risk of new vertebral fractures in postmenopausal women with osteoporosis. Calcitonin has also been shown to be effective in reducing the pain of vertebral fractures.

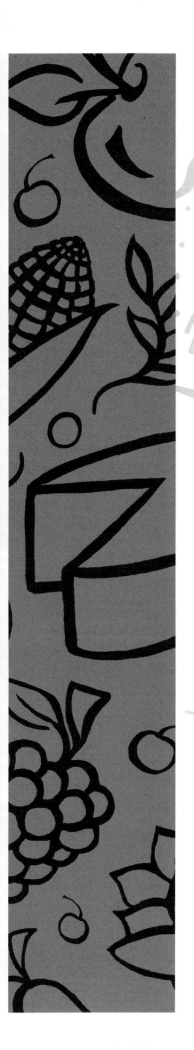
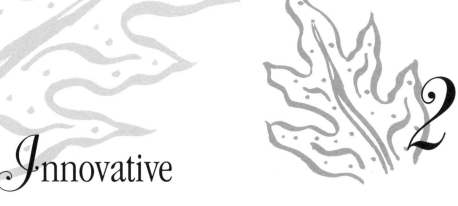

CHAPTER 2

Innovative TREATMENTS FOR THE 21st CENTURY

40

INNOVATIVE TREATMENTS FOR THE 21ST CENTURY
by James McKoy, M.D.

The management of arthritis is at an exciting crossroad with an increased focus on early diagnosis, intensive early use of disease modifying drugs, and intensification of treatment for resistant disease. We now have multiple new drug options for our patients. These new innovative treatments will put a stop to the suffering associated with arthritis. For the first time in nearly a decade, several new drugs are becoming available to treat the pain, stiffness, swelling, and destructive nature of arthritis.

Viscosupplementation

Two innovative treatments for osteoarthritis are Hyalgan (hyaluronan) and Synvisc (hyalgan G-F 20). These drugs are in a new category called viscosupplements or hyaluronic acid substitutes. Hyaluronate is a natural chemical found in the body and it is present in a particularly large amount in joint tissues and in the fluid that fills the joint space. The body's own hyaluronate acts like a lubricant and a shock absorber in the joint, and it is needed for the joint to work properly. In osteoarthritis, there may not be enough hyaluronate, and there may be a change in the quality of the hyaluronate in joint fluid and tissues.

Now we can replace this fluid, helping to relieve the pain and suffering of many patients with osteoarthritis. Synvisc is a series of three injections into the knee, one every five days. Hyalgan is injected into the knee once a week over a period of five weeks. The cost of these injections is approximately $630 for the series.

The beneficial effects of the hyaluronic acid substitutes are limited to symptomatic relief. Patients should avoid prolonged weight-bearing activities for 48 hours after injection. Pain relief may last up to eight months or longer and the treatment may be repeated. Side effects are local and minimal and may consist of some mild discomfort, swelling, and redness of the joint. A rash and itching might appear. Viscosupplementation does not affect the body systemically, avoiding the side effects of most current NSAIDs. This innovative treatment is very safe and effective for patients who have responded poorly to treatment and are not candidates for a total knee replacement.

COX-2 Inhibitors

Since its introduction in the United States in January, 1999, Celebrex—approved by the FDA for rheumatoid arthritis and osteoarthritis—has become one of the fastest selling new drugs in history. Vioxx is the second drug of this class and FDA-approved for the treatment of osteoarthritis, dysmenorrhea, dental pain, and post-op orthopedic pain.

COX-2 inhibition is an important treatment option for millions of people with arthritis. In clinical research, COX-2 drugs were shown to be as effective as the maximum prescription-strength non-steroidal anti-inflammatory drugs (NSAIDs) naproxen and ibuprofen in treating arthritis pain and inflammation. In osteoarthritis (OA) patients, COX-2 drugs improved pain, stiffness, and patient functions such as walking, bending, and getting in and out of a car. Importantly, COX-2 inhibition was associated with significantly fewer upper gastrointestinal (GI) ulcers than traditionally-used arthritis medications such as naproxen and ibuprofen.

This new class of drugs will reduce hospital admissions for ulcers and the number of ulcer-related deaths. Safety is obviously a key advantage to the COX-2 drugs, but their unique mechanism of action actually offers patients and doctors other benefits over existing therapies. It's a team player, demonstrating no clinically significant drug-to-drug interactions with other therapies commonly taken by arthritis patients. Unlike NSAIDs, COX-2s have no proven effect on platelet aggregation or bleeding time. The use of these newer agents is much safer than NSAIDs when used together with blood thinners like coumadin but still should be monitored closely..

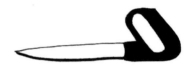

Offset-Handle Knife
The offset handle on this knife actually allows for a good cutting position and makes better use of hand strength. The knife is well balanced and avoids the development of pressure points.

Designed by using advanced molecular technology, a COX-2 drug is clearly differentiated from traditional NSAIDs because of its innovative mechanism of action. COX-2 drugs target and block the COX-2 enzyme that plays a role in causing arthritis pain and inflammation without blocking the COX-1 enzyme that protects the gastrointestinal system. Traditional NSAIDs inhibit both Cox-1 and Cox-2 enzymes. Blocking Cox-1 enzyme in some patients can cause stomach irritation, ulcers, kidney impairment and easy bleeding secondary to inhibition of platelet function.

The recommended therapeutic dose of Celebrex for OA is 200mg daily administered as a single dose. For rheumatoid arthritis, the recommended therapeutic dose is 200mg once a day or 400mg, once a day. Recommended dose for Vioxx is 12.5mg to 25mg a day. For non-arthritic pain control, 50mg for five days is generally recommended.

Many of the approximately forty million Americans with arthritis use the currently available NSAIDs. Use of these medications may lead to stomach ulcers and other serious complications, such as GI bleeding or perforation. In fact, a recent study estimates that these complications cause 107,000 hospitalizations and 16,500 deaths each year in the United States. The newer drugs can significantly reduce these statistics and associated suffering and cost.

In clinical studies, the most common gastrointestinal side effects of the COX-2 agents were dyspepsia, diarrhea, and abdominal pain. Discontinuation due to each of these side effects was less than one percent. Patients who have a known allergic reaction to sulfonamides should not use Celebrex. Patients who have a known allergic reaction to aspirin or NSAIDs should not use Celebrex or Vioxx. Although the COX-2s have a low potential for stomach ulcers, they are not totally safe. Physicians and patients should remain alert for signs and symptoms of GI bleeding. Until there is sufficient scientific evidence to prove otherwise, I would be cautious about using COX-2s in patients with moderate to severe cardiovascular disease.

Relieving the pain and inflammation of arthritis is very important for patients around the world. The COX-2 class of drugs will address some serious unmet medical needs in ulcer prevention. This is a very significant and exciting step forward because it's the first major advance in arthritis medication that we've seen in a number of years. Basically it means that people suffering from arthritis no longer have to fear the serious side effects of their medications. For many years that fear has been a major concern for both patients and doctors, so this is fantastic news.

Arava (leflunomide)

Arava (leflunomide) is the first new disease modifying anti-inflammatory rheumatic drug (DMARD) to become available in some twenty years. Leflunomide is a reversible enzyme inhibitor approved by the FDA for the treatment of rheumatoid arthritis and the first drug to receive specific labeling for retarding radiologic progression of the disease as evidenced by decreased erosions and joint space narrowing. It inhibits the pathway for synthesis of pyrimidine that prevents activation of cells, causing the signs and symptoms of RA. Leflunomide appears to have a faster onset of action and a longer duration or response than currently utilized DMARDs.

This drug can be used in combination with other drugs as well as used alone. The safety of leflunomide is comparable or superior to that of other DMARDs (including methotrexate and sulfasalazine), with GI effects and transient liver enzymes elevations the most frequently reported. This drug does not appear to involve the kidneys, lungs, or bone marrow. Leflunomide has been proven to improve signs and symptoms and slow the pro-

44   The Executive Chef's Arthritis Cookbook and Health Guide

gression of rheumatoid arthritis.

TNF-Blocking Agents

There is a new class of drugs called anti-TNF (tumor necrosis factor) that work by neutralizing a natural compound thought to be a major cause of joint destruction, pain, and swelling. This new class of drugs called a biologic-response modifier inactivates tumor necrosis factor, a substance involved in causing the inflammatory reaction and joint destruction.

Enbrel (etanercept)

Enbrel (etanercept), a soluble TNF-alpha receptor, is the first in this brand new class of drugs for patients with moderate to severe rheumatoid arthritis who haven't responded to one or more drugs like methotrexate. This drug has demonstrated more rapid, sustained, and superior results than some of the common drugs such as Plaquenil, Azulfidine and methotrexate. Mild injection site reactions were the only significant side effects. Patients who have been shown to be at risk for infections should not receive Enbrel. Enbrel is injected twice each week by the patient or someone else. Blood test monitoring may not be needed as frequently as present drugs like methotrexate.

Remicade (infliximab)

Infliximab is a chimeric (mouse/human) IgG monoclonal antibody that binds to alpha-TNF with high affinity and specificity. The drug is administered by intravenous infusion at four- or eight-week intervals with sustained clinical benefits. Combination with methotrexate demonstrated a high level of benefit in patients with active disease despite methotrexate. Infliximab with methotrexate at all doses and schedules significantly reduces progression of structural damage compared with methotrexate alone. Most common adverse events reported during clinical research were mild and consisted of headaches, nausea, coughing, abdominal pain, and upper respiratory tract infection. Most reactions respond to slowing the infusion rate, and/or medical treatment with antihistamines and/or Tylenol.

The long-term consequences of Enbrel and Remicade are not yet known and the possibilities of infection, induction of autoantibodies, and even drug-induced autoimmune diseases and malignancies must continue to be carefully considered.

Kineret (anakinra)

Kineret (anakinra) is the first FDA approved selective blocker of interleukin-1 (IL-1), a protein which is found in excess in rheumatoid arthritis. It is a genetically engineered medication that works against arthritis by inhibiting one of the most potent molecules, interleukin-1, causing inflammation, pain and joint destruction. Kineret should not be used with TNF blocking agents etanercept and infliximab until there is sufficient clinical research to prove safety with these agents. Preliminary data suggest a higher incidence of serious infections and the occurrence of neutropenia (low white blood cell count).

The cost is approximately $11,000 a year. This drug is being marketed to treat moderate to severe rheumatoid arthritis patients who have failed traditional treatments. Main side effects reported thus far have been injection site irritation and a small risk of serious infection. Kineret (anakinra) is given by daily injections of 100 mg beneath the skin.

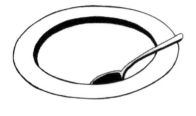

Inner-Lip Plate
The special inside edge keeps food from sliding off the plate which makes eating with one hand pretty easy.

DE2E7

D2E7 is a code name for a new drug, not FDA approved yet, that belongs to the new therapeutic class of treatment for rheumatoid arthritis like enbrel and remicade that inhibit tumour necrosis factor alpha (TNF-a), a key mediator of inflammation, pain and joint destruction.

The market name and cost of this drug are unknown at this time. The drug is injected only once in two weeks, while remicade requires an intravenous infusion, enbrel requires two injections weekly and anakinra requires daily injections. Reported side effects are similar to other anti-TNF blockers.

CDP870

CDP870 is a code name for another new drug, not FDA approved yet, that is also an anti-tumour necrosis factor blocker. This drug has polyethyleneglycol that makes it longer lasting. This will decrease the frequency of injections as compared to enbrel and ankinra.

Side effects reported include headaches, nausea, diarrhea, infections, injection site irritation. These are similar side effects as seen in the other newer medications.

Innovative Nonsteroidal Anti-Inflammatory Drugs (NSAIDs)

Drug [1]	Indications/MOA[2]	Onset of Action	Toxicity	Dosing	Cost per month/year
Celebrex (celecoxib) Pharmacia/Pfizer	RA, OA Inhibits COX-2 which decreases pain and inflammation. Does not inhibit COX-1 which causes gastric erosions and ulcers.	Onset in 30 to 60 minutes for pain, 2-3 hours for inflammation. Steady state 5 days.	Same as other NSAIDs but to a lesser degree. Common side effects are indigestion, diarrhea, abdominal pain, skin rash	For OA, 200mg once day. For RA, 200mg once a day or 400mg daily	Approx. $81/$972 for 200mg once a day. Approx. $140/$1,680 for 400mg twice a day.
Vioxx (rofecoxib) Merck	OA, dental pain, orthopedic pain, menstrual cramps Inhibits COX-2	Onset 30-45 minutes for pain. 2-3 hours for inflammation. Steady state 2-3 days.	As other NSAIDs but less. Common side effects are indigestion, headache, diarrhea, skin rash, hypertension, peripheral edema.	15 to 25 mg orally once a day for arthritis. 50mg per day for 5 days for pain.	Approx. $71/$852 for 15mg to 25mg.

(1) Drug - trade name, (generic name), drug matter, manufacturer
(2) MOA - mode of action

Chapter 2 Innovative Treatments for the 21st Century 47

Innovative Disease Modifying Anti-Inflammatory Rheumatic Drugs (DMARDs)

Drug[1]	Indications/MOA[2]	Onset of Action	Toxicity	Dosing	Cost per month/year
Arava (leflunomide)	Pyrimidine inhibitor Prevents proliferation of T cells. Retards joint destruction. Improves symptoms.	3-4 weeks	Contraindicated in pregnancy. Hepatotoxicity, hair loss, nausea.	Loading: 100mg daily for three days. Maintenance: 20mg daily. Can be used in combination with methotrexate.	$245/$2980
Enbrel (etanercept)	TNF inhibitor Reduces rate of joint destruction. Improves signs and symptoms. Better than methotrexate in slowing rate of new erosions.	1-2 weeks, sustained response in 4 weeks	Is well tolerated. Local minor skin reactions. Lower rate of side effects and fewer infections than methotrexate.	25mg injected beneath skin twice a week. Is effective as a single agent but can be used with methotrexate.	$1,000/ $12,000 Must fail methotrexate before most carriers will pay.
Remicade (infliximab)	TNF inhibitor Prevents structural damage. More efficient than methotrexate.	4-6 weeks	Is well tolerated. Headaches, nausea, coughing, abdominal pain, upper respiratory tract infections.	3mg/kg as a 3-hr infusion at week 0, week 2, week 6 and every 2 months thereafter.	$8000/yr.. Must fail methotrexate before most carriers will pay.
Kineret injected (anakinra)	Reduction of inflammation pain and joint destruction by blocking interleukin1	4 weeks	Injection site irritation, nausea, infections	100mg injected beneath the skin daily.	$11,000/yr

(1) Drug - trade name, (generic name), drug matter, manufacturer
(2) MOA - mode of action

Older Rheumatoid Arthritis Therapies

Drug[1]	Indications/MOA[2]	Onset of Action	Toxicity	Dosing	Cost per month/year
Rheumatrex (methotrexate)	Alters DNA synthesis, retards joint destruction, improves signs and symptoms for rheumatoid and psoriatic arthritis	4 weeks	Pregnancy, toxic to fetus, hepatotoxicity, hair loss, nausea, mouth sores, bone marrow suppression	7.5mg-20mg weekly, can be injected beneath the skin or in muscle. Folic acid 1mg/day helpful in reducing side effects.	$62/$740 brand name; $29/$345 generic; $22/$290 injected
Plaquenil (hydroxychloroquine)	Rheumatoid arthritis, lupus. Anti-inflammatory	3-6 months	Visual effects, dyspepsia, stomach cramps	200-400mg per day	$38/$451
Neoral (cyclosporine)	Inhibits T-cell activation, inhibits interleukin II	4 weeks	Kidney failure, bone marrow suppression	2.5-4mg/kg per day	$293/$3,518 oral $325/$3,896 injection
(prednisone) glucocorticoids	Anti-inflammatory immunomodulator	1-2 days	Susceptible to infections, bone thinning, high blood pressure, cataracts, skin changes	Oral, 5mg/day long term. Injection 3X/yr in single joint. Can use a short tapering course of high dose steroids.	$6.25/$75.00 for 5mg per day. Marked variation in price throughout the country.
Azulfidine (sulfasalazine)	Rheumatoid arthritis Anti-inflammatory	12-20 weeks	Low cell count, dyspepsia, rash, headache, nausea	2-3grams/day	$33/$394 brand name $15/$180 generic

(1) Drug - trade name, generic name, drug matter, manufacturer
(2) MOA - mode of action

Alternative & Complementary APPROACHES TO TREATING Arthritis

CHAPTER 3

50

ALTERNATIVE & COMPLEMENTARY APPROACHES TO TREATING ARTHRITIS
by James McKoy, M.D.

Arthritis is a chronic condition often requiring several treatment approaches. Americans spent $14.8 billion in 1997 on supplements, including herbs, vitamins, and minerals, just to name a few. This is big business. It is a cultural shift that more and more people are seeking an alternative approach to treating diseases. People are searching for ways to live longer and healthier lives. They feel that the natural approach to caring for their bodies is the best way to achieve this. The fear of drugs and the promise of miracle cures from alternative treatments are contributing to the booming business of alternative care.

The alternative or complementary approach that I am using to successfully treat arthritis is a highly personalized approach, which integrates mind, body, and nature. It is a well rounded approach which includes nutrition/lifestyle changes, weight management, exercise, mind/body medicine, energy healing, music therapy, aromatherapy, manual healing methods, and vitamin/herbal supplements along with traditional medical management. Here I will focus mostly on vitamin and herbal supplements. See the charts for examples of some of these other modalities.

Supplements can be very expensive. Health insurers in the past have refused to pay for alternative therapies, but that is changing as insurers realize they can serve patients and save money. Not only are changes going on with health insurers, many medical schools are beginning to include alternative care in their curriculum. More is being reported in the news and major medical journals about alternative approaches to treating diseases.

Advice for Those Seeking an Herbal Cure

Store shelves are loaded with different brands of the same supplements. It's difficult for the consumer to know what to buy. Reading labels is very confusing and they can be difficult to interpret with all the ingredients in very small print and unknown amounts. Many supplements are polluted and not natural even when labeled "natural." Many supplements are contaminated with heavy metals like mercury, lead, and arsenic. The amount of the active ingredient may vary as much as ten times from one brand to another. Many products have false claims and ingredients don't hold up to scrutiny. These things happen because there is no regulation or requirement to follow good manufacturing practices like drug companies.

1. Be a smart consumer. Do your homework prior to shopping for a natural approach to treat your arthritis. Supplements promising you a miracle cure are not telling you the truth. There is no herbal cure for arthritis. Don't buy based on testimonials. Find out whether there has been any research done on the product or see what experience alternative practitioners in your community have had. Many of these practitioners sell quality products in their offices.

2. There are some supplements used alone or in combination with others which might be helpful in treating arthritis and may allow you to lower the dose of your traditional medications. Some supplements are helpful for those who can't tolerate or don't want to take traditional medicine. But you must seek help from knowledgeable professionals before you begin any treatment.

3. Prior to shopping for a cure, find out what type of arthritis you have. Talk with your doctor and ask for advice on a more natural approach and on monitoring for potential side effects. There are over 100 different types of arthritis. Some supplements might be harmful in some forms of arthritis and helpful in others. Salespeople in the stores are not doctors. They may have very little experience or knowledge about the supplements being sold in their stores and the possible contraindications. Some may think all arthritis is the same and that all supplements are good for arthritis. For example, some may erroneously suggest that patients with lupus take alfalfa or echinacea, which can cause a flare-up of lupus.

4. Choose a product which is labeled "standardized." Standardized brands are thought to carry a consistent dose of the ingredients that make the formula work. Many brands often don't provide the levels of the active ingredient promised on the bottle.

5. The fewer ingredients in the product the better. Don't buy products with so many ingredients on the label they require a magnifying glass to read them. Try to buy supplements with one or two well-known ingredients. Make sure the milligram amount is listed. Just like the use of triple therapy (methotrexate, Plaquenil, and Azulfidine) to treat rheumatoid arthritis, it might require two or three herbal supplements. I have had them work better given as individual supplements in combination with others than all together in the same formula.

Adaptive Handled Cookware
These pots are designed for people with limited hand, wrist, and forearm strength and range of motion. Two easy grip handles for even weight distribution give you confident control of hot dishes.

Chapter 3 Alternative & Complementary Treatments 53

Natural products are drugs and are not necessarily safer than traditional drugs. Natural substances can contain powerful, potentially toxic chemicals. There is no research on many of these products to determine safe and effective doses. Many people tend to take more pills because it is natural and they think it is safer. There are many natural products being used to treat arthritis that can cause liver damage, gastrointestinal upset, and death, such as comfrey, black pearl, pennyroyal, hemlock, and kombucha tea. Many people with arthritis are already on medications that can potentially damage the liver, kidneys, and other organs. Care must be taken when combining supplements and medications to avoid unwanted drug interactions. As an example, ginkgo and Coumadin or garlic and vitamin E with non-steroidal anti-inflammatory drugs (NSAIDs) such as Motrin, Naprosyn, Relafen, Voltaren, etc. can contribute to greater thinning of the blood.

Patients who are taking supplements should tell their physicians because the supplements may interact with prescription drugs. The vast majority of patients are taking these supplements right along with their regular medicines. If there is a problem, it is blamed on the traditional medicine because most patients never tell their doctors that they are on supplements. Most supplements will not have a consumer warning on them describing drug interactions or cautions. Because we have no idea what effects these supplements can have if you are pregnant, breast feeding, young, or have a chronic illness, it is wise to stay away from them unless recommended by your physician.

6. Never stop your traditional medications and start some "miracle cure" because of an advertisement or testimonial. This could cause an acute flare-up of your arthritis and, in cases of lupus, could contribute to an early death. Consult your physician and the two of you can determine what should be done based on the seriousness of your illness.

There are many complementary treatments for arthritis. I have found the following to be effective in my practice over the past eighteen years for osteoarthritis, rheumatoid arthritis, osteoporosis, and fibromyalgia.

Please don't rush out and buy every supplement suggested. I recommend starting with only one or two supplements, depending on the severity of your condition. If you get no response after four to six weeks, you might try other supplements as directed by a knowledgeable alternative practitioner. Most of the time, doctors use three or four different prescription drugs (combination therapy) to treat arthritis. This also applies to herbal supplements. There is usually no single prescription drug that controls arthritis and there is no single supplement that does the job. There are many combinations of supplements that can be used. Some combinations will work better in some people than others. For example, I may start with glucosamine sulfate and MSM in combination for four to six weeks for a patient with osteoarthritis/degenerative joint disease. If optimal response is not achieved, I may then add bromelain and/or topical analgesic creams.

Remember, talk to your physician before starting any of these supplements or treatments.

Complementary Treatment For Osteoarthritis

1. Stress management: tai chi, qi gong, and yoga breathing exercises

2. Weight management and dietary modifications:
   Foods to add to your diet: artichokes, cherries, cabbage, grain cereals, cold water fish (salmon, mackerel, herring, sardines, tuna, anchovies), fresh fruits and vegetables, leafy greens, garlic, onions, olive oil, barley, parsley, and squash

   Foods to avoid: refined foods, saturated fatty foods from meat and dairy products, high gluten foods (corn, wheat), mustard, salty foods, chocolate, and nightshade family foods such as bell peppers, eggplant, and tomatoes. A three- to four-month trial may be helpful.

3. Water, 64 ounces a day if there is no kidney, heart, or liver disease

4. Glucosamine Sulfate, 1 gram (1000mg) three times a day for three weeks, then decrease to 500mg three times a day. May increase blood sugar in some diabetics.

5. Chondroitin Sulfate, 800 to 1200mg daily in divided doses.

6. MSM (methyl sulfonyl methane), 1000mg twice or three times a day with meals. Avoid if kidney or liver disease.

7. Bromelain, 750mg twice a day. Be sure that the product lists the units of activity on the label called MCUs.

8. Penetran Plus Analgesic Cream to the affected joints four times a day. Capsaicin cream can also be used, but may

sting or itch. Arnica Arthritis Cream (homeopathic medicine) three times a day to affected joints.

9. Devil's Claw, 750mg three times a day with meals

10. Vitamin B-6, 100mg twice a day. Do not exceed this dosage.

11. Boron, 1-3mg twice a day. A good high potency multivitamin may contain this amount of boron.

12. Acupuncture, massage, reflexology, and chiropractic

13. Mind-body medicine (meditation, music therapy, visual imagery, spiritual healing, prayer)

Complementary Treatment for Rheumatoid Arthritis

1. Stress management: tai chi, qi gong, yoga breathing exercises, and seven to eight hours of restful sleep

2. Weight management and dietary modifications:
Foods to add to your diet: cold water fish three times a week (salmon, tuna, herring, mackerel), onions, garlic, olive oil, watercress, cauliflower, squash, parsley, barley, and plenty of cruciferous vegetables such as broccoli, cabbage, brussels sprouts, turnips, collard greens, and kale. These vegetables have an abundance of vitamins, minerals, fiber, and protector nutrients. They also contain phytonutrients such as isothiocyanates and Indole carbinols responsible for beneficial anti-cancer effects, helping to lower cholesterol, boost the immune system, and neutralize toxins. Flavonoid-rich foods such as beets, red wine, cherries, green tea, cranberries, blueberries, raspberries, red and black grapes contain catechins, anthocyanins, proanthocyanidins, flavones, flavonones, and ellagic acid that boost the immune system, neutralize toxins, and help to control arthritis.

Foods to avoid: high protein and high fat diets, refined foods, pastries, and white bread, canned foods, all MSG-containing foods, all preserved foods, artificial sweeteners, white flour, saturated fatty foods from red meat and dairy products, high gluten foods (corn, rice), mustard, salty foods, chocolate, and nightshade family foods such as bell peppers, eggplant, and tomatoes

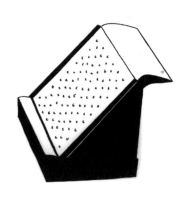

Grater with Suction Feet
Suction feet hold the grater in place for one-handed use while the bin holds the grated food for easy use and convenient cleanup. This grater comes with a reversible plastic plate for fine or coarse grating.

3. Water, 64 ounces a day if no heart disease, kidney disease, or liver disease

4. Mind-body medicine to control the psychological factors. Use prayer, meditation, visual imagery to affect your condition with your mind.

5. Exercise program. The stronger the muscles around the joint, the less instability and pain. Water exercises (aquatherapy), walking, and light weights are the best forms of exercise. Soak in heated water, heated mineral baths, or heated whirlpool baths as often as possible.

6. High potency multivitamins with minerals. A good product should have selenium 200mcg, zinc 20mg, boron 1-3mg. Vitamin C, 500mg twice a day.

7. Omega 3 fatty acids (fish oil), two capsules with each meal or eat at least three servings of cold water fish (such as salmon) each week. Adding 1-2 tablespoons of flax seeds daily to cereals or salads can be very helpful.

8. MSM (methyl sulfonyl methane), 1 gram (1000mg) three times a day with meals

9. Penetran Plus Analgesic Cream applied to the affected joints four times a day

10. Ginger, 1000-2000mg daily in divided doses

11. Boswellia, 200mg three times a day for two to three months. If no response, increase to a maximum dose of 400mg three times a day.

12. Ashwagandha (*Withania*) extract, 1 capsule a day. May increase effects of sedating medications.

13. Turmeric (curcumin), 400-600mg two to three times a day

14. Bioflavoids/carotenoids, 500-1000mg a day

15. Phytodolor (by Enzymatic Therapy/Phytopharmica), 20 drops taken internally daily. Can be increased to a maximum dose of 20 drops three times a day.

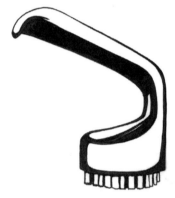

Uni-Turner
Retractable plastic prongs automatically conform to knobs or controls such as faucets, stove knobs, or radiator caps. The L-shaped handle increases leverage to aid in operating them.

Complementary Treatment for Fibromyalgia/Chronic Fatigue Syndrome

1. Vegetarian, low protein, low fat, high fiber diet

Chapter 3 Alternative & Complementary Treatments 57

2. Eliminate common food allergens: sugar, white flour, processed foods, caffeine, aspartame, alcohol, nicotine, red meats, wheat, and dairy products

3. Water, 64 ounces a day if no heart failure, renal disease, or liver disease

4. Psychosocial counseling (cognitive behavioral medicine, mind-body medicine, thought field therapy). Learn to modify self-limiting thoughts, beliefs, memories, and behaviors.

5. Graded exercise program

6. Aquatherapy

7. Guided imagery

8. Yoga, tai chi, qi gong

9. Music therapy

10. Massage therapy

11. Penetran Plus Analgesic Cream applied to the affected muscles

12. Malic acid/magnesium 1200-2400mg of malic acid and 300 to 600mg of magnesium for pain taken in divided doses daily

13. High potency multivitamins with minerals. Selenium, 200mcg at lunch. Vitamin C, 500mg twice a day.

14. Alpha lipoic acid, 100mg three times a day. Powerful antioxidant that helps reduce symptoms of fibromyalgia/ chronic fatigue if used regularly. Don't expect instant results. Best response is to take along with selenium, 200 mcg daily. Whey protein can potentiate the effects of these supplements.

15. For sleep, try these supplements but only one at a time: Melatonin, 2.5-5.0mg under the tongue one-half hour before bedtime. If moderate sleep disturbance, try "Knockout" (combination of herbs), follow directions on bottle. Valerian, 500mg of herbal extract one hour before bedtime. Kava, 150mg (30% kavalactones), take 2-3 capsules one hour before bedtime. Caution: do not take kava and alcohol together.

58   The Executive Chef's Arthritis Cookbook and Health Guide

16. SAM-e, 200mg twice a day, can be increased slowly by adding 200mg per day every two weeks to a maximum of 800mg a day (this should be directed by your physician). Do not take SAM-e if you are taking anti-depressant medications.

17. Co-Enzyme Q10 helps with muscle metabolism, energy, and pain. Take 100mg twice a day with meals.

18. NADH (nicotinamide adenine dinucleotide hydrogen) for energy. Start at 5mg a day and increase to twice a day in two weeks, depending on tolerance.

19. Vitamin B complex, follow directions on bottle.

20. Ginkgo biloba, 120mg to 160mg daily in divided doses. Avoid if taking anticoagulant medications such as warfarin, Ticlid, or Plavix. Can cause easy bleeding.

21. Omega-3 fatty acids, two capsules with each meal

22. MSM (methyl sulfonyl methane) helps with pain. Start with 1000mg three times a day.

23. Acetyl L-Carnitine, 1000mg four times a day helps improve energy.

24. Glutamine, digestive enzymes, and aromatherapy oil (peppermint) can improve digestion and irritable bowel symptoms associated with fibromyalgia.

25. DHEA 25mg to 100mg depending on blood levels. Measure DHEA-S blood levels and only start if levels are less than 75mg. Should only be taken with a physician's supervision. Do not take if you have breast, ovarian, prostate, or other hormone-related cancers.

26. Armour Thyroid 1/4 grain per day. Must be prescribed by a doctor and can be titrated higher. Thyroid therapy should be used only if under the care of a physician.

Note: I recommend starting out with only two to three supplements depending on the severity of your condition. If you see no response after four to six weeks, other supplements as directed may be added one at a time until fatigue and pain are controlled. Never stop any of your medications unless directed by a physician.

Caution: Avoid all supplements if pregnant or breast feeding.

Chapter 3 Alternative & Complementary Treatments

Educational Resources:

The Fibromyalgia Network Newsletter 1-(800) 853-2929

Jenny Fransen and Jon Russell. *The Fibromyalgia Help Book.* (www.fmnetnews.com)

Mind/Body Medicine
For optimal health we must find harmony with our environment and within ourselves. There must be a balance between the emotional, physical, intellectual, and the spiritual. Mind/body medicine covers activities and therapies that focus on the interrelationship of these four systems that can be integrated in all forms of disease and treatment programs.

The goal in all forms of mind/body medicine is to help deal with the fundamental cause or factors contributing to the disease process and provide effective therapies by combining both mental and physical approaches. The fact that the mind rules the body is the most fundamental fact that we know about the process of life. Sir William Osler said that he would rather know what sort of person has a disease than what sort of disease a person has.

Our bodies and minds are clearly not independent of one another. Our life experiences and the ways we process and hold those experiences in our minds can dramatically influence those mechanisms within the body-mind that are intended to keep us well. The immune system, it seems, is particularly susceptible. Traumatic experiences in our lives like divorce, death of a loved one, loss of a job, a stressful job environment, loneliness, unhappiness, and unfulfilling love relationships can affect our health. Just as our minds can send out messages that impact our bodies in negative ways, the very power to do that suggests the exact opposite: that perhaps our minds can also have a positive influence on our health.

Healing begins with a love for self and others, and for life itself. You bring all of you to the healing relationship—your general health, your state of mind, your beliefs, and images that you entertain concerning yourself and your future. Everything that you hold in your consciousness plays a valuable part in the healing relationship or destructive forces causing spiritual, mental, and physical ailments.

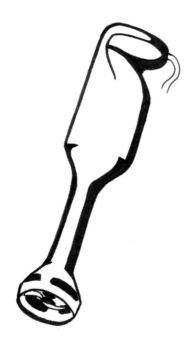

Hand Held Blender
Compact and light weight, this blender purees food quickly and easily with one hand. The shaft comes off for easy cleanup.

The following are a few modalities that can help to bring balance to the total person:

• Spirituality is a source of relaxation and comfort for many people, whether it involves practicing a particular religion or contemplating spiritual values outside a religious context. Praying and meditation on biblical principles that pertain to the mind and body can unite spirit, soul, and body to bring about a spiritual healing. Our values and life experiences have physical repercussions. As a man thinketh in his heart so is he. Our emotions influence everything else in our life. Spirituality constitutes who we are as individuals and can help us be at ease with ourselves, content, happy, and maximally productive. Spirituality helps us share, care, trust, and gives us the strength to have balance in all areas of our lives. When we are spiritual we can touch others with trust, innocence, and love. Disharmony in this area leads to disease and shortens life expectancy.

• Guided imagery teaches patients to imagine scenarios that may help influence certain physiological conditions. A cancer patient, for example, may imagine a tumor dissolving through the healing action of the immune system. While there are no conclusive studies on imagery, patients often report physical and psychological benefits.

• Aromatherapy is the use of natural plant essences or essential oils. Our bodies readily absorb the benefits of these highly concentrated plant and flower essences through inhalation or application to the skin. This natural approach can enhance physical health and emotional well-being. Aromatherapists believe that the fragrance of the oils has a soothing effect on the brain's limbic system, which is involved in memory, emotion, and hormone control. These oils work directly in the body to bring about healing, peace, purification, and joy.

• Meditation includes a number of different Asian and Western practices. All share the basic characteristics of sitting or resting quietly, often with the eyes closed, and performing mental exercises designed to relax the body and focus concentration.

• The relaxation response is a state of psychological and physiological rest characterized by lowered oxygen consumption and reduced heart rate. It can be induced by many different techniques, including meditation, yoga, tai chi, qi gong, and hypnotherapy. This deep relaxation can relieve stress and its many symptoms.

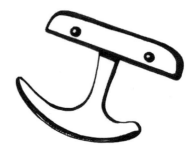

Rocker Knife
The rocker knife has a large wooden handle with a stainless steel, single-edged blade. Because pressure is applied directly from above the food, less strength and dexterity is needed by the user. With a carrying case, it's ideal to carry in purse or pocket.

Chapter 3 Alternative & Complementary Treatments   61

• Support groups bring people together who are suffering from the same disease or similar types of trauma. Within the group, experiences and feelings can be shared which may yield great psychological benefits and perhaps improve the functioning of the body's natural defenses as well.

• Music therapy can bring harmony to your soul. The sound environment is an auditory context that holds the experiences, thoughts, feelings, beliefs, and spoken and unspoken communications. The value of music as a therapeutic tool in altering one's state of mind and one's state of physical being has been researched and documented for many years.

• Yoga is a series of body positions and movements developed over thousands of years to calm the mind, relax the body, and ease the spirit. Yoga involves both physical movement and a meditative state of mind, which may serve the dual purpose of improving a person's physical condition and combating emotional problems, such as depression and anxiety. The two-way connection between mind and body is used in many ways to influence the hormonal, nervous, and immune systems. Meditation and breathing exercises lead into cycles of stretches and poses that may vary from session to session. Yoga can be learned and practiced at home; however, modified movements may be required during pregnancy or if a person has a condition such as heart disease. A yoga specialist can recommend the appropriate adjustments.

• Tai Chi is an effective exercise for health and well-being. Published studies by Dr Paul Lam, a world renowned instructor who specializes in Tai Chi for Arthritis, and others have shown that Tai Chi stretches and strengthens joints, muscles and ligaments and improves cardiorespiratory fitness. Seventy-eight percent of participants have experienced significant pain relief, and achieved a better quality of life and improved general health. This form of exercise is suitable for almost anyone and can be practiced anywhere. It integrates the body and mind. This form of exercise uses gentle and circular movements for all different skill levels.

62   The Executive Chef's Arthritis Cookbook and Health Guide

Alternative or Complementary Medicine for Rheumatoid Arthritis

Medicine [1]	Indications/MOA [2]	Onset of Action	Toxicity	Dosing	Drug Interaction
Phytodolor Liquid Extract by Enzy. Therapy/ PhytoPharmica	Rheumatoid arthritis Optimal muscle and joint function, anti-inflammatory	2-4 weeks	Very safe, nausea, diarrhea	20 drops 3 times daily	Aspirin, Ticlid, Plavix, warfarin
Ashwagandha (*Withania*)	Rheumatoid arthritis Anti-inflammatory	3-4 weeks	Some nausea, diarrhea but otherwise appears to be safe	Extract: 1 capsule a day Raw herb: 1-2 grams daily as a tea	May enhance the effects of both stimulants (amphetamines) and depressants
Yucca Extract saponins glycosides 4:1 extract	Anti-inflammatory Natural cortisone (phytosterol)	4-6 weeks	No serious side effects reported, mild diarrhea	500-1000mg per day	No known interactions except for laxatives
Feverfew (*Tanacetum parthenium*)	Inhibits prostaglandin synthesis, inhibits serotonin release from platelets and white blood cells	4-6 weeks	Mild GI upset, tachycardia (rare), nervousness, gas, hypersensitivity reactions	0.2-0.6mg of parthenolide per day; 50-200mg in tabs; tincture 5-20 drops	Closely monitor patients on warfarin. Contraindicated in pregnancy, lactation, and children under two.
Curcumin (*Curcuma longa*) Turmeric	Antioxidant Anti-inflammatory	4-6 weeks	No significant side effects reported	400-600mg three times a day	Poss. additive effects with blood thinners like aspirin, Ticlid, Plavix, warfarin. Avoid in pregnancy.
Ginger	Anti-inflammatory Peripheral circulatory stimulant	6-8 weeks	Occasional heartburn	2-4mg of the rhizome a day; 2.0gm of the powdered drug in divided doses	May interfere with cardiac, antidiabetic drug, or blood thinners like aspirin, Ticlid, Plavix, warfarin
Nettles (*Urtica dioica*)	Inhibits synthesis of pro-inflammatory prostaglandins	4-6 weeks	No significant side effects reported	300mg 1-2X a day. 750mg extract per day	No known interactions

(1) Medicine - chemical or herbal name, (*botanical name*)
(2) MOA - mode of action

Chapter 3 Alternative & Complementary Treatments 63

Alternative or Complementary Medicine for Osteoarthritis

Medicine [1]	Indications/MOA [2]	Onset of Action	Toxicity	Dosing	Drug Interaction
Glucosamine sulfate	Improves disease symptoms by repairing and rebuilding cartilage.	4-6 weeks, 12 weeks for full effect	Nausea, diarrhea	1 gram (1000mg) 2-3 times daily or 1500mg twice a day. 3X a day if over 150 lbs.	May require diabetes medication adjustment
Capsaicin	Interferes with the body's perception of pain.	1-2 weeks for full effect	Burns. Avoid applying to broken skin. Avoid rubbing eyes. Wash hands.	Apply to affected joint 4 times a day.	None known
Fish oil Omega-3 fatty acids	Decreases pain and inflammation. Shows benefits in both RA and OA.	4-6 weeks	Well tolerated. Fish taste in mouth.	1-2 grams with each meal	May interact with aspirin and blood thinners
MSM (methyl sulfonyl methane)	Has shown some benefit on both RA and OA.	2-3 months for positive results	Skin may develop sulfur smell. Otherwise safe.	1000mg 2-3 times a day with meals	None known
Bromelain (protein-digesting enzyme from pineapple)	Relieves pain and inflammation. Can be used in both RA and OA.	2-3 weeks	Nausea, diarrhea, otherwise very safe	750mg twice a day on empty stomach	May interact with aspirin and blood thinners
Devil's Claw (*Harpargophytum procumbens*) 3% Iridoid glycosides	Relieves pain and inflammation. Can be used in both RA and OA.	4-6 weeks	Avoid if you have stomach ulcers, pregnant, or breast-feeding.	750mg three times a day. Can be taken in tincture, tea, or capsule	May interact with acid inhibiting drugs.
Boswellia serrata extract standardized to 37.5% boswellic acids	May improve biochemical structure of cartilage. Improves circulation and fights inflammation. Can be used in both RA and OA.	Full effects may not be felt for 4-8 weeks	Avoid in pregnancy. Occasional mild allergic reaction or mild gastrointestinal distress.	400mg three times a day	No known interactions

(1) Medicine - chemical or herbal name, (*botanical name*)
(2) MOA - mode of action

64   The Executive Chef's Arthritis Cookbook and Health Guide

Alternative or Complementary Medicine for Osteoporosis

Medicine [1]	Indications/MOA[2]	Components	Toxicity	Dosing	Drug Interaction
Ipriflavone (synthetic isoflavone derivative)	Enhances bone density. Accelerates bone regeneration and calcium deposition.	Synthetic isoflavone derivatives	Heartburn, vomiting, constipation, diarrhea, skin rashes, pruritus. May lower white blood cell count.	300mg twice a day	Safe with minor side effects. Caution with blood thinners, oral contraceptives, and theophylline.
Phytoestrogens (soy products, green beans, nuts/seeds, flaxseed oil)	Mild estrogenic effect. May improve vaginal dryness. Mild effect on hot flashes.	Isoflavones genistein phytosterols saponins lignans	Nausea, flatulence (gas), intolerance of soy products	50-100mg of isoflavones a day. One cup of nuts/seeds to one cup of soy products a day. Exact optimum amount uncertain.	No known toxicity or side effects. Caution if patients with history of estrogen-related cancers.
Remifemin Black Cohosh (*Cimicifuga racemosa*)	Mild relief of hot flashes and improves mood.	Triterpenoid glycosides, isoflavones and aglycones	Large doses cause dizziness, nausea, headaches, stiffness, and trembling.	Remifemin, one tab twice a day	No drug interactions
Strawberry (*Fragaria*) (nuts, dried beans, wine, cider, beer, and many other fruits and vegetables)	May increase level of circulating estrogen. Helps in utilizing calcium and magnesium.	Boron	No known toxicities. Minor allergic reactions.	Limit the total dose of boron to 3mg a day. Strawberry has high content of boron. 1-2 cups a day or 5-8 servings of fruits and vegetables.	No known interactions
DHEA (Dehydroepiandosterone)	Improves mood and possible mild increase in muscle mass.	Converted to estrogen and testosterone	May include acne, hair growth, irritability, headaches. Long terms effects unclear. Possible cancer risk.	25-75mg a day depending on blood DHEA-S levels	Possible liver damage with Imuran and methotrexate. Use only under a physician's care.

(1) Medicine - chemical or herbal name, (*botanical name*)
(2) MOA - mode of action

Chapter 3 Alternative & Complementary Treatments 65

Alternative or Complementary Medicine for Fibromyalgia

Medicine [1]	Indications/MOA [2]	Onset of Action	Toxicity	Dosing	Drug Interaction
Vitamin B_{12}	Energy	4-6 weeks, with optimal effect 2-3 months	No significant side effects at recommended doses	2000mcg a day for first month, followed by 1000mcg sublingual daily	No known interactions
Alpha-lipoic acid	Necessary co-factor in two vital energy-producing reactions. Considered a vitamin. Has antioxidant properties.	4-6 weeks	No side effects reported	100mg a day to a max of 100mg three times a day.	No known interactions
MSM (methyl sulfonyl methane)	Pain. Odorless form of DMSO. Same anti-inflammatory qualities as DMSO, but safe.	2-4 weeks, may take 2-3 months for positive results.	Very safe. No significant side effects. Skin may develop a sulfur smell.	1000mg three times a day	No known interactions
NADH (nicotinamide adenine dinucleotide)	Stimulates energy production, improves mental clarity.	4-6 weeks	Reported to be very safe. No side effects reported.	5-10mg a day	No known interactions
Malic acid/ magnesium	Muscle pain, improves circulation and muscle function, counteracts stress.	4-6 weeks	Nausea, diarrhea, vomiting, flushing	1200-2400mg of malic acid and 300-600mg of magnesium	No known interactions at doses given
DHEA (dehydroepiandosterone)	Claims to improve mood, energy, and counteract stress hormones and improve estrogen/ testosterone.	4-6 weeks	Untested in long-term clinical trials. Acne, increased heart rate and palpitation, body hair, irritability, insomnia.	Dose should be based on result of low lab test DHEA-S. Usual starting dose is 25-50mg a day.	May increase breast cancer and heart disease risk in some women. May cause liver damage with Imuran or methotrexate.

(1) Medicine - chemical or herbal name, (*botanical name)*
(2) MOA - mode of action

66

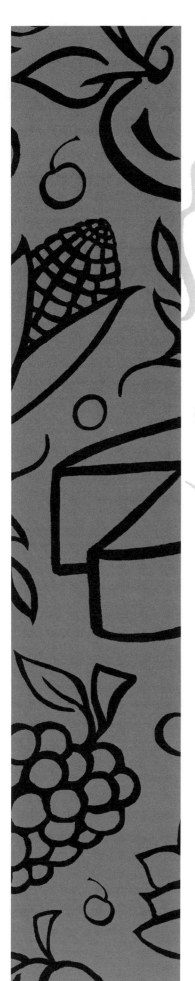

Arthritis
AND NUTRITION

CHAPTER 4

68

ARTHRITIS AND NUTRITION
by Executive Chef Prentiss Carl Haupt

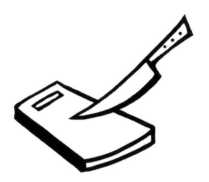

Millions of people suffer from some form of arthritis. Because arthritis is commonly believed to be incurable, the standard medical response has been simply to prescribe medication to reduce the symptoms. There are now new schools of thought that say the pain and disability caused by arthritis can be alleviated through diet, nutritional supplementation, stress education, and other alternative methods of therapy.

The Executive Chef's Arthritis Cookbook and Health Guide will show you some of these alternative methods. Then you and your doctor can decide if such treatment will benefit you.

There are some sound scientific reasons to think that foods you eat may affect certain kinds of arthritis. But there is not yet enough evidence to clearly understand how diet might help or might hurt specific types of arthritis.

The Executive Chef's Arthritis Cookbook and Health Guide is all about good, fresh, healthy, and wholesome food, not calorie counting.

This book has many healthy recipes, all tested, with a nutritional analysis added to each recipe. Included in the recipes are products which come from health food stores, and are increasingly available in supermarkets. We use no animal products such as milk, cream, cheeses, butter, and sour cream. Instead, we use the same products made from grains, beans, and so forth. We do not use any white sugar, white flour, or salt. Instead of salt I have invented a salt substitute that I will tell you how to make. Honey and whole wheat flour are used in the recipes, plus much more. Enjoy these recipes, enjoy good health, and enjoy life.

70   The Executive Chef's Arthritis Cookbook and Health Guide

CASE STUDIES

Diet played a major role in the treatment of my own arthritis. I have also worked with many arthritics, planning and following up on their own diet experiences. The results of the following four case studies were chosen to show you what diet can do over an extended period of time.

Study Group 1:

A group of twelve people from 35 to 68 years of age joined a group to try to alleviate their arthritis pain and live a healthier lifestyle. The objective was to test my hypothesis about the **NO foods**. When we started, we didn't have a lot of information except for my theory about the **NO foods** and eliminating those foods from their daily diet. (Chapter 5 explains the **NO foods**.) During this study, no one drank any alcohol or smoked. The first thirty days the participants wrote down everything they ate every day.

Garlic was added to many of their diets. Refined products were removed. Sugar and salt were totally eliminated. Each person drank at least 64 ounces of water daily. Exercise was added for everyone, especially walking. People ate good, fresh, wholesome food. They used my salt substitute instead of salt.

Results:

Of the twelve people who started the program, seven people finished. The five people who dropped out reported that they were not willing to stop eating their traditional foods. The seven people who stayed with the program reported the following benefits:

1. Eating better by eating fresh, healthy food
2. More flexibility from daily exercise
3. Eliminating heartburn
4. Having more vitality
5. Feeling rejuvenated
6. Experiencing less joint pain
7. Having less inflammation and, for some, the total elimination of inflammation
8. Gaining a better attitude toward life
9. Spending less money on pills and doctor bills

Case History 1

Tommy was a 68-year-old Hawaiian man in the group. He grew up by the ocean, fished every day, ate plenty of pork and other **NO foods** from Chapter 5. For one month before we started he wrote down everything he ate, as did everyone in the group. When he showed me his list I was horrified.

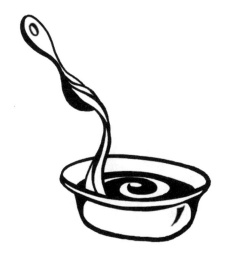

When I met him, Tommy walked with very small steps, just shuffling along. He could not fish anymore. He was heartbroken. After ninety days on his new diet, he walked as a normal 68-year-old man would. He walked by my place of work every day and thanked me for the changes. But the best result was that I got to eat plenty of the fresh fish that Tommy caught. Tommy died a few years ago, sitting on the ocean's edge, at peace with God, doing the thing he lived for—fishing. When he passed on he was 82 years old and a true friend.

Case History 2

A 52-year-old woman I know through church, who was developing arthritis to the point of joint pain all over, tried my plan. She had been a heavy meat eater. She eliminated 97 foods from her daily eating habits, including all the **NO foods**.

She only used the health food substitutes in this book, plus others she discovered. Now, she walks two to three miles, three to five days a week, and enjoys a newly revitalized sex life. She lives pain-free almost daily—she told me a few times she had tried some of the **NO foods**, and then she experienced joint swelling.

She thanks the good Lord every day for the help. In the beginning her husband said I was crazy. He told her to just take her pills and be glad she wasn't as bad as some really crippled people. Now he is happy to have his wife back. Incidentally, her husband is a doctor.

Study Group 2:

Study Group 2 consisted of seventeen people from the ages of 45 to 60 years. Like the first group, the participants wrote down everything they ate every day for the first thirty days.

I met with each individual, one on one. They had their thirty day lists, snacks included. It is really incredible how much meat is eaten here in Hawaii, especially pork products. No one drank any alcohol and no one smoked during this study.

Using the list of **NO foods**, participants eliminated thirty-seven to fifty-five items from their daily menus. A lot of these items had been eaten two to seven times per week.

They added garlic to many of their foods. Refined products were eliminated. Sugar and salt were totally eliminated. Instead of salt, they used my salt substitute. Everyone exercised—walking worked out the best—and ate good, fresh, wholesome food.

Results:

Eighty-five percent of the people who started finished. Three of the finishers experienced no improvement in health, except for the exercise they were now getting. All the other participants experienced much better health than when they started.

The people who stayed on the program experienced benefits similar to Study Group 1. They were eating better, becoming more flexible, avoiding heartburn, having reduced or no inflammation and less joint pain, along with feeling better about their lives.

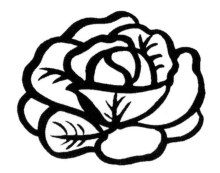

The main thing I noticed was how much better these people's attitudes toward life had become. They were much happier, being freer from pain than when they started.

Study Group 3:

This study involved a group of thirty professional people who all suffered from some kind of inflammation of their joints. In this group fourteen people smoked. They had to give up smoking in order to participate in the study. Thirteen of them had not returned to smoking as of one year later.

This group was younger than the other studies. They were 32 to 49 years old and better educated than prior study groups.

From the beginning, participants eliminated all the **NO foods** from their diet after thirty days of recording everything they ate. It was really unbelievable to see how many sweets and candies they consumed. For ninety days they ate only my recipes of good, fresh foods from health food stores.

They drank 64 ounces of water daily. At the end of the study many people reported that water tasted good to them, since almost no one drank plain water before they started.

The participants used my salt substitute instead of table salt. There is plenty of natural sodium in foods, so additional salt is

Chapter 4 Arthritis & Nutrition   **73**

not really needed. Salt does not flavor foods. It neutralizes the taste buds that sense bitterness, so your brain only thinks it flavors foods.

After ninety days of following the diet, all the people in the study—except two—benefited by eating better, becoming more flexible, avoiding heartburn, having reduced or no inflammation and less joint pain, and felt better about their lives.

Just remember: God put food on earth to nurture us, not harm us. So if your body is harmed by processed foods, eat the foods as fresh products, and if one does you harm, stop using it.

One of the sources I found really helpful in my own search for help with arthritis is *Back To Eden* by Jethro Kloss. I asked the Kloss family if I might quote the information I found most useful in this book and they graciously gave permission. Here are some valuable suggestions for treatment.

From *Back to Eden*, pp. 416-417:

Treatment: All unwholesome, devitaminized food must be strictly avoided. Tea, coffee, liquor, white flour products, cane sugar products, soda biscuits, fried potatoes, meat, pork and bacon especially. When fed on the foregoing foods, the blood cells will not be able to rid the system of impurities...All food should be eaten as dry as possible, and well masticated so that it is thoroughly mixed with saliva to help digestion. This will alkalinize the system as much as any one thing you can do. Wonderful results may be obtained from a prolonged fruit diet. After taking the fruit diet for two or three weeks, use potassium broth, French toast and mashed potatoes...Drink slippery elm tea; it is very nourishing, cleansing, and strengthening. Solid food must be taken sparingly at first, after the fruit diet.

Take a good sweat bath every day and drink two or three cups of pleurisy tea. Use a teaspoon of pleurisy root to a cup of boiling water and let steep for twenty minutes. Drink this while in the tub. Thorough massage after the bath is very beneficial. If there is *inflammation* of the joints, do not massage those parts.

Mix equal parts of the following herbs: black cohosh, gentian root, angelica, columbo, skullcap, valerian, rue, and buckthorn bark. Use a heaping teaspoon to a cup

74   The Executive Chef's Arthritis Cookbook and Health Guide

of boiling water; steep and drink three or more cups per day, as the case may require. Drink a half-cupful at a time.

An excellent poultice for swollen joints is made as follows: two tablespoons of mullein, three tablespoons of granulated slippery elm bark, one tablespoon of lobelia, and one small teaspoon of cayenne; mix thoroughly together, then mix with enough boiling water to make a stiff paste. Spread a layer of paste about one-fourth of an inch thick on a cloth. Cover the swollen joints with this poultice and it will bring great relief.

Another excellent way to relieve the pain is to mix equal parts of oil of origanum and oil of lobelia, then add a few drops of oil of capsicum or extract of capsicum (red pepper). This can be applied full strength or mixed with coconut oil. Massage thoroughly with this, as long as there is no inflammation of the joint.

The following herbs are also very beneficial in rheumatism and arthritis: bitterroot, buckthorn bark, burdock, saw palmetto berries, black cohosh, wintergreen, yellow dock, sassafras, skullcap, and bear's foot. Look up their descriptions and take those best suited to your case. Use singly or in combination.

From *Back to Eden,* pp. 835-836

ARTHRITIS TREATMENT

Alternate hot and cold treatments are many times very helpful in relieving the pain of arthritis. This treatment is mainly for arthritis in the hands, wrists, or feet. The treatment is simple to give and only minimal equipment is needed. You should have two containers large enough to accommodate hands or feet. One of the containers should be filled with hot water at 105° to 110°F. and the other should contain water at 60° to 70°F. This is about the temperature of water that comes from the cold water faucet.

1. There should be enough water in the container to reach nearly to the elbows or knees.
2. Use a bath thermometer to determine the water temperature.

3. The extremity should be placed first in the hot water for three minutes and then in the cold water for 30 seconds.
4. Seven complete changes should be made, ending with the hot water.
5. This can be done two or three times a day.
6. If the hot water causes increased swelling, the temperature can be decreased to 105°F. or the time in the hot water can be reduced to two minutes and the time in the cold water increased to one minute.
7. If there is poor circulation, the hot water should never be more than 105°F.
8. For extremely painful joints, an ice pack can be used until the swelling subsides and then the alternate hot and cold treatments may be used.

GOOD FUN

Arthritis affects each person in a different way, but we all know one thing: it can make life difficult! There are many new products available to make life easier for arthritis sufferers.

There are ways to help each other. After all, isn't that why God put us on the earth, to help mankind? People who have arthritis are more likely to be older, so go to senior centers and make friends. Many of us are looking for ways to enjoy our time. Get together in groups. Figure out recipes you want to try. Analyze these recipes. Figure out what part of a recipe each one of you can work on. Go to the store and buy the necessary ingredients for each recipe you want to cook. Go to a different person's house each day. In the long run I know you will find this an easier way, a cheaper way, and you will develop camaraderie and companionship. You will spend many enjoyable hours together, talking about life, laughing and joking, cooking and eating. Here in Hawaii we sit around the table eating and "talking story."

CARBOHYDRATES

The carbohydrates in foods are the source of most of our energy. About half of our daily calories come from carbohydrates, mostly grains and sugar, followed by potatoes, vegetables, fruit, and dairy products.

76   The Executive Chef's Arthritis Cookbook and Health Guide

Carbohydrates contain three basic elements—carbon, hydrogen, and oxygen. The way the elements are arranged makes sugars; everything from simple sugars such as glucose, to very complex carbohydrates such as starch. The carbohydrates we eat consist mostly of starch, sugar, and fiber.

All the carbohydrates we eat, simple or complex, must be broken down to simple sugars before they can be used by the body. Fiber passes through the body basically unchanged because we have no enzymes able to break it down to simple glucose.

Starting with saliva in the mouth, starches are reduced to simpler sugars as they pass through the digestive system until they are carried to the liver and changed to glucose. Glucose from the liver is delivered in the blood to all the cells of the body where it is used to produce energy. The by-products of energy production are heat, water, and carbon dioxide which the body eliminates through the kidneys, lungs, and skin.

The liver changes some glucose into a form of sugar called glycogen. It stores part of the glycogen for emergencies and the rest is stored in the muscles to use in contraction. Any carbohydrates not used by the body cells or stored as glycogen is turned into fat. Each gram of carbohydrate provides four calories and it takes about 3,500 calories to make one pound of fat. To control fat, we have to cut back on carbohydrates.

Cereals contain starch and fiber and various vitamins and minerals. Important nutrients are lost when cereals are refined. Foods that have been processed so that little remains except carbohydrates are said to contain "empty calories."

Carbohydrates in themselves are not nutritionally bad or fattening. But the carbohydrate should be of the most nutritious kind, rather than refined sugar and devitalized grains. Too much "empty calorie" carbohydrates can lead to health problems, notably obesity and tooth decay.

Here are some ways you can use carbohydrates to support your health.

- Eat whole grain bread and cereal.
- Eat raw fruits as often as possible.
- Cut back on processed foods.
- Eliminate refined sugar and refined cereals.
- Read food labels.

SUGAR

In 1999, the average American consumed 158 pounds of sugar, equivalent to fifty teaspoons a day! That's thirty percent higher than in 1983. This sharp increase is paralleled by a doubling in the rate of overweight and obesity in children and adolescents in the past twenty years.

The main problem with increased sugar consumption is that it crowds out nutritional foods. People who eat diets high in sugar consume less fruits and vegetables and get less vitamins and minerals, increasing their risk of osteoporosis, cancer, and heart disease.

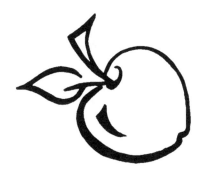

Tooth decay is clearly associated with sugar. Any sugar or starch that sticks to the teeth can increase acid levels in saliva leading to decay. Acidic "sports drinks" and fruit juices as well as candy, dried fruit, crackers—anything that sticks to the teeth—can put you at risk.

You can cut down on cavities by not eating between-meal snacks containing lots of sugar. Eat high carbohydrate foods only as part of a meal. Brush your teeth after eating, and floss your teeth every day. Have regular checkups with your dentist and a thorough twice-a-year cleaning by a dental hygienist.

Much of the sugar we eat comes in manufactured products where it is used to preserve foods or add bulk or density. You may think you are doing well by not putting sugar in your coffee, and still be loading up on sugar with the processed foods you eat.

Look at the nutritional labels on the food you buy if you want to discover how much sugar you are eating without realizing it. Look at the Nutritional Facts table under Total Carbohydrates. Multiply the number of grams by four to get the total calories from carbohydrates. If you don't really need these calories for energy, your body will use about 200 of them to make an ounce of fat.

Here is some useful information about the different sugars:

Glucose is the only form of sugar that can be used directly by the body for energy. All other forms have to be broken down in the digestive process first. Most fruits, some vegetables, honey, and corn syrup all contain glucose.

Sucrose (table sugar) is a combination of glucose and fructose and is found in sugar cane, sugar beets, maple syrup, fruit, and some vegetables, like sweet potatoes. Brown sugar is table sugar with a little molasses or burnt sugar added for color.

Fructose or **fruit sugar** is found in fruits, some vegetables, honey, and berries.

Lactose or **milk sugar** is found only in the milk of humans and other mammals and is composed of glucose and galactose.

Maltose or **malt sugar** is produced during the malting process of grains and is found in beer, malted foods, and sprouted grains.

Starch is the way most carbohydrates are stored in plants. Starch is slowly broken down by the body to the simple sugar glucose before it is absorbed. Starch is found in whole grains, legumes, nuts, potatoes and other tubers, lentils, sesame and sunflower seeds, yams, sweet potatoes, and some other vegetables.

ARTIFICIAL SWEETENERS

To avoid sugar, many people use artificial sweeteners. Here are comments on the most commonly used artificial sweeteners.

Saccharin has no calories, is inexpensive, and has a slightly bitter aftertaste. Saccharin is known to cause cancer of the bladder in experimental animals when very high doses are given. It has been approved for human use by the FDA with a label that reads, "Use of this product may be hazardous to your health. This product contains saccharin which has been determined to cause cancer in laboratory animals." It should not be used by children or pregnant women. Saccharin is sold as Sweet'n Low.

Cyclamate has no calories and is excreted unchanged by the kidneys. However, cyclamate is banned by the FDA pending review of studies that showed it caused cancer of the bladder.

Aspartame has the same caloric content as sugar but only a very small amount is needed, making the number of calories used very small. Aspartame cannot be used in cooking because it breaks down when heated. It is dangerous to a small group of people with phenylketonuria, so the package must be marked with a warning. The body produces methanol, formaldehyde, and formate when it metabolizes aspartame, although in small amounts. Methanol is found in higher amounts in citrus juices and tomatoes. It is marketed as Equal and NutraSweet.

Acesulfame K contains no calories, is not metabolized by the body, and has some aftertaste. More than ninety studies verify the sweetener's safety. It is sold as Sunett.

Sucralose tastes like sugar because it is made from table sugar, but it cannot be digested and adds no calories to food. Its safety has been supported by over 110 animal and human studies. It is sold as Splenda.

Stevia is a sweetener made from a South American shrub. The FDA considers it an unapproved food additive whose safety has been questioned by published studies. It can be sold as a dietary supplement but not promoted as a sweetener.

BREAD AND REFINED FLOUR

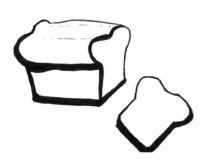

Importance of Bread

Bread baked with whole grain flours has been the staff of life from the earliest times. Bread made with milled white flour simply doesn't have the nourishment that is found in whole grain bread. Make sure that you purchase 100 percent whole wheat bread. From the earliest times more unleavened bread was used than leavened bread. If yeast of any kind is used in bread, it needs to be thoroughly baked

Oats make an excellent bread. You can also make a delicious bread by taking part whole wheat flour, whole corn flour, whole oat flour, and whole soybean flour. By adding a little malt, honey, or Karo syrup, you can make a bread anyone can live and work on by eating just a little fruit with it. A person can live very well on a diet of only whole wheat bread, whole rye bread, or whole barley bread, with vegetables and fruit added.

Refined or Milled Flour

Refining of cereal grain (wheat, rice, corn) removes many of the valuable nutrients and makes the grain less nutritionally valuable. Refined flour will not spoil and turn rancid and it is less likely to be infested with insects. This is an advantage to the producer but not necessarily to you, the consumer.

The essential vitamins and minerals in grains are located in the bran, aleurone, and germ layers. The portion remaining after the milling process contains only starch and a little protein. Whole grain contains the entire seed except for the outer layer or hull, which we can't eat so it is discarded. Whole grain cereals and breads should be kept in the refrigerator to keep the fat from turning rancid.

80   The Executive Chef's Arthritis Cookbook and Health Guide

The enrichment of refined white flour was made mandatory by the U.S. government to replace some of the lost nutrients. Enrichment consists of adding thiamine, riboflavin, niacin, and iron in sufficient quantity to bring the grain almost back to its original content; addition of calcium and Vitamin D was optional. The seventeen other minerals and vitamins, as well as fiber, that are removed during the milling process are not replaced and are absent even in enriched bread and flour.

When I read the ingredients in a loaf of locally baked whole wheat bread, I see it is made of enriched wheat flour (flour, malted barley flour, reduced iron, niacin, thiamine mononitrate, riboflavin, folic acid), water, whole wheat flour, honey, wheat bran, wheat gluten, oats, barley, brown sugar, raisin juice concentrate, wheat, rye, yeast, partially hydrogenated soybean oil, salt, wheat germ, mono- and diglycerides, calcium sulfate, sodium proprionate.

In comparison with the commercial loaf of bread, the ingredients listed on the loaf of sprouted whole wheat bread I bought at the health food store reads as follows: sprouted wheat, whole wheat flour, water, yeast, salt, honey, soy oil, malt, and lecithin.

The difference can make a difference to your health. Use 100 percent whole-grain bread. You will find it to be a good source of fiber, minerals, vitamins, and complex carbohydrates.

SALT

Salt is one way we get sodium which is essential to our metabolism. Sodium helps maintain the proper water balance, assists in muscle contraction, aids in the proper functioning of the nervous system, maintains the correct balance of acids in both the blood and urine, and aids in the absorption of nutrients through the cell membranes.

However, most of us get way more sodium than we need. Our bodies need only 500mg of sodium per day. Anything over 2500mg is probably too much. For some people excess sodium causes high blood pressure. For others, sodium is no problem. The body maintains a very careful balance of sodium and gets rid of the excess in the urine and perspiration.

The recommended daily allowance of salt is 3 to 8 grams, or 1100 to 3300mg of sodium. The average daily intake of salt is 6 to 17 grams, or 2300 to 6900mg of sodium. One teaspoon of salt has about 2000mg of sodium.

Here are some ways to reduce the amount of sodium in your diet.

From *Back to Eden*, p. 615

1. Remove the salt shaker from the dinner table. This may be done gradually over two or three weeks.
2. Cut down by one-half the amount of salt added to food while cooking.
3. Omit or limit salty foods.
4. Eat fresh fruit and vegetables whenever possible. Canned vegetables may have up to ten times as much sodium as fresh vegetables.
5. Eat unsalted frozen vegetables rather than canned.
6. Cut down on the consumption of prepared foods.
7. Avoid foods with MSG on the label. Oriental food is high in MSG (monosodium glutamate), which has been reported to cause mental confusion and/or headaches in some people. This has been termed the "Chinese Restaurant Syndrome."

Table salt is composed of sodium (40%) and chloride (60%). Sodium salts are plentiful in fruits and vegetables such as tomatoes, asparagus, celery, spinach, kale, radishes, turnips, carrots, lettuce, strawberries, and many others. A healthy diet will give you all the sodium you need. When no salt is added to food, a person soon learns to enjoy the real flavor of the food.

The word salt comes from the Latin word *salus,* meaning "health." Salt has been used as a preservative for centuries. Roman soldiers at one time received their pay in salt and from this custom the word *salary* originated. Salt has been so widely proclaimed as a health hazard that 40% of adults are now trying to cut down on their salt consumption.

Some processed foods contain quite large amounts of sodium. If you are concerned about the amount of sodium you are eating, be sure to check the food labels. If you must reduce your salt intake, look for foods with "low sodium," "salt free," or "no added salt" on the label.

From *Back to Eden,* pg. 616

Foods High in Salt

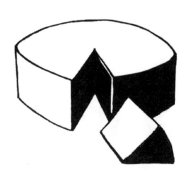

Cheese
"Fast foods"
Processed meat:
  luncheon meat
  corned beef
  franks
  sausage
  salami
  cured ham and bacon
Canned soups
Canned fish:
  herring
  sardines
  anchovies
Bouillon broth
Canned vegetables
Frozen dinners
Bread
Celery salt
Garlic salt
Onion salt
Salted snacks and nuts
Sauces:
    Worcestershire
    ketchup
    soy sauce
Pickles, olives
Frozen entrees
Sauerkraut
Drinking water, specially
    if water softener is used.

Reducing salt is best done gradually. Our salt substitute, which you will find below, will help you get off salt.

You can go a long way toward reducing your salt intake by avoiding salty commercially-prepared foods. Some canned soups contain the recommended daily allowance of salt in just one serving. While weaning yourself away from salt, try exploring some of the delicious herbs and spices God put on earth for us to use.

In recent years many major food processors have introduced "reduced salt" or "no salt added" products. Health food stores are a great source for these less salty products. In many cases, the workers in these stores are very knowledgeable about these products.

The United States Food and Drug Administration has established the following guidelines for foods that make claims about sodium.

Label Guideline

Sodium Free: Contains less than 5 milligrams (mg) per serving.

Very Low Sodium: Contains 35mg or less per serving.

Low Sodium: Contains 140mg or less per serving.

Reduced Sodium: Sodium content must be reduced by 75% or more below what would be in the product it replaces.

Unsalted, No Salt Added, Without Added Salt: No salt was added in processing to a food that would normally be processed with salt.

SODIUM COMPOUNDS

The following is a list of sodium compounds that are common additives to the foods you purchase. They should be prohibited on a sodium-restricted diet.

Sodium chloride: common table salt, used in cooking, canning, and processing

Monosodium glutamate (MSG): a seasoning used in home and restaurant cooking, and in many packaged, canned, and processed frozen foods

Baking powder: used in the preparation of breads and cakes

Baking soda: sodium bicarbonate, used in the preparation of breads and cakes, and in some styles of vegetable cookery. It's also used as an alkalizer for cases of indigestion.

Brine: salt and water solution used in processing foods, and in canning, freezing, and pickling

Disodium phosphate: used in some quick-cooking cereals and in processed cheeses

Sodium alginate: used in chocolate milk and ice cream to make them smooth

Sodium benzoate: used as a preservative in condiments

Sodium hydroxide: used in processing of some fruits and vegetables, and ripe olives

Sodium propionate: used in pasteurized cheeses and in some breads and cakes

Sodium sulfate: used as a bleach for some fresh fruits, and as a preservative of some dried fruits

SALT SUBSTITUTE

At first you will miss salt, but as time goes by your taste buds will change and you will learn to enjoy the natural flavors of your favorite foods.

There are many commercial salt substitutes available. Most contain some salt or other sodium that aggravates arthritis sufferers' conditions. READ THE LABEL.

Here is a salt substitute I developed and use frequently. Many of the people I've worked with or counseled swear by it. Only buy the "low sodium" or preferably the "no sodium" products for this recipe.

1 cup.	Nutritional Yeast
1/2 oz.	Granulated Sea Kelp
1/2 oz.	Garlic Powder
1/2 oz.	Mild Chili Powder
1/4 oz.	Dill Weed
1/2 oz.	Onion Powder

Method of Preparation
Your favorite health food store will have all the ingredients you need. Ask them to weigh it for you and put it in one bag. This should cost you somewhere between 60¢ and 75¢ depending on where you live.

Combine all of the ingredients in a small glass bowl and mix well. Buy yourself one of those large aluminum salt shakers you see in the supermarket. Put the salt substitute in there and shake, shake, shake over your foods. When first using this product, start with a little and add more if necessary. Compared to salt you don't have to use as much.

Enjoy.

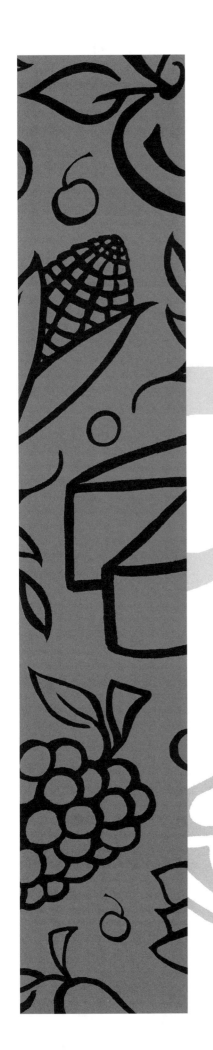
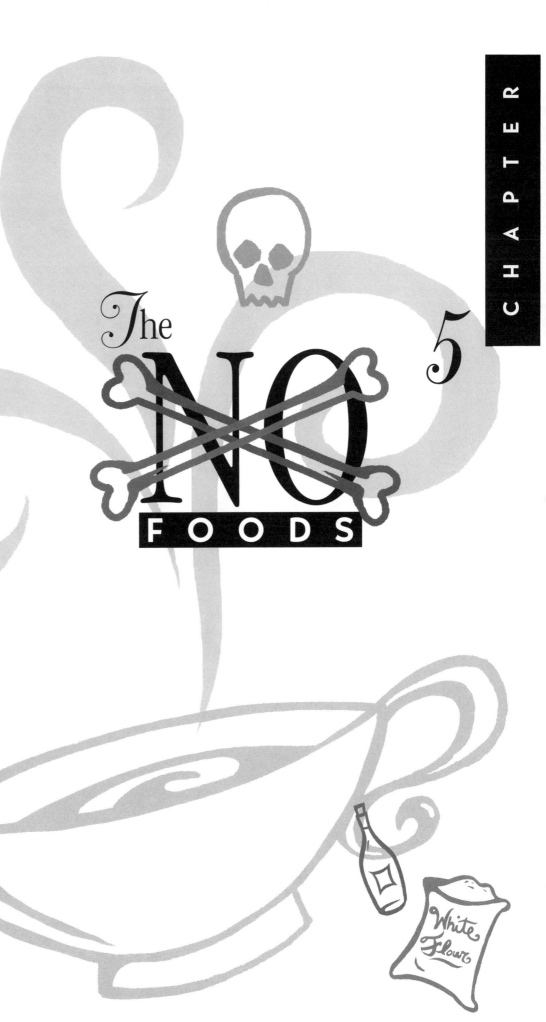

CHAPTER 5

The NO FOODS

THE NO FOODS

The **NO foods** are what this book is all about. We feel that by omitting these foods and eating a balanced diet of fresh, good, wholesome foods, your flare-ups will be eased and possibly go away. There are many people who believe that arthritis can be caused by allergic reactions to certain foods, by chemical additives in food, or a combination of the two.

The first group of foods to omit from your daily eating are the foods of the nightshade family. Common vegetables belonging to the nightshade family are:

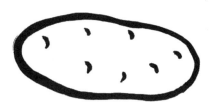

Eggplant
Bell Peppers: Green, Red, and Yellow
Tomatoes
Cherry Peppers
Potatoes
Red Clusters (a type of chili pepper)
Chili Peppers
Long and Red Peppers
Pimento
Paprika
Cayenne

From *Prescription for Cooking*, p. 49-50.

Nightshades

What are nightshades? As a botanical family, the *Solanaceae* comprise some ninety-two genera with over two thousand species. Its members include many stimulating, medicinal, or poisonous plants, such as *tobacco, henbane, mandrake,* and *belladonna* (also known as the deadly nightshade). The food plants of the nightshade family include some of our most popular vegetables: *tomatoes, potatoes, eggplant,* and *peppers* of all kinds (green, red, chili, paprika, cayenne, hot, sweet, and so on, except for black and white pepper). Research has found that when people with joint pains stopped consuming all varieties of nightshades, their condition improved dramatically.

It turns out that *nightshades* are *high in alkaloids,* chemical substances with a strong physiological effect. In the case of potatoes, storage conditions after harvest that include light and heat may, over time, increase their content of the alkaloid *solanine* up to toxic limits. Improperly stored old potatoes have been known to cause symptoms severe enough to require hospitalization, including gastrointestinal inflammation, nausea, diarrhea, and dizziness.

Earl Mindell in his book *"Unsafe at Any Meal"* stated the following concerning potatoes, "Solanine, present in and around these green patches and in the eyes that have sprouted, can interfere with the transmission of nerve impulses, and cause jaundice, abdominal pain, vomiting, and diarrhea."

These alkaloids act a little like a variation of vitamin D, in that they appear to affect the metabolism of calcium. Nightshade foods may, through a mechanism not yet understood, remove calcium from the bones and deposit it in joints, kidneys, arteries, and other areas of the body where it does not belong. Thus, they may contribute to arthritis.

Nightshades are consumed in appreciable quantities mostly in dietary systems that also include milk products. These foods often show up in pairs: tomato sauce and cheese, potatoes and sour cream, spicy Indian foods, yogurt, and eggplant parmigiana.

Nightshades, with their calcium disturbing alkaloids, have something to do with the digestion or assimilation of milk products, which have an excessively high calcium content. After all, cow's milk contains four times more calcium than a human mother's milk; that may turn out to be too much for the human metabolism to handle, and we may, therefore turn to nightshades in self defense.

In other words, when the nightshades are consumed in calcium rich diets, they help keep the calcium from depositing itself in the wrong places. Such is the case as long as the body is functioning properly. If it is not, then either the nightshades pull out calcium from all kinds of other places or the dairy calcium does not get utilized and collects in the joints, etc.

The symptoms include bone loss, tooth decay, and what is called the "naked tooth feeling" (a sensation of rawness or brittleness in the teeth). Solutions: if you are avoiding dairy foods and eating low fat, you may want to test eliminating the nightshade vegetables from your diet.

Dr. Collin H. Dong, a San Francisco physician created a diet called the "Dong diet." He believes arthritis is caused by allergic reactions to certain food and chemical additives in the food. His diet prohibits meat, fruits, tomatoes, all dairy products, all acids including vinegar, all types of peppers, hot spices, chocolate, roasted nuts, alcoholic beverages, especially wine, soft drinks, all foods containing preservatives, additives and chemicals, mainly MSG (monosodium glutamate).

His diet favors fish, which is good because fish oils appear to benefit arthritis. His diet cuts back on most of the nightshades. Eggs as well as vitamin A and D, in supplement form, or foods fortified with these vitamins, as found in margarine, should be avoided. The sun on the skin promotes sufficient vitamin D, the green leafy vegetables, the orange colored ones, such as carrots, sweet potatoes, and cantaloupes provide plenty of vitamin A in the diet.

Norman F. Childers, a former professor of horticulture at Rutgers University had severe joint pains and stiffness after consuming tomatoes in any form. He was aware of the nightshade family of plants and their toxicity. He observed livestock kneeling because their knee joints were painful to hold them up, after eating weeds containing solanine. He then started to test the nightshade foods one at a time and found that each one aggravated his arthritic pain. He eliminated everyone of the nightshade family from his diet and within months his pain vanished. He totally believes that those who are sensitive or allergic to the nightshade vegetables will cure the aches and pains of arthritis by avoiding those foods.

The macrobiotic diet that is noted for its healing properties forbids meat, eggs, dairy products, poultry, fruit juices, and nightshade vegetables.

If you have arthritis or think you might, if you have bone loss or aching muscles and joints, you should experiment with these foods to see if you improve.

The Executive Chef's Arthritis Cookbook and Health Guide is an **elimination diet**. Arthritis is basically a flare-up of inflammation in a joint. Where does this inflammation come from? What makes it happen? You're going about your usual daily routine, you have lunch, and a few hours later you have a flare-up. Why? What caused it?

Our hypothesis is that one of the foods you ate caused the flare-up to happen. What can you do? You can try our plan!! The prospect of easing or taking away your arthritis by simply giving up certain foods seems well worth a try.

The role of your food intake or diet is the most written about, talked about, and hotly debated subjects when discussing arthritis. There is much advice about this in many recent books. But there isn't much information on what people should not eat. Especially lacking are documented case studies involving what people should not eat.

Our elimination diet puts into action our theory that certain types or groups of food are more likely to cause an arthritic flare-up than others. Our theory is that certain foods will cause allergy-like reactions in people who are sensitive to these foods. We also know the reactions vary with each individual. So how do you know which foods might be causing your problems?

Putting The Plan to Work: The First Way

Exactly how a food sensitivity can affect arthritis isn't known. If it was known, a medical test could determine which foods cause your problems. Instead, a different sort of test is needed. If you write down what you eat before you eat it, you'll document which foods you ate before an arthritis flare-up. When one happens, you can go to our list of **NO foods** and see if one or more of the foods you ate that day is on our list. You will then be able to test which food caused your flare-up by simple elimination: one at a time, eat these foods on different days and see if a flare-up occurs. If one does, simply don't eat the food that is making life painful for you. It is very important to eat only one food at a time that you think is causing you a problem so you'll know what your reaction is to that single food. We usually eat meals that combine many different foods which can mislead you into thinking one kind of food causes a reaction, when it was actually another food you ate that caused it. This is the short way.

Putting The Plan to Work: The Second Way

The second way takes longer, but is good when a build-up of reactions causes your arthritis. For thirty days, write down everything you eat. Breakfast—lunch—dinner—snacks—drinks. Everything! Everything! Everything!

After that month, take your list and go through the **NO foods**. Mark down beside each **NO food** the number of times you ate it during the thirty-day period.

Now over the next ninety days try each food one by one. Did it cause a flare-up? If so, stop eating this food. Your body is telling you, "No, no, no!"

After ninety days of eliminating foods that hurt you, your body should start to feel better. If you eat new foods and they cause flare-ups, add them to your list of foods that you as an individual will eliminate. Enjoy better health!

The Executive Chef's Arthritis Cookbook and Health Guide has a few of the nightshade vegetables in some of the recipes because not everyone has a problem with them. Remember we are eliminating the foods one by one, so if they don't cause an arthritis flare-up, go ahead and enjoy them. You may notice we have a full chapter about potatoes. Why? Statistically only 4 to 5% of arthritis sufferers have a problem with potatoes, which means 95 to 96% of the people can eat them. So if you can, enjoy.

Foods High in Purines

Gout sufferers should avoid foods high in purines. Gout is a type of arthritis in which uric acid crystals are deposited within the joints and cause inflammation. Many protein foods contain purines from which uric acid is produced, causing a gout flare-up. If you have gout, stay away from these foods:

Anchovies	**Herring**
Scallops	**Red Meats**
Wild Game	**Mushrooms**
Cauliflower	**Lentils**
Dried Peas	**Turkey**
Sweetbreads	**Gravies**
Mackerel	**Liver**
Sardines	**Meat Extracts**
Asparagus	**Spinach**
Dried Beans	**Chicken**
Goose	**Brains**
Red Wine	**Too much alcohol in general**

Sometimes they can aggravate other types of arthritis as well, so all arthritis sufferers should observe their reaction to these foods.

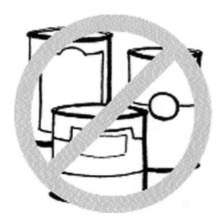

Other Foods

You might be surprised at what you will find at the health food store—many of them are run like supermarkets, and all of them concentrate on healthy foods. Buy fresh, fresh, fresh foods. See Chapter 23 for health food store products you can buy to improve the quality of the foods that you now eat. Don't forget to include plenty of raw vegetables (except the ones that cause reactions) in your daily intake of food.

Try to avoid all canned vegetables because they contain salt, white sugar, and chemical preservatives that aren't good for arthritis sufferers. We suggest you avoid the meats listed below.

FOODSERVICE CUTS OF BEEF

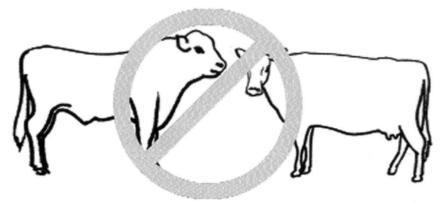

Cubed Steak
Swiss Steak
Rib Steak
Ribeye Roll Steak
Inner Skirt Steak
Outer Skirt Steak
Ground Beef Patties
Knuckle Steak
Top Steak
Bottom Steak
Porterhouse Steak

Chuck Roll
Beef Brisket
Short Ribs
Flank Steak
Ribeye Roll
Top Round
Outside Round
Bottom Round
Beef Rib Oven Prepared
Beef Foreshank
Beef Bones

Chapter 5 The NO Foods

Ready Rib Roast
Stewing Beef
Inside Round
Smoked Tongue
Top Round Roast Beef, Cooked
Roast Beef, Outside Round (Flat, Corned, Cooked Eye Round)
Beef Ribs
Beef Chuck
Chuck Tender
Beef Loin
T-Bone Steak
Strip Loin Steak
Top Sirloin Butt Steak
Bottom Sirloin Butt Ball Tip Steak
Boneless Deckle Off Corned Brisket
Corned Outside Round
Tri-Tip Steak
Tenderloin Steak
Shoulder Clod-Boneless Deckle
Beef Liver
Portion Cut Frozen Beef Liver
Calf Liver
Portion Cut Frozen Calf Liver
Veal Sweetbreads
Beef Tongue
Beef Oxtail

All Other Beef Products, moo moo moo

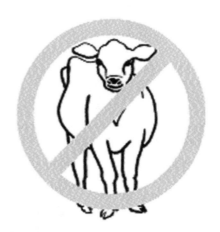

FOODSERVICE CUTS OF VEAL

Boneless Chuck
Hotel Rack
Rack, Ribeye
Veal Chops
Loin, Butt Tenderloin
Veal Cutlets
Foreshank
Osso Buco
Veal for Stewing
Shoulder Clod Roast
Rib Chops
Veal Loin
Strip Loin
Leg of Veal
Hindshank
Breast
Veal Cubed Steak
Ground Veal

All Other Veal Products, moo moo moo

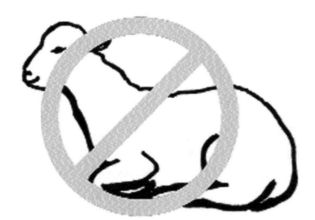

FOODSERVICE CUTS OF LAMB

Lamb Shoulder-Boneless
Rack of Lamb
Lamb Loin
Leg of Lamb
Denver Style Ribs
Lamb Breast
Ground Lamb

Shoulder Chops
Rib Chops
Loin Chops
Lamb for Stewing
Hindsaddle
Boneless Sirloin

All Other Lamb Products, baa baa baa

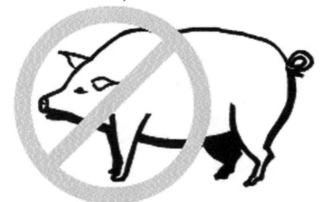

FOODSERVICE CUTS OF PORK

Pork Shoulder Boston Butt
Shoulder Butt
Shoulder Hocks
Pork Loin
Tenderloin
French Ham, Short Shank
Boneless Fresh Ham
Pork Filets
Butt Steaks
Ground Pork
Boston Butt Steaks
Pork Belly
Spareribs

Ham, Boneless, Skinless, Cured and Smoked, Fully Cooked, Special
Ham, Shankless, Skinless, Cured and Smoked, Tied
Ham, Semi-Boneless, Femur Bone in, Cured and Smoked, Skinned, Tied
Ham, Semi-Boneless, Femur Bone out, Cured and Smoked, Skinned, Tied
Ham, Shoulder, Cured, Smoked
Ham, Shoulder, Picnic, Cured and Smoked

Chapter 5 The NO Foods 95

Loin Chops
Pork Loin, Canadian Back
Boneless, Cured and Smoked, Tied
Loin, Cured and Smoked
Back Ribs
Diced Pork
Cubed Pork
Pork Loin, Chops
Ham, Short Shank, Cured and Smoked
Ham, Boneless, Skinless, Cured, Fully Cooked, Moist Heat
Shoulder, Cellar-Trimmed Butt
Ham, Boneless, Skinless, Cured and Smoked
Loin, Bladeless, Cured and Smoked
Canadian Back, Cured and Smoked, Unsliced
Canadian-Style Bacon, Cured and Smoked, Sliced
Hocks, Shoulder, Cured and Smoked

All Other Pork Products, oink oink oink

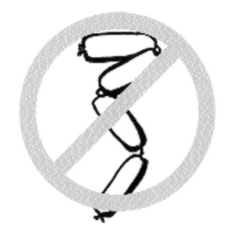

MEATS FURTHER PROCESSED/BY-PRODUCTS

Ring Bologna
Knockwurst
Polish Sausage
Beerwurst
Blood and Tongue
Hamburger Loaf
Pickle and Pimento Loaf
Thuringer
Liverwurst
Head Cheese
Fresh Pork Sausages
Bratwurst
Prosky
Mettwurst
Minced Ham
Bologna
Frankfurters
Pepperloaf
Smoked Sausage Links
Lebanon Bologna
Bologna
Pork Sausage
Pork Sausage, Patties
Pork Sausage, Patties, Precooked
Liver Sausage (Braunschweiger)
Salami, Cooked
Minced Luncheon Meat
Dry Salami
Cervelat
Breakfast Sausage
Smoked Sausage
New England Brand Sausage
Meat Loaves
Meat Food Product Loaves
Breakfast Sausage, Cooked

Remember, there are many **NO foods** that won't cause your own arthritis flare-ups. Each of us is affected by foods in a different way. If the food has no effect on you and you enjoy it, *eat it!*

Diet Tip
Too much red meat with the safety concerns of preservatives, bacteria, iron, fat, and other chemicals has been associated with the increase of arthritis symptoms in some patients. If red meat is eaten at all, it should be limited to less than three ounces a day. Better yet, red meat should be more of a side dish or garnish than the focus of all your meals.

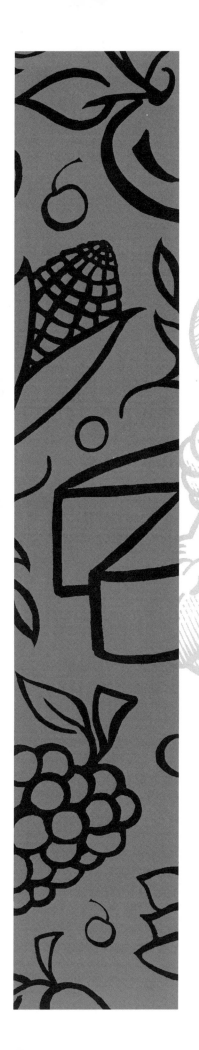
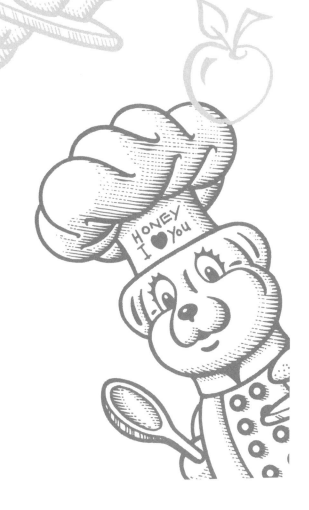

APPLES & HONEY

CHAPTER 6

98

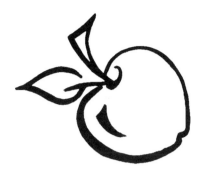

Diet Tip
For a great dessert, peel, core, and slice a couple of apples. Put them in a bowl, drip a tablespoon of honey over them, then sprinkle a small dash of cinnamon and eat. What a great, healthy dessert!

APPLES

Apples are the fruit of the earth many of us love to eat. Thanks to a man named John Chapman, America has and always will have plenty of this glorious God-given fruit. "Johnny Appleseed" was born in 1775 in Leominster, Massachusetts. He helped propagate apples across America. Chapman collected apple seeds from cider mills, dried them, put them in little bags, and gave them to all takers who were headed west. The fruits of Chapman's work can still be found. The apples of trees descended from seeds Johnny Appleseed planted still go into apple pies and many other apple-related products on American tables.

At one time there were probably more than 1,000 different American apple varieties. Most of them have now disappeared. Some were killed off by insects and different diseases when no controls existed. Some disappeared because they didn't ship well. Some trees were cut down by folks fighting the evils of cider and applejack. Unfortunately, there's not room enough to mention the many other reasons why all these varieties disappeared.

Varieties that survived and we still enjoy are: the mellow Baldwin, the Cortland, the yellow Golden Delicious, the Red Delicious, the Gravenstein (which is used for applesauce), the Red Lady, the Rome, the McIntosh, the Pippin and the Northern Spy, just to name a few.

Besides enjoying the fresh, raw fruit, apples are available canned as applesauce, or as juice or cider, plus many other ways of canning and cooking the product. An average apple contains only about 85 calories, and only a trace of sodium. An apple provides a small amount of a variety of vitamins and minerals, including calcium, iron, thiamin, and ascorbic acid. Of course, an apple contains no cholesterol, only living animals contain cholesterol. There is a saying among food service professionals that goes, "If it doesn't have a liver, it doesn't have cholesterol."

Apples, apples, apples. Eat plenty of them. They are good for you, they taste good, and they are good roughage. Remember the old saying, "An apple a day keeps the doctor away."

When buying apples, look for firm, crisp apples with no soft spots, bruises, or wrinkles. High color is an indication of maturity and only apples picked when mature will have good flavor and texture. Avoid apples that yield to pressure on the skin—they will have a soft, mealy flesh. Bruised areas are a sign of exposure to frost or to improper handling. To maintain apple quality, store them at refrigerator temperature. They like a relatively high humidity.

The material for the following section was provided by the National Honey Board.

TOP 10 REASONS TO USE HONEY

10. It keeps baked goods moist.
9. Its versatility—honey butter, spread, sweetener, condiment.
8. It's natural—gives customers a very good wholesome feeling.
7. Its convenience—no refrigeration, can sit on a table.
6. Its golden honey color—brings a sheen to food.
5. It's fat free—used to thicken salad dressings.
4. It's promotable for restaurants.
3. It's profitable—popular natural food.
2. Its taste—very upscale taste.
1. The bees need the work!

HONEY TIP SHEET

Honey adds beautiful golden color and delightful sweet flavor to bring out the best in so many foods.

Cooking Tips

- For best results, use recipes developed for using honey.
- When you substitute honey for granulated sugar in recipes:

    substitute honey for up to one-half of the sugar. With experimentation, honey can be substituted for all the sugar in some recipes.

    reduce the amount of liquid in the recipe by 1/4 cup for each cup of honey used in baked goods.

    add about 1/2 teaspoon baking soda for each cup of honey used in baked goods.

    reduce oven temperature by 25° F to prevent over-browning of baked goods.

    for easy removal, spray measuring cup with vegetable cooking spray before adding honey.

- Honey adds a sweet, smooth and distinctive taste to recipes. Honey also absorbs and retains moisture. These qualities retard drying out and staling of baked goods.
- A 12-ounce jar of honey equals a standard measuring cup.
- Because of its high fructose content, honey has greater sweetening power than sugar.

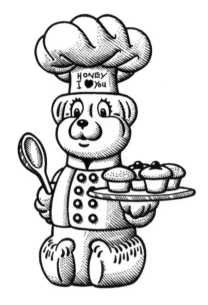

Lifestyle Tip

Medical research has shown that prayer is an effective addition to any treatment program. When you pray, count your blessings and give thanks and praise. Ask to be filled with love and inspiration. Request protection and guidance. Be sure to forgive yourself as well as others. Sing love melodies and hymns to yourself. Ask for your needs and the needs of all others to be met, especially those you perceive to be your enemies. Sit quietly after you pray and write down any feelings, thoughts, or images that come to mind. See how you can use them in your pathway to healing.

Chapter 6 Apples & Honey 101

Buying and Storage Tips

- Select mildly flavored honeys, such as clover, for use in cooking where delicate flavors predominate.

- Use strongly flavored honeys in spreads or other recipes where a distinct honey flavor is desired.

- Store honey at room temperature.

- If honey crystallizes, remove lid and place jar in warm water until crystals dissolve. Or, microcook 1 cup of honey in microwave-safe container at HIGH (100%) 2 to 3 minutes or until crystals dissolve; stir every 30 seconds. Do not boil or scorch.

NOTE: Honey should not be fed to infants under 1 year of age. Honey is a safe and wholesome food for older children and adults.

Look for the Honey Bear logo on products containing a substantial amount of honey.

HONEY NUTRITION FACTS

Honey is the only natural sweetener known that needs no additional refining or processing to be utilized. Its unique flavor is attributable to the floral source from which the honey bees gathered nectar—there are more than 300 such sources in the United States.

Honey is an invert sugar composed of 38 percent fructose, 31 percent glucose, 1 percent sucrose and 9 percent other sugars along with water and small amounts of vitamins, minerals and acids.

As a carbohydrate, honey is a good supplier of energy at 64 calories per tablespoon. Honey contains small amounts of riboflavin, thiamine, ascorbic acid and small amounts of minerals. The nutrients supplied by honey and other sweeteners are too low to be considered as practical sources of these nutrients.

Because of honey's unique composition, it is digested a little differently than other sweeteners. When compared to table sugar, honey has less of an effect on blood glucose and insulin levels primarily due to its higher fructose content.

Health Tip

Approximately 42% of Americans used some form of complementary and alternative medicine in 1997 and paid more visits to complementary and alternative practitioners than to conventional primary care physicians. Complementary and alternative treatment should be used not as a replacement for, but in conjunction with conventional medicine. Discuss all complementary and alternative treatments with your primary care physician.

HONEY FORMS AND FLAVORS

Consumers can look for honey at grocery stores and farmers' markets in these forms:

Liquid Honey
Free of visible crystals, liquid honey is extracted from the honey comb by centrifugal force, gravity or straining. Because liquid honey mixes easily into a variety of foods, it is especially convenient for cooking and baking. Most honey produced in the United States is sold in liquid form.

Creme or Spun Honey
While all honey will crystallize in time, creme or "spun" honey is brought to market in a finely crystallized state. The crystallization of creme honey is controlled so that, at room temperature, the honey can be spread like butter. Outside the United States, creme honey is the preferred form.

Comb Honey
Comb honey is honey that comes as it was produced—in the honey bee's wax comb. The comb, along with the honey, is edible.

Cut Comb
Cut comb honey is honey that has been packaged with chunks of the honey comb.

Lifestyle Tip
Obtain working aids for household tasks and simplify your work. Eliminate all unnecessary steps. Organize your storage space. Weed out all the articles that you do not use more than a few times per year. Place all items that are used regularly near the places where they are used. See to it that saucepans, frying pans, kettles, spices, and other food ingredients are placed near the stove and are as light as possible.

Chapter 6 Apples & Honey 103

HONEY COLOR AND FLAVOR—
IT ALL DEPENDS ON WHERE THE BEES BUZZ

The color and flavor of honeys differ depending on the nectar source (the blossoms) visited by the honey bees. Honey color ranges from nearly colorless to dark brown, and its flavor varies from delectably mild to distinctively bold, depending on where the honey bees buzzed. To learn more about available types of honey in your area, contact a local beekeeper, honey packer or distributor, or the National Honey Board.

Following is a look at some of the most common honeys and their floral sources.

Health Tip
Patients with rheumatologic conditions such as osteoarthritis, fibromyalgia, and rheumatoid arthritis frequently use complementary and alternative treatments. Patients should readily tell their physicians about complementary and alternative treatments they are using, because of potential side effects, incompatibility with some of their medications, or determining what supplements aren't useful for their particular illness.

Alfalfa
Alfalfa honey, produced extensively throughout Canada and the U.S., is light in color with a pleasingly mild flavor and aroma.

Basswood
Basswood honey is often characterized by its distinctive "biting" flavor. Basswood honey is generally water white in color and strong in flavor.

Buckwheat
Buckwheat honey is dark and full-bodied. The production of buckwheat, and therefore buckwheat honey, has declined in the United States. It is still produced, however, in Minnesota, New York, Ohio, Pennsylvania and Wisconsin as well as in eastern Canada.

Clover
Clover honey has a pleasing, mild taste. Clovers contribute more to honey production in the United States than any other group of plants. Red clover, Alsike clover and the white and yellow sweet clovers are most important for honey production. Depending on the location and type of source clover, clover honey varies in color from water white to light amber to amber.

Eucalyptus
Eucalyptus honey comes from one of the larger plant genera, containing over 500 distinct species and many hybrids. As may be expected with a diverse group of plants, eucalyptus honey varies greatly in color and flavor but tends to be a stronger flavored honey. Eucalyptus is the major source of honey in Australia. It is also produced in California.

Fireweed
Fireweed honey is light in color and comes from a perennial herb that affords wonderful bee pasture in the Northern and

Pacific states and Canada. Fireweed grows in the open woods, reaching a height of three to five feet and spikes attractive pinkish flowers.

Orange Blossom

Orange blossom honey, often a combination of citrus sources, is usually light in color and mild in flavor with a fresh scent and light taste reminiscent of the blossom. Orange blossom honey is produced in Florida, Southern California and southern Texas.

Tulip Poplar

Tulip poplar or tulip tree honey is dark amber in color. The flavor, however, is not as strong as one would expect of a dark honey. Tulip poplar honey is produced from southern New England west to southern Michigan and south to the Gulf states east of the Mississippi.

Tupelo

Tupelo honey is a premium honey produced in northwest Florida. It is heavy bodied and is usually light golden amber with a greenish cast and has a mild, distinctive taste.

Wildflower

Wildflower honey is often used to describe honey from miscellaneous and undefined flower sources.

Honey Blends

While different types of honey are available, most honey, especially honey supplied in bulk, is blended to create a unique and consistent taste and color.

For more information, contact:
Mary Humann
Marketing Director
National Honey Board
390 Lashley Street
Longmont, CO 80501-6045
1-800-553-7162

(Thank you very much, Mary!)

Health Tip

Remember that everybody gains when you do not tire yourself out with unnecessary chores. Rest between chores. See to it that you have a comfortable resting place for lying and sitting within easy distance. Teach yourself to cut down your own demands for perfection.

CHAPTER 7

FACTS ABOUT Water

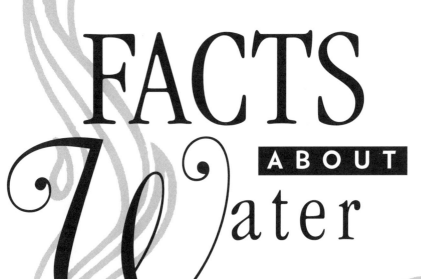

MEETING THE CHALLENGES OF LIFE WITH WATER
by James McKoy, M.D.

In our quest for optimal health and longevity, we simply overlook many of the important steps that can make this happen. America is suffering from chronic water deprivation, sleep deprivation, clean air deprivation, poor nutrition, lack of exercise, and too much stress. I believe these account for 80 to 90% of all illnesses.

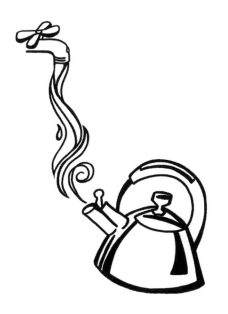

Health Tip
Regular training in a heated swimming pool is a pleasant and effective way to maintain flexibility, strengthen your muscles, and improve your general condition.

We have become too lazy to do what it takes to walk in good health. We abuse our bodies and expect clinics and hospitals to patch us up. Sometimes health professionals can help and sometimes we only wish we could do something. Many people are committing suicide slowly by neglecting their bodies. One of the major neglects is not giving the body the amount of water it needs for survival.

We may never climb Mt. Everest but we still have to face the challenges of life, which at times can loom before us larger than mountains. God therefore wants us to enjoy the best of health so we can better cope with these challenges. One of the ways we can do this is to take advantage of the precious gift He has given us of pure clean water. Water is the most versatile medium for all kinds of chemical magic and constitutes the major portion of our bodies. Water functions to dissolve substances in the body. It is a medium for chemical reactions, aids in temperature control and digestion, boosts our metabolism, helps to clear the body of toxins, and is a lubricant. It is the most important element we can put into our bodies besides oxygen. Without water, our life processes would cease in a few days.

Water makes up approximately 60% of our total weight. Lean muscle tissue contains about 73% water. Fat tissue is about 20% water. Thus, as fat content increases and the percentage of lean tissue decreases in the body, the percentage of body water content declines. Drinking enough water can help you to lose weight better and safer than fen-phen, diet drinks, pills, and potions which people are using unsuccessfully in the battle of the bulge.

Lack of water can contribute to weight gain by slowing your metabolism, decreasing clearance of toxins from the body, decreasing energy levels, and causing electrolyte shifts that are important for cellular function. A large glass of water 15-30 minutes prior to eating can decrease appetite and stomach capacity for food.

Water is so vital that a loss of even 20% of the total volume of fluid can result in death. About two-thirds of the water volume of the body is actually in the cells, with the other one-third outside the cells, namely in the blood and the fluid that circulates around the cells themselves. Virtually every activity that takes place within the body is through the medium of water.

For example, a thin film of fluid is constantly bathing the eye to protect it and to enable us to blink. If it were not for this lubricant, the surface of the eye would dry out, making it very difficult and painful to open and close the eyelids. It would also make it very difficult for us to see. Water lubricates the muscles and joints and allows them to function the way they are designed to function. The brain is made up of 80% water. If you don't drink adequate water, the neurons of the brain will die and you will become forgetful, depressed, and stressed out with mood swings. We age more quickly with inadequate water.

Cells deteriorate because waste products are being accumulated. Can you imagine a house that is allowed to throw out only 99.9% of its garbage that it produces every day? Within a few months, the house will have very bad odors. The accumulation of waste products and toxins can damage every organ in our body and cause a myriad of diseases. Water has been proven to reduce your blood pressure, lower your cholesterol level, decrease pain, prevent anxiety, help to handle stress, maintain your youthful skin, regain the sexual powers of your earlier years, increase your mental power and alertness, prevent heart disease, and give you the energy of your youth. Diseases are one of your body's many cries for water.

Like air, water is something that we take for granted, until it becomes very scarce. Unfortunately, many people today have gotten out of the habit of just drinking plain water. It is a common practice to drink a lot of tea, coffee, and carbonated drinks, especially those which contain caffeine and a lot of sugar. In the long term this often proves very detrimental to a person's overall physical condition. For this reason, I encourage everyone to develop the healthful habit of drinking plain pure water.

We should never wait until we are thirsty to drink water. Signs of thirst indicate that we are dehydrated and doing damage to our bodies. The thirst mechanism is not always reliable.

The average American drinks one and a half glasses of water a day. Think what would happen if you only put one quart of oil in a car which required eight quarts and you drive it to the max. It will soon fall apart and stop working. We are falling

Diet Tip
For optimal weight management try to minimize consumption of saturated fat (cheese, beef fat, lard, egg yolks, butter, whole milk) as well as trans-fatty acids (french fries, potato chips, margarine). The body needs fat, but eat more unsaturated fat instead (olive oil, avocados, nuts, etc).

Chapter 7 Facts About Water **109**

apart and will soon stop working because of our own neglect, discipline, and learned taste. A good rule of thumb is to drink one-half of your body weight in ounces evenly distributed throughout the day. I encourage everyone to drink two to three quarts of water a day. The body requires a minimum of approximately 64 ounces to function properly.

Drinking the appropriate amount of water throughout the day is a nominal investment in your health that provides rewards lasting a lifetime. The only things you have to lose are low energy, premature aging, disease, and death.

The following six things are components given to us by God so we might enjoy a more abundant and healthful life:

Pure air which we don't get enough of because of shallow breathing and lack of exercise,
Sunlight,
Rest,
Proper diet,
The use of water, and
Trust in divine power that these are the true remedies.

Your elixir for life is water. Start taking this tonic today for buoyant health and longevity!

COOL, CLEAR, AND PURE WATER

Make it a habit to drink water even when you are not thirsty. It is important to drink eight or more glasses of quality water each day. Your kidneys and bladder function better with plenty of water to help wash out the waste products that you do not need or that can harm you. Water is your best medicine.

Drinking water, breathing fresh, clean air, and eating quality fresh foods that add fiber to the diet are the things that will prevent or ease many diseases. Without air, we will die in 6-10 minutes. Without water, we will die in 3-5 days, but we can go without food for 30-40 days. So, for a long, healthy, disease-free life, get plenty of water, fresh air, and quality fresh foods. Add to this, stress management, daily exercise, and a positive mind-set, and you have the secrets to a healthy and happy life.

How Safe Is Your Water?

The Water Quality Association's "National Consumer Attitude Survey" found that almost half of American consumers are worried about contaminants in their water.

Lifestyle Tip
Choose your footwear very carefully. Adapted soles (insoles) are often necessary for comfort. Orthopedic shoes individually designed are often advisable to prevent corns and painful feet.

- 60% of adults believe the quality of their water affects their health.

- One in three believes their water supply is not as safe as it should be. Their top-rated concerns are bacteria, proper purification, lead, chlorine, carcinogens, and agricultural run-off.

- Only 29% of consumers have ever had their water tested.

- Use of home treatment systems reached an all time high with 38% of consumers using some treatment device. Consumer use of home treatment devices equals that of bottled water.

Sources Of Drinking Water

The average American uses almost 100 gallons of water per day for bathing, cooking, drinking, cleaning, toilet flushing, and lawn watering. People get safe drinking water in three ways:

- from a public utility
- from a private source, like a well
- from bottled water

All sources of water contain some contaminants. These include chemicals, pesticides, animal and human wastes, bacteria and other microorganisms. We spend almost $5 billion annually cleaning up our water.

Municipal water systems

Almost 85% of us get water from a municipal source. Rain from clouds falls on the ground, then runs into streams or ditches (surface water) or percolates down through the earth to underground aquifers (ground water). The municipal water utility collects the surface water into reservoirs and sends it through treatment plants. Ground water is pumped up through wells and treated.

Public water is reliable and cheap, with some exceptions. Municipal water is treated by filtration, sedimentation, flocculation, and disinfection. Pesticide residues are removed with granulated activated carbon filters. Public water is usually disinfected with chlorine to protect it from contamination in the municipal distribution system and home piping. Chlorination does a good job but creates by-products that have been associated with a risk of cancer or other adverse health effects over time. On average, municipal water costs $2 per 1,000 gallons.

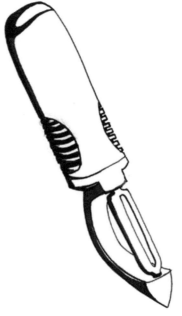

Lifestyle Tip
When you grip small objects, it puts a strain on the base joints. If you have arthritis in the hand with pain on gripping, build up the handles on your tools. Have the handles built up on household tools with narrow handles: whisks and beaters, openers, pens or pencils, thin knitting needles, and so forth. An occupational therapist can be very helpful in this area.

However, treatment plants have breakdowns. Both federal and state agencies require water suppliers to test their water. The water company is required to tell customers, within 24 hours, if there is a problem and what to do. The Safe Drinking Water Act requires water systems to issue annual *Consumer Confidence Reports* and send a copy to every user. The report tells where the water comes from, levels of pollutants, violations of regulations, and what the supplier is doing to fix them.

A *USA Today* study revealed that 40,000 U.S. water systems violated testing and purity requirements in a recent year. State and federal officials took action against only 10% of the violators. More than 25% were repeat offenders and had been out of compliance for three years. About 45 million Americans drink water that is polluted with fecal matter, parasites, disease-causing microbes, and pesticides at excessive levels that increase their risk of cancer, gastrointestinal disease, and miscarriage according to the Environmental Working Group in Washington.

The Environmental Protection Agency (EPA) recommends that the five million Americans who are infected with HIV, cancer patients on chemotherapy, and anyone taking immunosuppressive drugs should avoid tap water.

Water wells

Lifestyle Tip
Relieve strain on your hip by using a cane held in the hand on the opposite side. It is important that the cane is of the right length and that the handle is formed taking into account any changes which may have occurred in the small joints of the hand.

Water wells serve 15% of Americans and may or may not be safe depending on the underground source and homeowner care. Wells are not regulated by state or federal governments. After an initial inspection, the homeowner is on his own to ensure water quality. Wells may be contaminated by pesticides, fertilizers, and animal waste. If you get your water from a well, get it tested often.

Bottled water

Bottled water is almost always safe but may not be pure. Bottled water is processed and bottled in plants that are inspected by the FDA every five or six years. The International Bottled Water Association commissions NSF International to conduct annual surprise inspections of its members' facilities.

Bottled water is expensive, costing anywhere from 88 cents to $4 per gallon, about 500 times as much as public water. About 25% of bottled water is simply taken from public water supplies, processed, and bottled. The bottler takes out the chlorine that the municipal system put in. Then, most bottlers disinfect with ozone to avoid the taste of chlorine. The rest of bottled water comes from protected underground springs or wells that are naturally free of contaminants.

112 The Executive Chef's Arthritis Cookbook and Health Guide

Americans bought about thirteen gallons of bottled water per person last year, supporting a $4 billion industry. Water quality varies between brands. The FDA has not approved any health claims for bottled water.

Major Contaminants

The EPA issues drinking water standards for more than eighty different contaminants. These standards are set to limit the risk of disease from a lifetime of drinking two liters of water per day. Community water systems must test for these contaminants and report violations. About 8% of all water systems report violations annually. The major contaminants are:

Coliform Bacteria
Coliform bacteria are common in the environment and are generally not harmful. The presence of coliform bacteria in drinking water, however, indicates that the water may be contaminated with organisms that can cause disease. Fecal coliforms in drinking water are usually associated with sewage or animal wastes.

Cryptosporidium
Cryptosporidium is a one-celled animal, small enough to slip through most filters and resistant to chlorine. In 1993, "crypto" caused more than 100 deaths and made 400,000 people ill in Milwaukee. Between 65% and 97% of surface waters may be contaminated. There is no safe or effective cure for crypto, which can be deadly to older people and people with suppressed immune systems. The solutions offered by experts are:

- boil your water
- switch to bottled water
- use a reverse osmosis system with an "absolute" 1 micron filter

Arsenic
Arsenic produces skin lesions and is toxic to the nervous system. Arsenic comes from natural deposits and orchard runoff.

Copper
Copper contamination occurs mostly within the home from copper piping. High concentrations produce gastrointestinal irritation.

Lead
Lead can raise blood pressure, increase the risk of stroke and kidney disease, lower children's IQ, and cause delays in their physical development. The EPA estimates forty million

Health Tip
Many elderly people are using ginkgo biloba to increase memory but this supplement should not be used if you are on Coumadin, aspirin, or using NSAIDs. Ginkgo can cause bleeding when used in conjunction with these other medications.

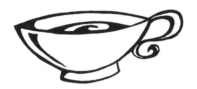

Americans use water that contains excessive lead. Lead contamination occurs mostly within the home from lead solder and acidic water. Over fifteen parts per billion is considered dangerous.

Nitrates
Nitrates can cause a potentially fatal disease called methemoglobinemia, or blue baby syndrome.

Radon
Radon-222 occurs in certain types of rock and can get into ground water. People get exposed to radon by drinking or bathing in the water. Radon is a suspected carcinogen.

Chlorination By-Products
Chlorination kills germs but reacts with organic material in the water to form chloroform and trihalomethanes which are suspected carcinogens. The safety limit is eighty micrograms per liter. Pregnant women exposed to water containing more than seventy-five micrograms show an increased risk of miscarriage.

Six Ways To Get Safe Water

If you are concerned about the quality of your household water, there are several options to increase its safety.

Reverse Osmosis
Reverse osmosis (RO) systems use a prefilter, activated carbon filter, and a semi-permeable membrane through which water flows under pressure into a storage tank. RO systems remove dirt, pesticides, insecticides, metallic tastes, odors, colors, arsenic, asbestos, benzene, iron, lead, mercury, nitrates, trichloroethylene, total trihalomethanes, radium, radon, and cryptosporidium. Units cost between $600 and $900, with annual cartridge replacement costs of $120 to $170.

Distillation
Distillation systems use a tank in which water is boiled into steam and condensed into almost pure water. Some contaminants can vaporize and recondense into the collecting jar unless there is a carbon filter. Distillation removes metallic tastes, odors, colors, arsenic, asbestos, benzene, lead, mercury, nitrates, trichloroethylene, total trihalomethanes, radium, radon, coliform bacteria, and cryptosporidium. Units costs from $250 to $1,450.

Filtration
Activated carbon filters fit a cartridge mounted under the sink or on the faucet. Only solid block filters remove crypto and

Lifestyle Tip
If you have arthritis of the hips and knees, there is less stress walking down stairs if you walk backwards. Make sure you practice this and always hold onto a guardrail.

114 The Executive Chef's Arthritis Cookbook and Health Guide

lead. Some remove chlorination by-products, cleaning solvents, and pesticides. The filters must be replaced regularly. Contaminated filters may actually be more dangerous than tap water.

Carafe or pour-through pitchers usually contain a granular carbon filter. Filtration removes metallic tastes, odors, asbestos, benzene, lead, mercury, trichloroethylene, radon, and cryptosporidium. Some filters, using brass fittings, have been found to add lead to the treated water.

Faucet-mounted filters cost from $9 to $25 with cartridge costs running $27 to $90 per year. Carafe filters runs from $5 to $13 and filters cost $28 to $78 per year.

Boiling
Boiling is good for killing bacteria and other microorganisms, but not practical for daily living. Boiling removes bacteria, cysts, and cryptosporidium.

Bottled Water
Bottled water is tap water or well water that is processed, bottled, and delivered to home or store. Bottling removes metallic tastes, odors, colors, arsenic, asbestos, benzene, lead, mercury, nitrates, trichloroethylene, total trihalomethanes, radium, radon, and cryptosporidium. A person using bottled water for drinking and cooking could spend over $700 per year.

Testing Your Tap Water

The U.S. Environmental Protection Agency supplies a phone number to help you locate the office or lab near your area that does certified water testing. Call the EPA's toll-free number:

Safe Drinking Water Hotline   1-800-426-4791

You can get a self-addressed container from a lab that allows you to put the filled bottle into a local mailbox. Test costs start as low as $15 to $20 a tap and results are usually available in two to three weeks. Call these labs to check out their offers:

National Testing Laboratories   1-800-458-3330
Suburban Water Testing Laboratories   1-800-433-6595

Health Tip
Feverfew, one of many supplements used to treat arthritis, can interact with anticoagulants such as Coumadin and increase bleeding risk.

To get information on safe drinking water and educational material on water quality issues, contact:

National Sanitation Foundation
P.O. Box 130140
789 N. Dixboro Road
Ann Arbor, MI 48113-0140
734-769-8010
1-800-NSF-MARK

or the

Water Quality Association
4151 Naperville Rd.
Lisle, IL 60532
630-505-0160

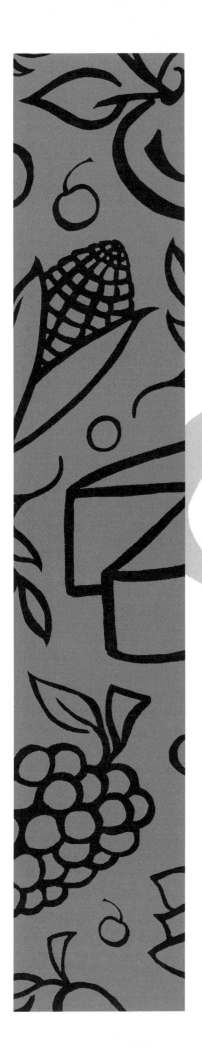

FACTS ABOUT Fats & ROUX

CHAPTER 8

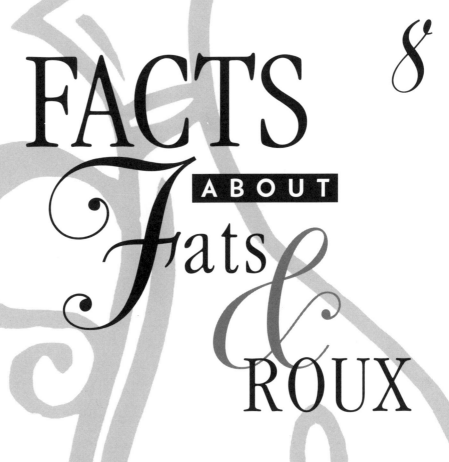

FACTS ON FATS

We need fats in our diet because they are a source of energy and carry the fat-soluble vitamins A, D, E, and K. Vitamin K is important in the treatment of arthritis. But there are good and bad fats, some essential to good health, others unhealthy. Getting the right types of fat into your diet can actually improve your performance, mentally and physically. A lack of certain fats your body can't produce has been associated with depression and other health problems. So, it's a balance we're after.

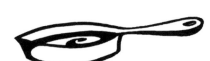

Lifestyle Tip
If you have arthritis of the hips, learn to work while sitting on a work chair of correct height that allows for straight or slightly out-turned hip and knee joints.

The typical American diet gets about 34% of its calories from fat. The American Heart Association recommends a diet which restricts total fat to less than 30% of calories, and saturated fats like meats and cheeses to less than 10% of calories. You can reduce your fat intake to a healthful level by choosing fewer fatty meats, greasy chips, and added fats.

Fats and oils are better sources of energy than protein or carbohydrates because fats are calorie dense, at nine calories per gram. Both protein and carbohydrates contain four calories per gram. Fat that fits within your daily calorie allowance gets burned. Excess fat might turn up on your hips. Fat satisfies and curbs the appetite because it takes longer to digest than carbohydrates and helps keep you from feeling hungry.

There are three types of fats found in oils: monounsaturated fats, polyunsaturated fats, and saturated fats. Polyunsaturated fats and their near relation, monounsaturates, are the good fats.

You'll want to eat the unsaturated liquid fats found in plants, nuts, oil, and fish rather than hard saturated fats found in meats, butter, and other animal foods. The right kind of fat is good for your health, but most people eat way too much of the wrong kind. Excess fat is stored in the liver, in arteries around the heart, and in all tissue. High fat diets show links to obesity, an increased risk of heart attack, and cancer of the breast, prostate, and colon.

Saturated Fats
You'll find saturated fat in all animal products and many vegetable oils:

Butter/lard	Milk/cream
Poultry (mainly skin)	Processed cheeses
Beef	Cheese
Chocolate desserts	Bacon/pork
Palm kernel oils	Coconut oils

120 The Executive Chef's Arthritis Cookbook and Health Guide

Saturated fats are the bad fats associated with heart disorders, hardening of the arteries, elevated serum cholesterol, heart disease, and cancer. Stay away from processed foods such as crackers, commercially baked goods, and stick margarines that list partially hydrogenated vegetable oils on their food labels. Hydrogenation converts the "good" oil into a harder fat, which acts like saturated fat. When you hydrogenate (harden) fat, it destroys some essential fatty acids. This process is used to prolong shelf life. Hydrogenated, or hardened oils, are difficult for the body to assimilate.

So, how do you spot saturated fats? Read the labels on the food you buy. The worst fats to consume are coconut oil and palm oil. These are called "vegetable oils" on labels and contain almost as much "bad" fat as lard. Palm oil is 49% saturated fat and coconut oil is 87% saturated. Saturated fat is associated with elevated cholesterol.

Soybean oil is the most common hydrogenated oil. Unaltered soybean oil is only 15% saturated, so it goes on the list with other good fats like safflower, corn, and olive oils. But partially hydrogenated soybean oil, which is used in a shortening like Crisco, increases the fat to 25%.

Polyunsaturated Fats

Polyunsaturated fats are liquid and stay that way. You'll find these fats in:

Nuts	Seeds
Vegetables	Fish
Walnut oil	Soybeans

Foods highest in polyunsaturated fats are:

Safflower oil	Primrose oil
Wheat germ oil	Cod liver oil
Pine nuts	Corn oil
Cottonseed oil	Sesame oil
Sunflower seeds	Flaxseed
Some soft margarines (usually from health food stores)	Pecans

When these foods are heavily processed, many of their benefits are lost. Try to use cold or expeller pressed oils.

Fish are the best source of polyunsaturated fats. Fish from cold, deep waters have a high content of these oils. Atlantic mackerel, Atlantic herring, salmon, and albacore tuna are the highest in

Health Tip
Echinacea stimulates the immune system and should be used when exposed to viral infections such as colds or influenza. It should not be used to treat autoimmune diseases such as lupus. Echinacea may stimulate the abnormal immune cells to do more damage to tissue. Do not use echinacea for more than two weeks at a time.

Health Tip
Herbs considered unsafe or ineffective are borage, calamus, chaparral, comfrey, germander, life root, pokeroot, sassafras and ephedra (ma huang).

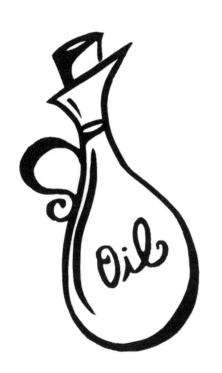

the "omega 3" fatty acids (polyunsaturated). These fatty acids help prevent clots from forming in the arteries. They lower cholesterol levels and reduce joint inflammation in arthritis.

Buy the freshest fish you can find. Fish should not smell "fishy." When a fish smells, the fatty acids have started to break down, becoming rancid.

Monounsaturated Fats
Monounsaturated fats are found in many foods, but not in red meat. Monounsaturated fats do not affect blood cholesterol levels and are useful in the diets of people with cholesterol problems.

Monounsaturated fats are found in:

    Olive oil   Peanuts
    Avocado   Cashews
    Pecans   Almonds
    Canola oil   Hazelnuts

Diets high in monounsaturated fats help to lower "bad" LDL cholesterol without lowering "good" HDL. Oils like olive oil are favored over polyunsaturated fats like corn oil.

Virgin olive oil is the best oil and is great for salad dressing. Olive oil helps lower cholesterol and control blood pressure and diabetes. It does not become rancid without refrigeration. However, unrefined olive oil should be kept refrigerated.

One tablespoon of olive oil averages almost ten grams of monounsaturated fat. You can get the same ten grams of monounsaturated fat from these other nutritious oils:

    4 teaspoons unrefined canola oil
    1-1/2 tablespoons raw almond butter
    1/2 fresh avocado
    1/4 cup raw almonds
    3 tablespoons raw hazelnuts
    2 tablespoons raw macadamia nuts
    1/4 cup raw pecans
    1/4 cup raw pistachios

Canola oil is low in saturated fat and is high in monounsaturates. Canola has 10% linolenic acid, a polyunsaturated and essential fatty acid, and is also rich in omega 3s. Canola is 6% saturated, 36% polyunsaturated, and high in monounsaturates (58%).

122 The Executive Chef's Arthritis Cookbook and Health Guide

Toxic Substances in Oils

Pesticides, herbicides, and other toxic chemicals are stored in the fatty tissues of animals. When these fats are eaten or converted to cooking fats, some of the chemicals get absorbed by our bodies. It makes sense to avoid foods that may be contaminated.

Be careful not to use rancid oils. Refrigerate the oils you use and try to buy oils in dark containers that protect them from light. Heating oils to high temperatures produces free radicals which damage the body.

ROUX— HEALTHY VARIATION

Roux is the base for many sauces, made by cooking fat and flour together. Most people use clarified butter for fat, but chicken fat, vegetable oils, and fats rendered from different roasts may also be used.

The standard ratio of fat to flour is 1:1 by weight, although the proportion may have to be slightly adjusted, depending on the type of fat or flour. Cooked roux should be moist but not greasy.

There are three basic types of roux, which differ according to the length of time they are cooked. White roux is cooked for the shortest length of time, brown roux for the longest, and pale (or blond) roux in the middle.

Health Tip
Vitamins extracted from natural sources are sometimes more beneficial (biologically active) than synthetic vitamins.

WHITE ROUX

8 oz.	Butter; use the health food kind, 94% fat free, made from canola oil
8 oz.	All-Purpose Whole Wheat Flour

Method of Preparation
Heat the butter over medium heat in a pan.

Add the flour, stirring constantly, cooking over low heat for about 8-10 minutes.

If the roux will not be used right away, cool it and store tightly wrapped in the refrigerator.

BLOND ROUX

Continue cooking 4-5 more minutes, stirring constantly, until roux becomes golden in color.

BROWN ROUX

Continue to cook the roux until it is browned and has a strong nutty aroma, stirring constantly.

Health Tip
Keep your body weight down. This will take the stress off your joints and will lessen pain and stiffness.

Cooking Ratios for Roux Used as Thickening Agents for Soups and Veloutés

Certain stocks thickened with roux are called veloutés. The stocks are chicken, turkey, fish, or veal.

To make a light velouté for soup stock, use 10-12 ounces of roux per gallon, for a medium velouté use 12-16 ounces per gallon, and for a heavy velouté use 18-20 ounces per gallon.

In order to thicken your stocks for cream soups, add cold roux to hot liquid, or hot roux to cold liquid. The temperature difference prevents lumping. Return liquid to a boil, or if cold liquid is being used bring it to a boil, then reduce heat to a simmer, whisk occasionally, and cook about 30 minutes to remove the flour taste. Strain through a sieve.

Add 1 quart of heated heavy cream (scalded) per gallon of thickened velouté. Now you are ready to use it for your soups and sauces. This recipe breaks down very well to 3/4, 1/2, or 1/4. Just use your basic math to figure out the necessary amounts.

This may sound like a lot of work, but it is a very, very simple task to perform in the kitchen.

KITCHEN TOOLS

CHAPTER

9

126

KITCHEN TOOLS

Here's a list of kitchen tools which will help you tremendously. There's no need to go out and buy all of them at once. If you really enjoy cooking, purchasing many of these over the years will make your time in the kitchen much easier.

The following list of tools wasn't easy to put together. There are literally thousands of tools for kitchen use. Today we live in a technology-conscious world where even the simplest tasks can now be done by machine in a second or so. A professional chef uses far fewer tools than most amateurs, but I genuinely feel some of these products will be useful to you.

Knives are the most important item you will choose. Don't be afraid of sharp knives, they don't slip. Only a dull knife cuts you.

Techniques for using kitchen tools can be found in many cookbooks, and there are other books that specialize in cooking tools and how to use them. Another great source of knowledge is a chefs' meeting. The American Culinary Federation ("The Authority on Food in America") has many local chapters and visitors are always welcome. Chefs are great talkers! And almost all of them love to share their knowledge.

Remember, the tools you choose will reflect your way of life. If you really enjoy cooking, go to a local community college and take a course. It is usually very inexpensive, quite rewarding, a great source of knowledge, and you'll meet new friends.

Enjoy cooking!

TOOLS OF THE KITCHEN

1. A combination of your brain, your eyes, and your hands. A good dose of common sense helps immensely.

2. **Knives**
   - Taper ground
   - Fluted
   - Serrated
   - Paring
   - Boning

   Pick sizes that fit you: go to the store and try different knives. Make sure they have a comfortable feel for your hand. Cooks' knives come in 4", 8" and 10" sizes, but larger ones are also available.

3. **Sharpening stone and oil**
   Used to sharpen your knives.

4. **Sharpening steel**
   A steel acts like a file on the knife's edge. It removes the burr.

5. **Carving fork**
   A fork to hold your product while you slice it. It keeps the food from skidding.

6. **Electric carving knife**
   It never needs sharpening, you just replace the blade. A great product for serious home cooks.

7. **Spreaders**
   Great for buttering a whole slice of bread at once.

8. **Oyster and clam knives**
   Used exclusively to open these shellfish.

9. **All purpose scissors**
   Used for trimming various products and strings.

10. **Peelers**
    Practical and economical for trimming broccoli, celery, carrots, etc., peelers are also reversible for left-handed use.

11. **Canelle knife**
    Used to pare strips of citrus fruits and cut thin grooves in cucumbers and carrots.

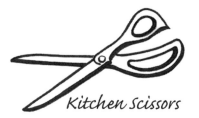
Kitchen Scissors

Chapter 9 Kitchen Tools 129

12. Zester
Used for zesting (peeling small strips from) oranges and lemons.

13. Egg slicer
This aluminum-framed instrument with ten fine wires slices eggs very neatly.

14. Box graters
They come in all shapes and sizes. Choose the one that's best for you.

15. Fish scalers
Used like a brush as you work your way from the tail to the head.

16. Pounders and tenderizers
To beat food that needs to be crushed, cracked, or flattened.

17. Mortar and pestle
Used to grind small quantities of spices and herbs.

18. Chinois
Another name for a fine wire sieve for straining.

19. Ladles
Used to measure and pour out soups, sauces, and stocks; also used to mash items so they pass through a chinois.

20. Citrus juicer
Removes juice from all different citrus products.

21. Garlic press
Presses garlic through fine holes; if used gently, only the juice of the clove will be extracted.

22. Nutcracker
A good one cracks the shell gently and neatly, while keeping the contents intact.

23. Coffee mill
Used to grind coffee beans for a fresher taste.

24. Salt shaker and pepper mill
For the dispensing of these products.

25. Cutting board.
Plastic ones are easier to clean and keep sanitary. They'll dull a knife faster than a wooden one, but that's why you get knife sharpening equipment.

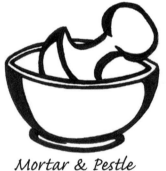

Mortar & Pestle

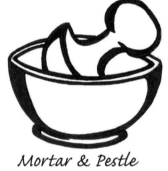

26. Rolling pin
Used for rolling dough and pastry. Also great for crushing peppercorns and other small items (wrap them in cloth or plastic wrap first).

27. Wooden forks and spoons
For stirring, beating, and creaming. Won't scratch.

28. Corn cob holders
Stick in each end of the cob to hold it.

29. Ice pick
Used to break up large blocks of ice, and to extract crabs and lobsters from their shells.

30. Skewers
Holds food firmly. Used for kebabs and many other dishes.

31. Toothpicks
Used for fastening, cake testing, and even tooth picking.

32. Trussing needles
Used to tie the legs and wings of birds: ducks, chicken, turkeys, etc.

33. Wooden spatulas
For folding mixtures together; doubles as a turning and lifting tool.

34. Scrapers and spatulas
Rubber or plastic bladed ones get everything out of the bowl.

35. Metal spoons
Used for stirring, mixing, and basting. The sturdiest ones are made of one piece of metal.

36. Rice paddle
Used for serving rice, or mixing cooked rice with various products.

37. Slotted spoon and skimmer
Designed to lift foods from boiling water or fat, and to remove scum from stocks, soups, and sauces.

38. Ice cream scoop
Used to scoop ice cream.

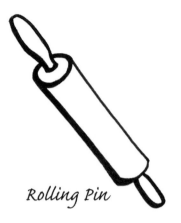

Rolling Pin

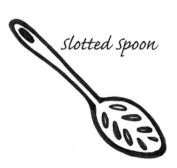

Slotted Spoon

39. Flour scoop
Scoops out flour so it doesn't spill all over the place.

40. Lifters and turners
For scooping food up quickly and turning it. Great for pancakes, bacon, fried eggs, etc.

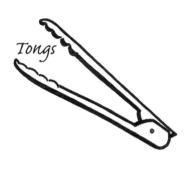
Tongs

41. Cooking tongs
Used for picking things up, turning them over, and setting them down.

42. Knife holder
Good product if you are used to keeping knives in a drawer—when they bump together, they can put nicks in the edge. Magnetic bar holders work well. Upright wooden ones work best.

43. Wine rack
Store your cooking wine on a rack in a cellar or other cool place when possible.

44. Storage containers
The more you have, the better.

45. Thermometers
- Oven
- Meat
- Freezer
- Deep fryer
- Multipurpose
- Candy

46. Scale
A pound scale that measures in ounces is a great help in the kitchen.

47. Timers
There are many kinds on the market. Choose one that suits you.

48. Measuring cups and spoons
- 1/4 teaspoon through 1 tablespoon
- 1/4, 1/3, 1/2 and 1 cup

49. Liquid measuring cups
Pyrex ones last a long time. One pint and one quart sizes are most popular.

50. Cheesecloth
A must if you are finely straining sauces, soups, stocks, and broths, unless you have a chinois.

51. Coffee maker
There are so many kinds on the market it's unbelievable. Choose the one you like. You can also brew tea in them.

52. Corkscrew
Used to open your cooking wine.

53. Can opener
Choose your own model from the hundreds that are available.

54. Colander
For straining pasta products, vegetables, or making spaetzli.

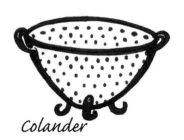
Colander

55. Chopsticks
They work like tongs once you know how to use them— a great addition to your cooking skills.

56. Whisks and beaters
Wire whisks come in many different sizes. Usually 6" to 12" long, made from very thin stainless steel. Sauce whisks are rigid and elongated in shape; they range from 6" to 10" in length. A must for every kitchen. Rotary whisks make your work easier.

57. Bulb baster
A plastic tube marked in ounces. Squeeze it and put it in liquid and it fills up. Squeeze it over your food to baste. A ladle or spoon will also do the same.

58. Bowl shaped sieve
Very versatile. Used for straining or lifting foods out of hot liquid.

59. String
A ball of white cotton string always comes in handy around the kitchen.

60. Food processor
Simple to use, they are strong, durable machines that make a lot of work very simple. If you go to a store and read about this great machine, I bet you get one.

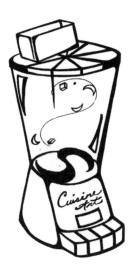

61. Mixing bowls
Sizes range from 4 ounces to 2 gallons. Choose the ones that work best for you.

62. Serving bowls
These come in all shapes, sizes, and colors. Choose what your eyes fancy.

63. Cake, bread, and pastry tins
They are so numerous you should browse through a catalog, then buy what you need.

64. Molds and presses
Many are very beautiful and what can't you make in these? Another product you should be able to find in a catalog. .

65. Pasta machine
Used to make fresh pasta with a minimum of fuss. A must for a good cook.

66. Casserole dishes
Get a few so you can make a meal in one and store the leftovers. The many kinds of earthenware pots with lids are too numerous to mention them all. A few are slow cookers, marmites, clay cooking pots, terrines, and bean pots.

67. Gratin dishes
Dishes which go from the oven straight to the table. They come in copper, porcelain, earthenware, or cast iron.

68. Roasting pans
You can do many things besides roasting in these pans. Sizes vary from 10" to 20". Make sure they'll fit in your oven before you buy them.

69. Plastic wrap
Plastic wrap is very necessary for any kitchen, especially if you have a microwave oven. And you can see what that left over is when it's covered.

70. Cake decorating equipment
Pick what you need from the thousands of items available in the stores.

71. Toaster
The pop-up ones seem to be most people's choice.

72. Sauce pans
From one pint to eight quarts in size, usually 4 to 6 in a set, which stack inside each other. Pans are made of copper, stainless steel, and white porcelain. Stay away from aluminum.

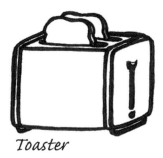

Toaster

73. Two handled pots
These are usually stockpots, used in making stocks, soups, and reducing sauces. They need to have two handles because they are heavy when full.

74. Steamer
All shapes and sizes are available. The expanding basket type is the most popular. Bamboo steamers are also great, the three-tiered ones being most common.

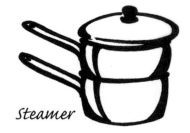
Steamer

75. Sauteuses
Great pans for reducing sauces. They're usually very heavy and expensive if they are copper, but they're worth their weight in gold.

76. Chinese wok
A thin-bottomed steel cooking instrument used over extremely high heat for rapid cooking. Can also be used as a deep fat fryer. Get one!

Many of these tools are made so arthritis sufferers can easily handle them. There are also many resource manuals for products available to arthritis sufferers. Here are the addresses for two sources of arthritis-friendly tools:

C.R. Newton
1575 S. Beretania Street, Suite 101
Honolulu, HI 96826
Phone Toll Free 1-800-545-2078
Phone (808) 949-8389
Fax (808) 955-4721

Sammons Preston
P.O. Box 5071
Bolingbrook, IL 60440-5071
Phone Toll Free 1-800-323-5547
Fax 1-800-547-4333

You can also find these manuals and catalogs through your doctor, the local Arthritis Foundation chapter, or your local library. The Internet is another great source for learning. And take a look at our Recommended Reading section in the Appendix. So get up, get out, find these resources, and make life simpler for yourself.

HERBS & SPICES

CHAPTER 10

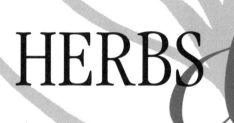

HERBS AND SPICES

Herbs and spices are as old as civilization. They are talked about in the Bible. The increased availability of fresh herbs has become a great plus for all people attempting to cut back on salt and sodium. Not only do herbs and spices make food taste better, they also help with the digestion of our foods, as discovered by the Chinese 6,000 years ago. Many of these products can be traced back to China.

Herbs are the leafy or soft portions of certain annual or biennial plants. The leaves are usually aromatic and are used to add flavor to foods. Spices are the roots, bark, buds, flowers, fruits, or seeds. True spices are the parts of plants that usually grow in the tropics, whereas herbs are always the leaves of plants which grow in the temperate zones.

There are so many herbs and spices found throughout the world today that it would take an encyclopedia to tell you about all of them, what they taste like, and what foods are best seasoned with them. Here we will first tell you about a dozen or so herbs and then some spices that can be used in everyday cooking.

HERBS

Basil

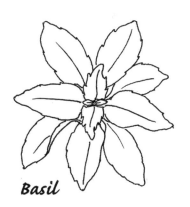

Basil

The leaves and stems of an herb grown in the United States and northern Mediterranean, basil has an aromatic, leafy flavor which is rich and spicy. It blends well with garlic, lemon, and thyme and is used for flavoring tomato dishes, salad dressings, sauces, French, Italian, and Thai dishes, and turtle soup. It goes well with poultry, or sprinkled on lamb chops. Basil is the main ingredient in pesto.

Cilantro

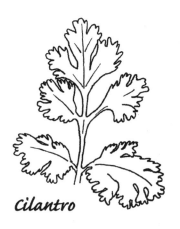

Cilantro

The leaves and stems are chopped to give off a bold sage flavor with a citrus taste. Cilantro gives a distinctive zap to ethnic foods, curries, salsas, guacamole, rice, and noodle dishes. The Portuguese use it for many of their ethnic dishes. It's also known as Chinese parsley and coriander leaf.

Bay Leaf

The dried leaves of an evergreen grown in the eastern Mediterranean countries, bay leaves have a woodsy, perfumed flavor with a trace of cinnamon. They are used in stews, sauces, and soups, in a bouquet garni, and for pickling, as well as in a variety of meat, fish, and game dishes.

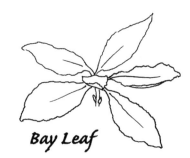

Dill

Dill has a mild, faint anise taste. It is used in pickling recipes, cold salmon, sauerkraut, potato salad, macaroni dishes, cucumber salad, beets, and hard-boiled eggs. It enhances poultry dishes, goes well with seafood, and is used in marinades.

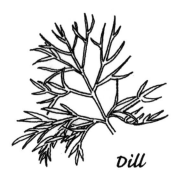

Parsley

One of the biennial herbs, parsley has a fresh, green, vegetable taste. Chew on a fresh stem, and bad breath will disappear. The ancient Greeks and Romans believed that chewing and swallowing the juices helped in a manly way. Parsley is used in soups and sauces, in pasta, potato, vegetable, and egg dishes. It's used as a garnish because its so pretty when fresh.

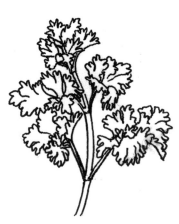

Watercress

Green watercress leaves are peppery and crunchy. Watercress salad is a great, healthy dish. It adds color and texture to stir fry dishes and soups, and is used as a garnish on red meat dishes.

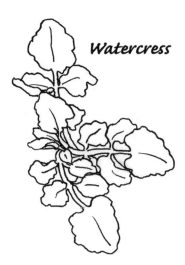

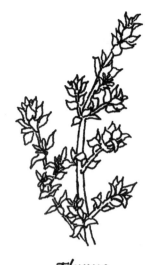

Thyme

Thyme
The leaves and stems of a shrub grown in Spain and France, thyme has a strong, distinctive, earthy flavor with a slight clove aftertaste. It is used in poultry seasonings, and blends well with lemon, garlic, and basil. Thyme is a great addition to seafood chowders, sausages, meatloaf, stews, and salads.

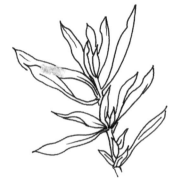

Tarragon

Tarragon
Believed native to Siberia, tarragon has a strong, pungent flavor with hints of licorice and vanilla. Tarragon goes well with sautéed or roasted chicken, salad dressings, seafood entrées, and sauces, Bearnaise sauce, tartar sauce, and omelets. Start with small amounts, then add more when necessary because of its distinctive flavor.

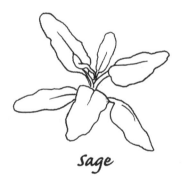

Sage

Sage
Sage has an aromatic and pleasantly bitter flavor that is camphoraceous and minty. It is the leaf of a shrub originally grown in Albania, Yugoslavia, and Greece. Sage goes well with orange, garlic, and lemon, and is used in meat and poultry stuffings, in sausages, stews, salads, and vegetable dishes.

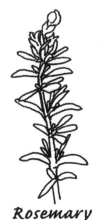

Rosemary

Rosemary
Used as a ground cover in many places, rosemary is an herb native to the Mediterranean region. It has a sweet, fresh taste with a piney and tea-like flavor. It is used in lamb and poultry dishes, soups, stews, and with roasted potatoes.

Mint
This perennial herb with a cool, sweet, refreshing taste comes in more than 30 different varieties. Mint is used in iced tea, mint juleps on race day at the Kentucky Derby, and mint jelly for lamb dishes. It's also used in and as garnish for fruit salads and newly created yogurt dips.

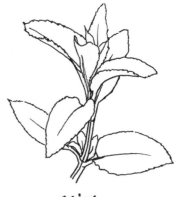
Mint

Oregano
Related to mint, oregano has a strong, peppery, marigold-like taste. It combines well with garlic, thyme, and parsley, and is used on garlic bread and pizza, in Italian tomato sauce, Greek salads, egg and cheese combinations, stews, and grilled fish.

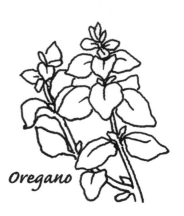
Oregano

SPICES

Spices are generally strong in flavor. They are made from the nuts, seeds, fruit, bark, or roots of selected plants, and are usually available either whole or ground. Every spice depends on delicate volatile oils for its aroma and flavor. Flavor loss in spices can be caused by high heat (don't store them above the range), excess humidity which causes caking, infestation by bugs, or exposure to sunlight which makes the color change.

When cooking food for a long time, ground spices should be added near the end. In uncooked dishes, the spiced liquid should be kept standing for several hours to develop good flavor.

Paprika
This spice has a hot, rich, earthy flavor. Native to Central and South America as well as the West Indies, its been used as a colorful garnish on many culinary dishes. It's good in goulashes, chicken paprika, braises, stews, and many sauces.

Pepper
Native to India and one of the earliest known spices, pepper is a universal seasoning with a hot and biting flavor. It's used in sauces, stocks, meats, vegetables, and wherever that pepper flavor is enjoyed.

Allspice
The dried, nearly ripe berry of the pimento, allspice is native to the western tropics. Its flavor resembles blended cinnamon, nutmeg, and clove. Allspice is used to flavor braises, stuffings, fish, pickles, relishes, barbecue sauce, baked lamb, soups, and gravies.

Cloves
From the Spice Islands in Indonesia, cloves are one of the very strongest spices. It is used in perfumes, medicines, and ointments as well as cooking. What is a roast fresh ham without a few cloves stuck in or a little ground clove on top? Cloves are used in puddings, spice and chocolate cakes, pumpkin pie and mince pie, in stocks, sauces, marinades, curries, and pickling. Use it in tomato sauce and tomato soup, pot roast, fish stock, and duck. An essential when making gingerbread and ginger cookies, cloves are a great spice in my opinion.

Ginger
Ginger root has a sweet, biting flavor. It enhances the flavor of desserts and baked goods, fish, soups, and ales. Candied ginger is a great addition to fruit cakes. Ginger is used in pickling and curry dishes. It brings out the flavor of roast lamb or pot roast.

Fennel
Originally from southern Europe and Asia Minor, fennel's sweet, licorice-like taste brings out the flavor in pies and baked fruit. It is used in bouillabaisse, potato salad, sausage, fish, tomato dishes, and marinades.

Nutmeg
The seed of a tropical evergreen, nutmeg is another native of the Spice Islands. It is used in sauces and cream soups, veal, chicken, sausage, and beef tongue, in punches, wines, egg nog at Christmas time, in desserts (especially custards), in fresh spinach, sautéed mushrooms, and in a wide variety of baked goods.

Celery Seed
Grown in France, India, and the United States, celery seed has a kind of bitter, refreshing, celery-like taste. It is used in pickling, dressings, fish, and relishes, salads (especially cole slaw), soups, stews, and tomato dishes.

Chili Powder
Chili powder is used in Mexican dishes, chili, curries, chili con carne, sausage, Mexican goulash, Spanish rice, steaks, and stews. Chili goes well with seafood cocktail sauce and creamed salmon.

Cinnamon

The inner bark of an evergreen native to Sri Lanka, cinnamon has a sweet, warm, nutty taste. It was known in China as far back as 2700 B.C. and the Romans burned it as an incense to their gods. Cinnamon is the second most commonly used spice, after pepper. It is used in custards, mince and pumpkin pies, sweet potatoes, hot beverages, curries, puddings, cakes, and breads. Apples are great with a little cinnamon sprinkled on top.

How To Store Herbs And Spices

In today's world, herbs and spices are available in both fresh and dried forms. Fresh herbs now also come in a freeze-dried package that you keep in the freezer. Take out and use the amount you need, then put back in the freezer.

Fresh herbs should be stored by wrapping them loosely in a damp paper towel or a damp cloth. Putting them in a plastic bag after wrapping helps retain the freshness and reduce wilting. They should be refrigerated at a temperature between 36-40°F. Fresh herbs that have been bought freeze-dried can be stored at 0°F, for up to one year.

Dried herbs, and both ground and whole spices should be stored in a cool, dry, dark place away from heat sources in your kitchen. Once a year or so, take a whiff of the dried herbs and ground spices to see if you can identify them by smell. If not, throw them away and replace with new ones. Whole spices will retain their flavor and aroma almost indefinitely.

How To Select Herbs And Spices

Aroma is a good way to tell the quality of both fresh and dried herbs and spices. A weak or stale aroma will usually indicate that they are old and less potent. You can tell the scent of herbs by using your fingers to crush a few leaves and then smelling those leaves and fingers. Fresh herbs may also be judged by looking for good color and fresh-looking leaves and stems without wilting, sun, or pest damage.

How To Properly Use Herbs And Spices

Herbs and spices can be used to give a better flavor and aroma to just about any dish. They should not overpower a dish's flavors; they should enhance and balance the dish. When an herb or spice is used properly, it can make that same old dish something special. If you use too much of any herb or spice, you will have a taste disaster on your hands.

Chapter 10 Herbs & Spices   143

For dishes that cook for a long time, whole spices give you a better result than ground ones and should be added at the beginning of cooking. Tie them in a cheesecloth bag for easy removal.

Ground herbs and spices do not hold up well during lengthy cooking processes, so add these about 20-30 minutes before the dish is done cooking. For uncooked preparations, fresh herbs should be added well in advance of serving time in order to give the different tastes in the recipe a chance to blend together. Fresh herbs should be chopped or minced before you put them in a dish.

Your local health food store can help you with purchasing and packaging your herbs and spices. Buy them in small quantities. Most quality stores have the great new freeze-dried herbs that will last a long time.

144

CHAPTER

11

COOKING
METHODS

146

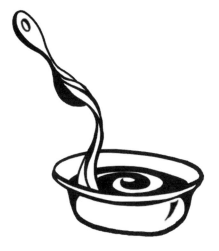

COOKING METHODS

Dry Heat Using Fat

To *sauté* literally means "to jump." In cooking it means to cook food quickly in a small amount of fat.

For sautéing, preheat the pan before the food is added. The food items must be seared quickly or they'll simmer in their own juices. Don't overcrowd the pan. By placing too much food in the pan, the temperature drops and the food begins to simmer, not sear like we want it to.

To **pan fry** means to cook food in a moderate amount of fat in a pan over moderate heat. More fat is used in pan-frying than sautéing and the cooking time is usually longer. Larger items are usually pan-fried and they are turned over rather than flipped around like in sautéing. The amount of fat to be used is determined by the size of the dish. Sometimes larger cuts of foods are pan-fried first then removed from the pan and finished in the oven.

Deep-fat frying means to cook foods submerged in some kind of hot fat. The quality of the finished product is characterized by the following properties: minimum fat absorption, minimum moisture loss, a crisp surface or coating, and an attractive golden brown color. So the quality of the fat is of the utmost importance—there should be no flavors imparted to the food by the fat used for frying. Most foods are cooked between 350°F and 375°F. When foods are greasy, they are usually fried at too low a temperature.

Moist Heat

To **braise** means to cook food covered with a lid and with a small amount of liquid added. Usually the product to be braised is browned first. Braising takes place at lower temperatures than sautéing. Usually the tougher cuts of meat are cooked this way because it takes a long time to dissolve the connective tissue. This method of cooking usually ends with a superb tasting sauce made from the leftover liquid.

Boiling means to cook in a liquid that has a rolling surface and is vigorously bubbling. Water boils at 212°F at sea level. Boiling is usually done with vegetables and starches. The water or other liquid used is usually seasoned or flavored.

148 The Executive Chef's Arthritis Cookbook and Health Guide

To **simmer** means to cook in a liquid that is bubbling very gently, at a temperature somewhere between 185°F and 205°F. Most foods cooked in a liquid are simmered.

To **poach** means to cook in a small amount of liquid that is hot but not bubbling, somewhere between 160°F and 180°F. Poaching is usually done with delicate foods such as eggs out of the shell and various fish and shellfish. When poaching fish and shellfish, the liquid is sometimes turned into a sauce.

To **blanch** means to cook an item partially by very briefly boiling it in a hot liquid, and then plunging it into ice water to stop the cooking process. The item may also be blanched by placing it in cold water, bringing it to a boil, then simmering it. This will dissolve out blood, salt, and other impurities from certain meats and bones.

To **steam** means to cook foods by exposing them directly to steam. Steaming of foods can achieve higher temperatures without the agitation of boiling. Steaming also refers to tightly wrapping or placing food in a covered pan, so it cooks in the steam created by its own moisture.

En papillote is a method where food items are wrapped in paper and sealed so they cook in their own steam. Sometimes foil is used instead of paper.

Dry Heat

To **broil** means that the food is cooked with radiant heat from above. Broiling is a rapid, high heat cooking method that is used when you are cooking tender meats, fish, poultry, and a few vegetable dishes. A salamander is a low-intensity broiler that is used in browning or melting the top of some foods before serving them.

Roasting and **baking** mean to cook foods by surrounding them with hot, dry air, usually in an oven. Roasting usually applies to meat and poultry items. Baking usually applies to breads, vegetables, fish, and pastry products. When roasting, you cook uncovered. The flavor usually comes from the browning process achieved during roasting.

Barbecuing means to cook with the dry heat that is created by burning wood and cooking over the hot coals. In barbecuing, food can be placed on a rack directly above the fire, or an open pit may be used with the fire below the food which is constantly turning on a spit, the way the first settlers learned from the Native Americans.

Grilling is much the same as barbecuing over hot coals. A heat source is used and a rack is placed above the source. Charcoal, electric elements, or gas-heated elements are used in grilling. The cooking is regulated by moving the food to different heat areas on the rack.

Griddling is done on a solid surface called a griddle, usually with a small amount of fat to prevent sticking. The temperature of a griddle is usually kept at about 350°F. Foods such as pancakes and eggs are cooked on a griddle.

Pan-broiling is like griddling, except it is done in a skillet or a sauté pan, instead of on a flat surface like a griddle. Fat must be removed as it accumulates or the process would be pan-frying. No liquid is added and the pan isn't covered or the food would steam. The products are usually cooked over moderate heat; sometimes an oven is used.

Smoking is done by any one of several methods for preserving and flavoring foods by exposing them to smoke. In hot smoking, the items are cooked. In cold smoking, the items aren't fully cooked. **Smoke roasting** is a method for roasting foods that are placed on a rack in a pan containing wood chips that smolder, emitting smoke, when the pan is placed over a fire or in an oven.

Poeleing, also known in some circles as butter-roasting, is a technique mostly associated with game birds and white meats. Meats are put in a covered pot on top of a bed of aromatic vegetables where they cook in their own juices. The vegetables then usually become part of a garnish for the sauce.

Microwave cooking refers to the use of a specific tool, a microwave oven, rather than moist-heat or dry-heat methods of cooking or reheating foods. You might want to spend some time at the library and read about this style of cooking to determine if you want to use it or not.

STOCKS & BROTH

CHAPTER 12

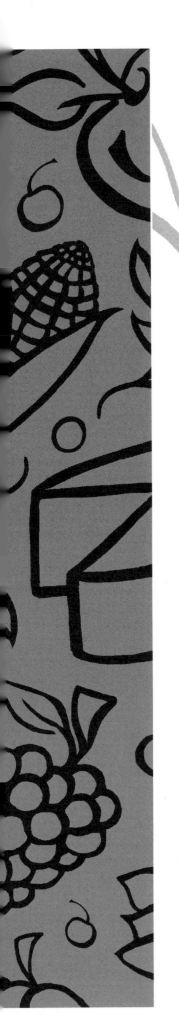

152

Chapter 12 Stocks & Broth 153

STOCKS AND BROTH

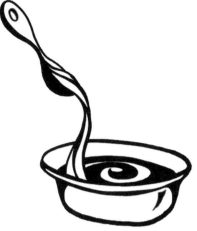

George Auguste Escoffier, the King of Chefs and the Chef of Kings, stated:

> "Stock is everything in cooking. Without it, nothing can be done. If one's stock is good, what remains of the work is easy."

VEGETABLE BROTH

For certain soups, a delicately flavored vegetable broth is preferred. Vegetables contain their own natural sodium, so season with the salt substitute at the end of the cooking process if necessary.

2	Carrots, cut small
2 cups	Celery, cut small
2	Medium Onions, cut small
6 oz.	Mushrooms, sliced
2	Medium Leeks, cut small
1 cup	Turnips, cut small
2	Bay Leaves
2	Stems of Parsley
2 qts.	Water
	Salt Substitute to taste (if necessary)

Method of Preparation
In a large pot, combine all the ingredients. Bring them to a boil, reduce the heat to a gentle simmer, and continue cooking for about two hours, or until the stock develops a good flavor.

Strain the broth and season to taste with salt substitute if necessary. Cool and refrigerate. You can freeze the broth for further use.

Yield
About 1-1/2 quarts

Hint
Now you will be able to use this recipe to make the incredible variety of soups which start from a vegetable broth. There are literally thousands of recipes out there—grab a cookbook and read!

Cooking Methods
Boil, simmer

Nutritional Analysis

Per Recipe
Energy   34 calories
Protein   1.2 gm
Fat   0.2 gm
Carbohydrate   7.7 gm
Fiber   1.7 gm
Cholesterol   0 mg
Iron   .9 mg
Sodium   32 mg
Calcium   31 mg
Sugar   3.4 gm

Recipe Cost: $3.43

Lifestyle Tip
Keep a "to do" list ready for times you feel ambitious.

Diet Tip
"Let thy food be thy medicine and thy medicine be thy food."
  Hippocrates (the father of medicine, 460-377 B.C.)

CHICKEN STOCK

Remember, folks: the only part of the chicken you can't use for cooking is the "cluck!" The bones are free if you save and freeze them from other meals.

3 lb.	**Chicken Bones**
1 gal.	**Cold Water**
4 oz.	**Onion, chopped small**
2 oz.	**Celery, chopped small**
2 oz.	**Carrots, chopped small**
1	**Bay Leaf**
1/8 tsp.	**Thyme Leaf**
1/8 tsp.	**Crushed Black Peppercorns**
1	**Whole Clove**
1-2	**Stems of Parsley**

Method of Preparation
Wash and rinse the bones in cold water. Place the bones in a large pot, add the cold water, and bring to a boil. Skim the scum. Simmer over low heat for one hour.

Add the rest of the ingredients and continue simmering over low heat for two more hours.

Strain, cool, and refrigerate for future use. You can also freeze this broth.

Yield
Approximately 2-1/2 quarts

Hint
This recipe can be cut in half with the same results.

Cooking Methods
Boil, simmer

Nutritional Analysis

Per Recipe
Protein	*9.7 gm*
Fat	*17.6 gm*
Carbohydrate	*1 gm*
Fiber	*0.25 gm*
Cholesterol	*67 mg*
Iron	*1.2 mg*
Sodium	*47 mg*
Calcium	*16 mg*
Sugar	*.55 gm*

Recipe Cost: $.63

Lifestyle Tip
Prioritize your chores: "must be done," "should be done," and "nice to get done."

Lifestyle Tip
Aerobic exercise, such as running, walking, biking, and swimming, performed continuously for thirty minutes with a sustained target heart rate is effective for fat burning because it increases the body temperature and oxygen flow. Anaerobic exercise such as weight lifting improves strength, bone density, muscle tone, and increases metabolic rate.

Chapter 12 Stocks & Broth 155

Nutritional Analysis

Per Recipe

Energy	*5.5 calories*
Protein	*0.15 gm*
Fat	*0.05 gm*
Carbohydrate	*1.5 gm*
Fiber	*0.25 gm*
Cholesterol	*0 mg*
Iron	*0.15 mg*
Sodium	*3.5 mg*
Calcium	*4.5 mg*
Sugar	*.5 gm*

Recipe Cost:	$.57

Lifestyle Tip
Self-sticking notes are great for helping you remember things.

COURT BOUILLON (FISH POACHING LIQUID)

Poaching fish gives it a unique flavor, leaves it very moist, and is fun to do!

1-3/4 pt.	Water
2 oz.	Cider Vinegar
1 oz.	Onion, chopped small
1/2 oz.	Celery, chopped small
1/2 oz.	Carrots, chopped small
1/4 tsp.	Cracked Black Peppercorns
1	Bay Leaf
1	Stem of Parsley
2	Thin Slices of Lemon
	Salt Substitute to taste

Method of Preparation
Combine all of the ingredients and bring to a boil over low heat. Simmer for 30-35 minutes. Strain. Cool and save for poaching fish.

To poach, reheat enough liquid to just cover the fish. Cook over medium heat until fish feels firm to the touch. Read about poaching in Chapter 11 on Cooking Methods.

Yield
Approximately 1-1/2 pints

Hint
You can place this in reclosable plastic freezer bags and freeze. It will last at least 6-8 weeks without losing flavor.

Cooking Methods
Boil, simmer, poach

FISH STOCK

From bones, veggies, herbs, and water comes this wonderful flavored liquid. Now you have the base for great soups, sauces, and whatever else you want to make from this recipe.

3 lb.	**Fish Bones with heads**
1 oz.	**Butter Substitute**
2 oz.	**Onions, chopped small**
1 oz.	**Celery, chopped small**
1 oz.	**Carrots, chopped small**
8 oz.	**White Wine**
1	**Bay Leaf**
1/4 tsp.	**Thyme Leaf**
2	**Stems of Parsley**
1/4	**Lemon**
3 qt.	**Cold Water**

Method of Preparation

Clean bones and heads under cold running water. Remove any dark skin, blood spots, and gills.

In a large pot, melt the butter substitute and sauté the onions, celery, and carrots. Cover and cook over low heat for 5 minutes, so they'll sweat their juices.

Add the fish bones, wine, bay leaves, thyme leaf, parsley stems, and lemon. Cover and sweat over a low heat for 6-7 minutes.

Add the cold water and bring to a slow boil. Skim off the white scum, and simmer for only 45 minutes. If you cook it longer, it will get bitter.

Strain the stock through a towel or cheesecloth, cool, and refrigerate for future use. You can also freeze it.

Yield

Approximately 2-1/4 quarts

Hint

If you go to your local fishmarket, they'll probably give you the bones for free, since they pay to have them hauled away.

Cooking Methods

Boil, simmer

Nutritional Analysis

Per Recipe

Energy	*65 calories*
Protein	*10.7 gm*
Fat	*1.2 gm*
Carbohydrate	*.8 gm*
Fiber	*0.1 gm*
Cholesterol	*27 mg*
Iron	*0.4 mg*
Sodium	*61 mg*
Calcium	*14 mg*
Sugar	*0.3 gm*

Recipe Cost: $1.42

Lifestyle Tip

Electronic appointment calendars are helpful when writing is difficult.

Lifestyle Tip

Upraised chair seats make it easier for you to get up without causing a lot of stress to joints. Slide your buttocks to the front edge of the chair prior to getting up.

TURKEY STOCK

Remember folks: the only part of the turkey you can't use for cooking is the "gobble, gobble, gobble!"

2-1/2 lb.	Turkey Bones
1 gal.	Cold Water
4 oz.	Onion, chopped small
2 oz.	Celery, chopped small
2 oz.	Carrots, chopped small
1	Bay Leaf
1/8 tsp.	Thyme Leaf
1/8 tsp.	Crushed Black Peppercorns
1	Whole Clove
2	Stems of Parsley

Method of Preparation
Wash and rinse the bones in cold water. Place them in a large pot, add the cold water, and bring to a boil. Skim the scum. Simmer over low heat for one hour.

Add the rest of the ingredients and continue simmering over low heat for two more hours.

Strain, cool and refrigerate for further use. You can also freeze the product.

Yield
Approximately 2-1/2 quarts

Cooking Methods
Boil, simmer

Nutritional Analysis

Per Recipe

Energy	134 calories
Protein	15.6 gm
Fat	7.1 gm
Carbohydrate	1 gm
Fiber	0.25 gm
Cholesterol	46 mg
Iron	9 mg
Sodium	38 mg
Calcium	17 mg
Sugar	6 gm

Recipe Cost: $1.30

Lifestyle Tip
Large chalkboards are a great way to keep track of appointments.

Health Tip
Before getting out of bed in the morning and after sitting for prolonged periods of time, move your joints through a range of motions several times. This will help to prevent some of the stiffness and discomfort when you first get up to move.

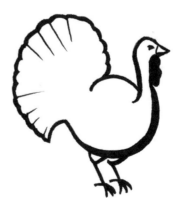

158

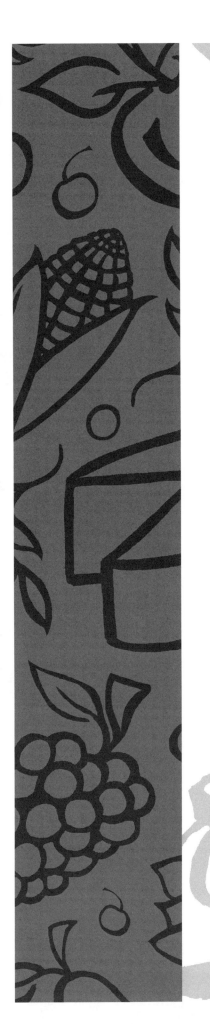

SAUCES
MARINADES
& BUTTERS

CHAPTER 13

160

SAUCES

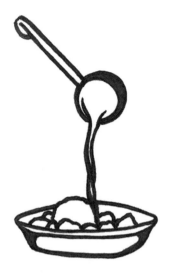

In this chapter I will tell you about sauces, about a great chef whose eyes always twinkled, and how he helped me with the building blocks of my future while I was at the Culinary Institute of America. Chef White was a man who left World War II with a skill, which he taught at a small under-funded cooking school in New Haven, Connecticut.

Chef White taught Introduction to Theory, Demonstration and Skill Development, the first kitchen course. He raised his mellow, soft-spoken voice only once while I was his student, in the very first five minutes of class. I'll never forget what he said.

"This is the most important course in your education," he said very simply, and he said it twice. It was, without a doubt, the reason I went on to become a Certified Executive Chef.

Chef White was a true old master. He loved to teach, he loved his students, and he loved educating them. Remembering him brings a few tears to my eyes because he was a great chef who understood the reason God put him on earth.

Three weeks before I was to graduate, Chef White summoned me to his kitchen. He asked, "Carl, do you have a job yet?" "No," I said, "but I have quite a few offers." He said, "Forget the offers. You are going to stay here and receive a fellowship to teach." I asked him what a fellowship was. He was dumfounded. He told me that it was what all students were working for. I had gone from class to class, taking it one day at a time, and I really didn't understand what he was talking about. He joked, "You Marines always only live one day at a time!"

Chef White made it possible for me to teach, to learn, and to become a better human being. Thank you, Chef White.

About Sauces

The following information and recipes come from my notes as a student at the Culinary Institute. Chef White used the school's textbook, *The Professional Chef*, 4th revised edition (1974) as his guide. I would personally like to thank Ferdinand Metz, CMC, President of the Culinary Institute of America, and Tim Ryan, CMC, Vice President of the Culinary Institute of America, for allowing me to use the materials. I have changed each of the recipes to adapt them to our arthritis diet guidelines.

162 The Executive Chef's Arthritis Cookbook and Health Guide

From *The Professional Chef,* pp. 309-310

A sauce is a fluid dressing for meat, poultry, fish, desserts, and other culinary preparations. Sauces enhance the flavor and appearance of the food they accompany. They may also add nutritional value.

A sauce may present a contrast in flavor, color and consistency. It should not, however, prevail over the food with which it is associated. It should be so prepared that it forms a part of the food it accompanies.

In most cases a sauce should be of proper consistency to flow readily and provide a coating for the food but not thick or heavy enough to saturate the food or cause difficulty in digestion.

A sauce must not mask or cover the flavor of a dish. Poor meat or poultry cannot be disguised by a sauce.

It is essential that the seasoning be correct so that the food product will not be flavorless or excessively flavored. Seasoning is an art learned only through experience, and extreme care must be exercised in the use of spices and herbs until this knowledge is mastered.

Many sauces are derived from the same basic stocks that are used in soup making. Sauce stocks are often reduced in volume by boiling to increase their strength.

Categories of Sauces

There are thousands of sauces varying in name and content. They fall into two basic categories: warm sauces and cold sauces.

The warm sauces comprise the largest group and are served with all types of food. The cold sauces are served with both hot or cold food and include various butter preparations that are often associated with shellfish.

The warm sauces are derived from a few leading sauces that are used as a basis for nearly all others. The leading sauces are sometimes referred to as mother sauces. Sauces that are derived from them are termed small sauces.

Chapter 13 Sauces, Marinades, and Butters 163

The leading sauces are:

1) Espagnole or Brown
2) Bechamel or Cream
3) Tomato Sauce
4) Velouté
   (chicken or fish)
5) Hollandaise

Espagnole or Brown Sauce is made from brown stock and brown roux and is used extensively in the preparation of all types of meat and poultry dishes.

Bechamel or Cream Sauce, while originally prepared from veal stock, is a term now used interchangeably with cream sauce. It is derived from milk and/or cream with the addition of white roux. This sauce is used with all types of vegetables and creamed dishes, including soups, fish, poultry, dairy and macaroni products. While white sauce is made of roux and milk, the term cream sauce is often used interchangeably.

Tomato Sauce is prepared from tomato products, white stock, seasonings and roux. It is used with various meat, poultry, fish, vegetable and macaroni dishes. It is also used for producing other products with a tomato character.

Velouté Sauce may be either chicken, veal or fish, although chicken is the usual ingredient. A velouté is derived from stock with the addition of light roux and is associated with the product from which it is derived. Fish velouté is specifically derived from a fumet (an essence or rich fish stock or court bouillon in which fish has been cooked). The term fumet is also used for reduced stocks derived from game.

Hollandaise Sauce Although hollandaise is not a basic sauce as such, it is included here because many of the drawn butter sauces are prepared in the same manner. Other sauces are derived from hollandaise, and it is used in combination with various culinary preparations to obtain a variety of sauces popular in fine eating establishments.

Hollandaise and its derivatives must be handled with extreme caution. Because of their high butter and egg content, these sauces must never be exposed to high heat because they will curdle.

The temperature at which they must be held (not over 180°F.) is a natural and prolific breeding ground for bacteria which thrive and multiply best under these conditions. These sauces should be made only in very small quantities and should not be held over from one meal to another. Maximum retention time should not exceed 1-1/2 hour. Practice proper sanitation procedures and avoid danger of food poisoning.

Stainless steel cookware must be used for preparation of hollandaise sauce, as aluminum discolors eggs.

Hollandaise and its derivatives are often used with fish, vegetables and eggs.

Meat Glaze or glace de viande is a gelatinous reduction of brown stock. This quality is due to the gelatinous content of the bones used in preparing brown stock. It is used to strengthen the flavor and consistency of sauces and other culinary preparations. It is also used to coat special dishes before serving, to improve their flavor and appearance.

Meat glaze is made by reducing brown stock in a large sauce pan or pot on the range. The stock should be allowed to simmer slowly and then be transferred to smaller sauce pans or pots as it reduces. The pot should be selected to hold the amount of stock used. At each change it should be carefully strained.

Each successive reduction will become heavier in consistency. The heat should be reduced as the product becomes heavier so that it will not burn. If heavy-bottom pots are available, their use is recommended.

When sufficiently reduced, the glaze should be thick enough to coat a spoon. It should be cooled and stored for future use and should be tightly covered to prevent dehydration or drying out. It may be kept for an indefinite period without spoilage. When small amounts are made, it does not require refrigeration.

It should now become clear why salt is not used in preparing stock. As the liquid is reduced by evaporation, its salt content remains the same and the finished product would be disagreeable to taste.

Chapter 13 Sauces, Marinades, and Butters 165

Demi-Glace Sauce is obtained by reducing a combination of equal quantities of espagnole and brown stock to half. It is used with small brown sauces.

Recipes for the Leading Sauces

All of the following sauce recipes can be refrigerated and stored for several days. They can be frozen and stored for a longer period. If the quantities are larger than you can conveniently use, the recipe quantities can easily be reduced by 1/2 or more.

Nutritional Analysis

Per Recipe
Energy	*142 calories*
Protein	*2.9 gm*
Fat	*7 gm*
Carbohydrate	*17 gm*
Fiber	*1.2 gm*
Cholesterol	*0 mg*
Iron	*0.9 mg*
Sodium	*160 mg*
Calcium	*19 mg*
Sugar	*2.3 gm*

Recipe Cost: $1.75

Lifestyle Tip
Shopping by mail or over the Internet is a great way to save time and energy.

Health Tip
Always discuss and obtain approval from your primary physician or a physician who practices holistic medicine BEFORE beginning any nutritional supplements. Some supplements may interact with your medications. Never stop any of your medications to go on a "miracle cure" without consulting your physician.

BROWN SAUCE
(Espagnole)

8 oz.	Onions, diced medium
4 oz.	Celery, diced medium
4 oz.	Carrots, diced medium
5 oz.	Soy Margarine
5 oz.	Bread Flour
2-1/2 qts.	Brown Stock or Beef Stock, hot
4 oz.	Tomato Puree
1	Whole Bay Leaf
	Salt to taste
	Pepper to taste

Method of Preparation
In a heavy sauce pot, sauté all the vegetables in margarine until the onions are transparent. Add flour and cook 10 minutes over low heat. Add hot brown stock and tomato puree, stirring until slightly thickened and smooth.

Add the bay leaf, salt, and pepper, and cook at a simmer for 1-1/2 hours. Adjust flavor and consistency. Strain and hold for service.

Yield
2-1/4 quarts

166 The Executive Chef's Arthritis Cookbook and Health Guide

BECHAMEL
or White Sauce No. 1 (Light)

This light white sauce is generally prepared for use in creamed vegetables.

3 oz.	Soy Margarine
3 oz.	Bread Flour
2 quarts	Milk
1/2 Tbsp.	Salt

Method of Preparation
Melt butter in thick-bottomed sauce pot. Stir in flour to make a roux. Cook over low heat, stirring constantly for 8-10 minutes. Don't let roux brown.

In a large saucepan, heat milk to boiling. Stir into roux gradually, beating briskly until sauce is thickened and smooth. Simmer for 5 minutes, stirring occasionally. Bring to a boil. Strain.

Yield
About 2 quarts

Hint
To make cream sauce, use cream or a mixture of cream and milk instead of plain milk.

White Sauce No. 2 (Medium)

4 oz.	Soy Margarine
4 oz.	Bread Flour
2 quarts	Milk
1/2 Tbsp.	Salt

Method of Preparation
Melt the butter in thick-bottomed sauce pot. Stir in the flour to make a roux. Cook over low heat, stirring constantly for 8 to 10 minutes. Don't let the roux brown.

In a large saucepan, heat the milk to boiling. Stir into the roux gradually, beating briskly until sauce is thickened and smooth. Simmer for 5 minutes, stirring occasionally. Bring to a boil. Strain through china cap.

Yield
About 2 quarts.

Nutritional Analysis

Per Recipe

Energy	99 calories
Protein	4.7 gm
Fat	5.5 gm
Carbohydrate	9.8 gm
Fiber	0 gm
Cholesterol	10 mg
Iron	0.3 mg
Sodium	332 mg
Calcium	152 mg
Sugar	5.2 gm

Recipe Cost: $2.42

Lifestyle Tip
Keep frequently used phone numbers handy so you don't have to use a heavy phone book.

Nutritional Analysis

Per Recipe

Energy	111 calories
Protein	4.7 gm
Fat	5.2 gm
Carbohydrate	11 gm
Fiber	0 gm
Cholesterol	10 mg
Iron	0.3 mg
Sodium	349 mg
Calcium	153 mg
Sugar	5.2 gm

Recipe Cost: $2.18

Lifestyle Tip
Keep your address and phone number attached to each telephone in your home. In case of an emergency, a visitor would be able to summon help quickly.

Nutritional Analysis

Per Recipe
Energy	*136 calories*
Protein	*5.4 gm*
Fat	*6.6 gm*
Carbohydrate	*14.1 gm*
Fiber	*0 gm*
Cholesterol	*10 mg*
Iron	*.55 mg*
Sodium	*383 mg*
Calcium	*154 mg*
Sugar	*5.1 gm*

Recipe Cost: $2.45

Lifestyle Tip
Use roller ball pens. They glide the easiest of all pens and pencils.

Diet Tip
Some foods may be contributing to a flare-up of your arthritis. To identify and eliminate food intolerances, start by eliminating ALL dairy products, including eggs, for six weeks. Then start using them again and observe your symptoms. If you experience no change, consider stopping nightshade vegetables (bell peppers, eggplant, tomatoes, and potatoes) for six weeks, then start using them again. Experiment with other common allergens causing arthritis symptoms such as wheat, gluten, corn, peanuts, and chocolate.

WHITE SAUCE No. 3 (Heavy)

6 oz.	Soy Margarine
6 oz.	Bread Flour
2 quarts	Milk
1/2 Tbsp.	Salt

Method of Preparation
Melt the butter in a thick-bottomed sauce pot. Stir in the flour to make a roux. Cook over low heat, stirring constantly for 8 to 10 minutes. Don't let roux brown.

In a large saucepan, heat the milk to boiling. Stir into the roux gradually, beating briskly until sauce is thickened and smooth. Simmer for 5 minutes, stirring occasionally. Bring to a boil. Strain through china cap.

Yield
About 2 quarts

168   The Executive Chef's Arthritis Cookbook and Health Guide

TOMATO SAUCE

2 tsp.	Garlic, chopped fine
6 oz.	Soy Margarine
8 oz.	Onions, chopped fine
4 oz.	Celery, chopped fine
3 oz.	Bread Flour
1-1/2 qts.	Brown Stock, hot
16 oz.	Tomatoes, peeled
1 qt.	Tomato Puree
1	Bay Leaf
1/2 tsp.	Ground Thyme
1/2 tsp.	Crushed Peppercorns
1	Whole Clove
	Salt to taste

Method of Preparation
Sauté garlic in melted butter until garlic is lightly browned. Add onions and celery, sauté until soft. Add flour to make a roux; stir until well blended. Cook 5 minutes. Add brown stock. Stir until slightly thickened and smooth, add peeled tomatoes, puree, and spices. Simmer for 1-1/2 hours. Strain, season.

Yield
2-1/2 quarts

BASIC SAUCE VELOUTÉ

5 oz.	Soy Margarine
5 oz.	Bread Flour
2 quarts	Chicken Stock, hot
	Salt to taste
	Pepper to taste

Method of Preparation
Melt the butter in a sauce pan, stir in the flour to make a smooth roux. Cook slowly for 5 to 6 minutes; don't brown. Slowly whip in stock until thickened and smooth. Check the seasoning. Continue to cook sauce for 30 more minutes. Strain.

Yield
About 2 quarts

Hints
Sauce Supreme: Make 1/2 of the recipe, and add 3 oz. scalded heavy cream.

Dill Sauce: To one quart of finished Sauce Supreme, add 1/2 cup finely chopped fresh dill. Cook over low heat for 15-20 minutes, then strain through a fine strainer.

Nutritional Analysis

Per Recipe
Energy	82 calories
Protein	1.9 gm
Fat	3.9 gm
Carbohydrate	10.9 gm
Fiber	1.7 gm
Cholesterol	0 mg
Iron	.9 mg
Sodium	101 mg
Calcium	17 mg
Sugar	1.3 gm

Recipe Cost: $3.25

Lifestyle Tip
Buy self-addressed return address labels.

Nutritional Analysis

Per Recipe
Energy	73 calories
Protein	1.9 gm
Fat	2.2 gm
Carbohydrate	7.5 gm
Fiber	0 gm
Cholesterol	0 mg
Iron	0.4 mg
Sodium	88 mg
Calcium	3 mg
Sugar	0 gm

Recipe Cost: $.60
(when the bones for the stock are already saved)

Lifestyle Tip
Use a rubber grip to hold a pen or pencil.

Chapter 13 Sauces, Marinades, and Butters   169

Nutritional Analysis

Per Recipe
Energy	*740 calories*
Protein	*3.7 gm*
Fat	*82 gm*
Carbohydrate	*7.5 gm*
Fiber	*0 gm*
Cholesterol	*425 mg*
Iron	*.75 mg*
Sodium	*18 mg*
Calcium	*47 mg*
Sugar	*0.1 gm*

Recipe Cost: $2.65

Lifestyle Tip
If you need someone's attention in the cellar, switch the lights off and on instead of climbing up and down the stairs.

Health Tip
When it comes to vitamins and minerals, dosage does make a difference. To prevent deficiencies you will need to take the recommended daily advisory (RDA) amount. When used therapeutically the dosage might be several times RDA quantities, often referred to as "High Potency" formulations.

HOLLANDAISE SAUCE

6	Egg Yolks
1 oz.	Cold Water
1-1/4 lb.	Butter, clarify and keep warm
1	Lemon, juice only
	Cayenne Pepper to taste
	Salt to taste

Method of Preparation
In a stainless steel bowl, whip the egg yolks and water together. Place the bowl over a pot of boiling water (like a double boiler), but make sure the bowl does not touch the water (results in overcooking).

Whip yolks lightly until cooked to a soft peak. Stir down from the edges and up from the bottom of the bowl. Remove from range.

Slowly pour butter into the eggs, whipping lightly to blend. Add lemon juice, cayenne pepper, and salt if needed. Don't overheat.

Yield
24 ounces

Additional Information on Hollandaise
Hollandaise sauce is one of the few sauces that cannot be successfully refrigerated to retard bacteria growth or boiled to kill organisms. This is because refrigeration hardens the butter in the sauce and causes the mixture to become solid, while overheating the sauce coagulates the eggs and causes the mixture to become lumpy.

When hollandaise is prepared, and later in serving it or adding it to other sauces, follow these sanitation and holding procedures:

1. Use only fresh eggs and fresh butter.

2. Sterilize all equipment, such as wire whip, spoons, pots, and other materials by scalding.

3. Serve all of the sauce within 1-1/2 hours after it is prepared. Never hold the sauce any longer.

4. Never add leftover hollandaise to a new batch of freshly prepared sauce.

CHEESE SAUCE

1-1/2 qts.	Milk
8 oz.	Cheddar Cheese, cubed
8 oz.	American Cheese, cubed
1 tsp.	Paprika
1 tsp.	Dry Mustard
1/2 Tbsp.	Worcestershire Sauce
1/2 tsp.	Salt
3 oz.	Butter
3 oz.	Bread Flour

Method of Preparation
Combine milk, cheeses, paprika, mustard, Worcestershire, and salt in top of double boiler. Heat until cheese is melted and milk begins to form a skin on top. Prepare roux with butter and flour. Cook 4-5 minutes, but do not brown.

Add roux to milk-cheese mixture, a small amount at a time, whipping until smooth. Then cook for 10-15 minutes longer. Bring almost to a boil, then remove from heat. Strain through china cap.

Yield
2 quarts

MUSHROOM SAUCE

1 lb.	Mushrooms, washed and sliced
1-1/2 Tbsp.	Shallots, finely chopped
8 oz.	Butter, melted
4-1/2 oz.	Bread Flour
2 quarts	Brown Stock, hot
2 oz.	Burgundy Wine
	Salt to taste

Method of Preparation
In a sauce pot, sauté mushrooms and shallots together in butter. Stir in flour to make a roux. Cook 10 minutes, stirring constantly. Add hot stock and stir until slightly thickened and smooth. Add wine. Salt to taste. Bring to boil and remove from range.

Yield
About 2 quarts

Hint
If holding for service, spread small amount of melted butter over top to prevent formation of skin.

Nutritional Analysis

Per Recipe

Energy	225 calories
Protein	10.4 gm
Fat	16.6 gm
Carbohydrate	8.7 gm
Fiber	0.05 gm
Cholesterol	53mg
Iron	0.5 mg
Sodium	462 mg
Calcium	302mg
Sugar	5.7 gm

Recipe Cost: $2.75

Lifestyle Tip
Use a large 24 to 30 point typeface when creating or reading a document on the computer.

Nutritional Analysis

Per Recipe

Energy	176 calories
Protein	1.9 gm
Fat	12.4 gm
Carbohydrate	8.2 gm
Fiber	0.4 gm
Cholesterol	31 mg
Iron	.75 mg
Sodium	123 mg
Calcium	0.5 mg
Sugar	0.05 gm

Recipe Cost: $3.10

Lifestyle Tip
If using the telephone directory is difficult, you may be eligible for free directory assistance. Check with your local phone company.

Chapter 13 Sauces, Marinades, and Butters **171**

Nutritional Analysis

Per Recipe
Energy *93 calories*
Protein *0.5 gm*
Fat *1.2 gm*
Carbohydrate *19.6 gm*
Fiber *0.1 gm*
Cholesterol *0 mg*
Iron *0.1 mg*
Sodium *1178 mg*
Calcium *8 mg*
Sugar *6.2 gm*

Recipe Cost: $0.69

Health Tip
Get plenty of rest.

Nutritional Analysis

Per Recipe
Energy *84 calories*
Protein *8 gm*
Fat *10.2 gm*
Carbohydrate *21 gm*
Fiber *1.5 gm*
Cholesterol *12 mg*
Iron *1.4 mg*
Sodium *1039mg*
Calcium *28 mg*
Sugar *0.6 gm*

Recipe Cost: $1.25

Lifestyle Tip
If you have a hard time getting to the mailbox, there is a hardship delivery where the Post Office will deliver directly to your door.

SWEET AND SOUR SAUCE

1 qt.	Chicken Stock
1 oz.	Vinegar
2 Tbsp.	Sugar
2 tsp.	Salt
1/4 tsp.	White Pepper
6 Tbsp.	Cornstarch

Method of Preparation
Reserve 4 oz. of chicken stock. Place the rest in a sauce pan and bring to a boil.

Combine the reserved cool stock, vinegar, sugar, salt, pepper, and cornstarch. Reduce heat and add the cornstarch mixture to hot stock, stirring until thickened and smooth.

Yield
1 quart

BARBECUE SAUCE

2 oz.	Onions, minced
1 Tbsp.	Garlic, minced
2 oz.	Salad Oil
2 oz.	Bread Flour
24 oz.	Brown Stock, hot
1 oz.	Sugar
1/4 Tbsp.	Dry Mustard
1/2 tsp.	Black Pepper
2 oz.	Cider Vinegar
16 oz.	Tomato Sauce or Puree
3/4	Lemon, juice only
2 oz.	Worcestershire Sauce
1/4 Tbsp.	Barbecue Spice or Chili Powder
	Salt to taste

Method of Preparation
In a sauce pot, sauté the onions and garlic in oil. When transparent, add the flour to make a roux. Stir until well blended. Next, add hot stock, stirring until smooth.

Dissolve sugar, mustard and pepper in vinegar. Add tomato sauce, vinegar mix, and lemon juice to the pot. Add Worcestershire sauce and barbecue spice or chili powder. Simmer 30 minutes. Salt to taste.

Yield
2 quarts

172　The Executive Chef's Arthritis Cookbook and Health Guide

SAUCE POULETTE

2 oz.	Soy Margarine
1/2 oz.	Shallots, chopped fine
1 lb.	Fresh Mushrooms, washed, sliced fine
1-1/2 qt.	Chicken Velouté (recipe on page 168)
4 oz.	Light Cream, scalded
	Salt and Pepper to taste
1/2 oz.	Parsley, chopped

Method of Preparation

In a sauce pan, melt the butter, add shallots; smother until tender (do not brown). Add the mushrooms and cook until tender. Stir in the velouté and simmer for 20 minutes, stirring frequently. Add the cream and bring to boil. Season. Add parsley.

Yield

2 quarts

TERIYAKI SAUCE AND MARINADE

My friend Douglas Tihada taught me this. I know he is very pleased, watching from above, that I'm sharing his recipe.

8 oz.	Low Salt Soy Sauce
24 oz.	Water
5 oz	Honey
2 Tbsp.	Sherry
1 Tbsp.	Sesame Seed Oil
2 Tbsp.	Ginger, chopped fine
3	Cloves Garlic, smashed
1/2	Orange, thinly sliced
1/2	Lemon, thinly sliced

Method of Preparation

Mix all ingredients well. Put in the coldest part of your refrigerator for 2 days. To marinate: pour enough over to cover the food and refrigerate for 2-4 hours. It's a great way to prepare meat for outdoor barbecuing.

Yield

1 quart

Hint

For teriyaki sauce, bring liquid to a boil, thicken with cornstarch and water, then cook for 10 minutes. It will last 1-2 weeks when properly stored in the refrigerator.

Cooking Methods

Boil, simmer

Nutritional Analysis

Per Recipe

Energy	*96 calories*
Protein	*1.8 gm*
Fat	*6.8 gm*
Carbohydrate	*7.3 gm*
Fiber	*0.4 gm*
Cholesterol	*8 mg*
Iron	*.7 mg*
Sodium	*141 mg*
Calcium	*11 mg*
Sugar	*0.2 gm*

Recipe Cost: $2.70

Lifestyle Tip

An easy way to vote is to register for a permanent absentee ballot, so you can cast your vote by mail.

Nutritional Analysis

Per Recipe

Energy	*107 calories*
Protein	*1.6 gm*
Fat	*1.6 gm*
Carbohydrate	*22.7 gm*
Fiber	*0.2 gm*
Cholesterol	*0 mg*
Iron	*.7 mg*
Sodium	*861 mg*
Calcium	*9.5 mg*
Sugar	*19.2 gm*

Recipe Cost: $1.57

Lifestyle Tip

Ask your bank how they can help you do your banking from home.

Chapter 13 Sauces, Marinades, and Butters   173

Nutritional Analysis

Per Recipe

Energy	*178 calories*
Protein	*0.4 gm*
Fat	*18.4 gm*
Carbohydrate	*3.5 gm*
Fiber	*0.1 gm*
Cholesterol	*0 mg*
Iron	*0.1 mg*
Sodium	*384 mg*
Calcium	*10 mg*
Sugar	*2.9 gm*

Recipe Cost: $1.52

Lifestyle Tip
Get a closet organizer so you don't have to root around.

Nutritional Analysis

Per Recipe

Energy	*513 calories*
Protein	*0.7 gm*
Fat	*55.1 gm*
Carbohydrate	*6.5 gm*
Fiber	*0.2 gm*
Cholesterol	*17 mg*
Iron	*0.3 mg*
Sodium	*240 mg*
Calcium	*5 mg*
Sugar	*0.4 gm*

Recipe Cost: $2.57

Lifestyle Tip
Keep a reacher inside your closet to pick up items on the floor.

ORANGE MUSTARD SAUCE

This sauce makes a tangy coating for just about any fresh steamed vegetable.

4 oz.	Soy Margarine
1 oz.	Olive Oil
4 oz.	Fresh Orange Juice
1	Orange, zested
2 Tbsp.	Fresh Chopped Garlic Chives
1 Tbsp.	Dijon Mustard
	Salt Substitute to taste

Method of Preparation
In a small pan, slowly melt together the soy margarine and olive oil. Turn heat on high, add the rest of the ingredients, and sauté for two minutes. You can use a large pot and stir your vegetables around in it till they are coated, or you can spoon the mixture on top of your vegetables.

Yield
Enough to cover four vegetable servings

Hint
If you like garlic, add 1 tsp. chopped with the olive oil and margarine, and let it simmer for a few minutes until you have a good garlic aroma. Then finish the recipe.

TARTAR SAUCE WITH CAPERS

Use this for better fried fish. If you ever taste a better recipe, please send it to me!

2 cups	Soy Mayonnaise
1/2 cup	Pickle Relish
1/4 cup	Chopped Onion
1 oz.	Lemon Juice
1 Tbsp.	Capers, chopped fine
1 tsp.	Caper Juice
1/8 tsp.	Ground White Pepper
	Salt Substitute to taste

Method of Preparation
In a bowl, mix all the ingredients well, and refrigerate.

Hint
You can double or triple this recipe very easily. In the restaurant business, we make it a gallon at a time.

Yield
Serves 4-8 (3+ cups)

MARINADES AND BASTES FOR FISH

Marinades and bastes add moisture and flavor to foods that will be barbecued or broiled. The following recipes will help you start discovering how marinades and bastes work with fish. They will provide enough marinade for four to five 6 oz. pieces of fish.

LEMON BUTTER WITH GARLIC BASTE

The combination of lemon, butter, and garlic makes a great all-time flavor to use with fish.

3 oz.	Butter, melted
2 oz.	Lemon Juice
1 tsp.	Chopped Dill
1 tsp.	Chopped Garlic

Method of Preparation
Melt all ingredients together. Brush liberally over fish while broiling or grilling.

Yield
Baste for five 6-oz. portions of fish

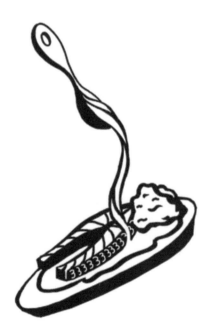

Nutritional Analysis

Per Recipe
Energy	63 calories
Protein	0.2 gm
Fat	6.6 gm
Carbohydrate	1.3 gm
Fiber	0 gm
Cholesterol	0 mg
Iron	0 mg
Sodium	163 mg
Calcium	5 mg
Sugar	0.3 gm

Recipe Cost: $0.77

Lifestyle Tip
Store mittens, scarves, and hats in a hanging shoe bag inside your coat closet.

Diet Tip
Vitamins, minerals, and other natural supplements are not a substitute for healthy dietary habits.

Chapter 13 Sauces, Marinades, and Butters 175

Nutritional Analysis

Per Recipe
Energy	*84 calories*
Protein	*1.3 gm*
Fat	*5.7 gm*
Carbohydrate	*6.4 gm*
Fiber	*0 gm*
Cholesterol	*0 mg*
Iron	*0.5 mg*
Sodium	*774 mg*
Calcium	*6 mg*
Sugar	*3.7 gm*

Recipe Cost: $0.84

Lifestyle Tip
Organize household items by storing them together near where they will be used.

Nutritional Analysis

Per Recipe
Energy	*244 calories*
Protein	*3.6 gm*
Fat	*23.5 gm*
Carbohydrate	*6.2 gm*
Fiber	*0.5 gm*
Cholesterol	*6 mg*
Iron	*1 mg*
Sodium	*135 mg*
Calcium	*144 mg*
Sugar	*0.1 gm*

Recipe Cost: $1.47

Health Tip
Take a good hot shower then make the water cool. When you cool off you'll feel better.

GINGER SOY MARINADE

Here in Hawaii in our regional cuisine we often use this combination of ginger-soy. Try it and enjoy.

1 tsp.	Fresh Ground Ginger
1/2 tsp.	Chopped Garlic
1 Tbsp.	Honey
1/2 tsp.	Grated Lemon Peel
1/2 cup	Soy Sauce, low sodium
1 oz.	Dry Sherry
1 oz.	Salad Oil
1 oz.	Lemon Juice
	Salt Substitute to taste

Method of Preparation
Mix ingredients together. Soak fish 10-12 minutes, turning a couple of times. Save the marinade to use for basting.

Yield
Marinade for five 6-oz. portions of fish

TANGERINE-BASIL-PARMESAN MARINADE

I promise this will excite your taste buds!

2/3 cup	Fresh Basil Leaves
1/4 cup	Chopped Parsley
3 oz.	White Wine Vinegar
3 oz.	Salad Oil
1 Tbsp.	Chopped Garlic
1 oz.	Parmesan Cheese
1/8 tsp.	White Pepper
4 oz.	Fresh Tangerine or Orange Juice
	Salt Substitute to taste

Method of Preparation
Combine all ingredients in a food processor. Soak fish for 30 minutes, turning several times. Use the marinade for basting.

Yield
Marinade for four 6-oz. portions of fish

176   The Executive Chef's Arthritis Cookbook and Health Guide

FISH MARINADE FOR BAKING

Here is a nice recipe that will impart a good flavor into the fish.

1 cup	**Salad Oil**
1 oz.	**White Wine**
1	**Bay Leaf**
1	**Sprig Fresh Parsley, chopped**
1/8 tsp.	**Dried Thyme**
1 oz.	**Lemon Juice or Tangerine Juice**
	Salt Substitute to taste
	Pinch White Pepper

Method of Preparation
Mix all ingredients together. Let fish marinate 25-30 minutes, turning 2-3 times.

Yield
Marinade for four 6-oz. portions of fish

Nutritional Analysis

Per Recipe
Energy	*490 calories*
Protein	*0.1 gm*
Fat	*54.5 gm*
Carbohydrate	*1.1 gm*
Fiber	*0.1 gm*
Cholesterol	*0 mg*
Iron	*0.3 mg*
Sodium	*2 mg*
Calcium	*5 mg*
Sugar	*0.2 gm*

Recipe Cost: $0.92

Lifestyle Tip
Shoe boxes make great storage for small items.

BASTING MIXTURE FOR BROILED OR BARBECUED FISH

Enjoy this recipe with your friends at your annual summer barbeque.

4 oz.	**Butter**
1 oz.	**Chopped Onion**
2 oz.	**Lemon, Lime, or Tangerine Juice**
1 tsp.	**Dried Tarragon**
1 tsp.	**Paprika**
1/8 cup	**Chopped Parsley**

Method of Preparation
In a sauce pan, melt butter until soft. Let cool, add the other ingredients, and smear over fish. Let sit 20-25 minutes, turning 2-3 times.

Yield
Baste for four 6-oz. portions of fish

Nutritional Analysis

Per Recipe
Energy	*597 calories*
Protein	*0.6 gm*
Fat	*65.6 gm*
Carbohydrate	*3.4 gm*
Fiber	*0.5 gm*
Cholesterol	*0 mg*
Iron	*0.7 mg*
Sodium	*278 mg*
Calcium	*21 mg*
Sugar	*0.7 gm*

Recipe Cost: $1.14

Lifestyle Tip
Store tools on a pegboard.

Chapter 13 Sauces, Marinades, and Butters 177

Nutritional Analysis

Per Recipe

Energy	*124 calories*
Protein	*3.9 gm*
Fat	*12 gm*
Carbohydrate	*2.1 gm*
Fiber	*0.5 gm*
Cholesterol	*4 mg*
Iron	*1.3 mg*
Sodium	*94 mg*
Calcium	*103 mg*
Sugar	*0.7 gm*

Recipe Cost: $5.21

Lifestyle Tip
Wrap the handles of household and outdoor tools with foam pipe insulation for easier gripping.

Health Tip
Vitamins and minerals work together to provide optimum nutrition. Too much of one, or not enough of another, may limit their effect or even create toxicity.

PESTO

Here is a recipe you can use over pasta, combine with hot vegetables, or stir into soup. You can also do what I do sometimes —just eat it straight.

2 cups	Fresh Basil Leaves, lightly packed
1 tsp.	Chopped Garlic
3/4 cup	Grated Parmesan Cheese
1/2 cup	Pine Nuts, toasted
3-4 oz.	Olive Oil
1/8 tsp.	Ground Black Pepper
	Salt Substitute, to taste

Method of Preparation
In a blender or food processor, place the basil and garlic. Blend till finely chopped. Stop and scrape the sides. Add the cheese and nuts and blend till nuts are chopped fine and the mixture is well combined.

Add the rest of the ingredients and blend well; scrape the sides and blend again.

Yield
Enough for 10-12 pesto meals

Hints
This pesto can be frozen. To serve, thaw and bring to room temperature.

Here in Hawaii we use half pine nuts and half macadamia nuts, toasted, which gives this a much better flavor.

178

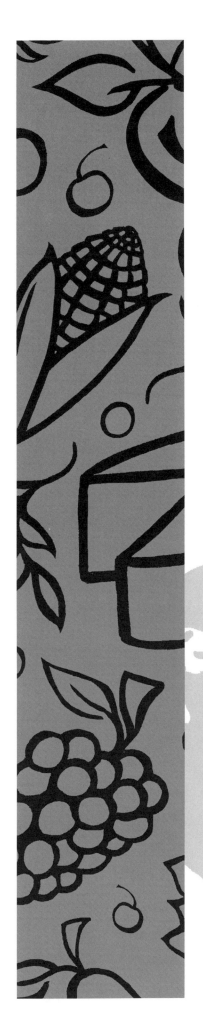

APPETIZERS

CHAPTER 14

180

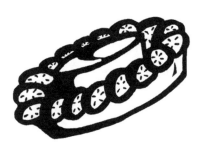

APPETIZERS

Little nibblers to go with wine or beer, colorful canapés to be served on a tray, thousands of beautiful appetizers to be served as a first course for dinner. All of these reflect the professionalism of the chef and his or her staff. Appetizers create an elegant setting for every occasion.

In Italian cooking, antipasto is the appetizer or hors d'oeuvre that comes before the pasta course—it can be a snack with drinks or the base of an entire luncheon. Is there anything in the art of cooking more beautiful than a platter of antipasto? Appetizers are served with many delightful garnishes. Crackers and breads can be dressed up into enjoyable additions to just about any appetizer, appetizer tray, or your appetizer table.

The most common single food used in appetizers are eggs. They play a varied role—just think of all the different ways we see eggs used in appetizers. There are deviled eggs, plain hard-boiled eggs, pickled eggs, sweet and sour eggs, caviar eggs, curried eggs, and about 10,000 more eggs that I don't have room to write about.

As I've said before, get out of the house (which is exercise in itself), go to the library, and read some books about appetizers. Use your imagination, make all you want, and enjoy them.

MUSHROOMS STUFFED WITH CRABMEAT

Since becoming a chef, I have eaten way too many of these small tidbits of ecstasy, my very favorite appetizer.

1 lb.	Crabmeat, thawed if frozen
1 cup	Soy Mayonnaise
1/2 tsp.	Dry Mustard
2 Tbsp.	Brandy
2 oz.	Fresh Tangerine or Orange Juice
1/2 cup	Crushed Macadamia Nuts, or whatever nuts you like
	Salt Substitute to taste
1/8 tsp.	Ground White Pepper
1/4	Whole Pimento, chopped fine (use only if you have no trouble eating them, since they're a member of the nightshade family)
1 tsp.	Pimento Juice, optional
2 lbs.	Medium Button Mushrooms, stems removed
1 lb.	Cheddar Cheese, health food kind, ground

Method of Preparation
Mix together all ingredients, except mushrooms and cheese. In a large dish or sheet pan, place all the mushrooms, stem side up. Put an equal amount of stuffing in each cap, and cover with cheese. Bake in a preheated 350°F oven for 12-15 minutes, or until hot.

Yield
Serves 4-6 persons as an appetizer.

Hint
This is excellent with some toasted garlic bread.

Cooking Method
Bake

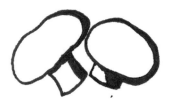

Nutritional Analysis

Per Serving
Energy	656 calories
Protein	36.7 gm
Fat	51.6 gm
Carbohydrate	11.6 gm
Fiber	2.2 gm
Cholesterol	59 mg
Iron	3.1 mg
Sodium	110 mg
Calcium	366 mg
Sugar	0.7 gm

Recipe Cost: $14.62

Health Tip
Exercise the best you can, even if it's just a little. Exercise, exercise, exercise!

Diet Tip
Fasting appears to reduce disease activity in rheumatoid arthritis. Fasting induces rapid changes in the endocrine and central nervous systems and in the lipids and proteins. Some people suggest that fasting can moderate the sensation of pain and related phenomena. But fast sensibly —consult your doctor.

Nutritional Analysis

Per Serving

Energy	*219 calories*
Protein	*6 gm*
Fat	*5.9 gm*
Carbohydrate	*33.4 gm*
Fiber	*1.4 gm*
Cholesterol	*2 mg*
Iron	*1.3 mg*
Sodium	*397 mg*
Calcium	*55 mg*
Sugar	*0.3 gm*

Recipe Cost: $2.43

Diet Tip
Food is best eaten the way the Almighty manufactures it for us. Many refined products we eat aren't good for us.

Diet Tip
We should be eating lots of fruits and vegetables and whole grain-based foods rich in fiber, vitamins, and minerals and low in calories. Four-ounce portions of well trimmed meat (or no meat), skinless poultry, or fish a day, and low-fat and nonfat dairy foods, are a healthy addition to the diet.

Chapter 14 Appetizers 183

GARLIC BREAD

Garlic bread is such a versatile item. Who doesn't like to dip this in a nice hot bowl of soup?

1	**Loaf French Bread**
	Olive Oil
	Chopped Garlic
	Soy Parmesan Cheese

Method of Preparation
Cut the loaf of French bread on the bias about 3/4 inch thick. Sprinkle each piece with a little bit of olive oil, some chopped garlic, and some soy parmesan cheese. How much you use depends on your taste, so we didn't suggest any quantities.

Preheat your broiler at the broil setting. Put the bread on a broiler pan and place on the second shelf down. It will get nice and toasty, with the cheese melting and browning just like it's supposed to. Yummy, yummy, yummy!

Yield
Serves 4-6

Hint
If you enjoy more garlic flavor, sauté your garlic in olive oil for a few minutes first, then follow the recipe.

Cooking Methods
Sauté, broil

CITRUS SALSA

Here in Hawaii we do a lot with fruit and fish. Simply broil a piece of fish and put half of a cup of this salsa on top. Another tastebud exploder!

2/3 cup	Orange Sections
1/4 cup	Lemon Sections
1/4 cup	Lime Sections
1 Tbsp.	Fresh Chopped Cilantro
	Jalapeno Peppers (Use only if you have no trouble eating them since they are a member of the nightshade family.)

Method of Preparation
In a bowl, toss all ingredients well.

Yield
Approximately 1-1/4 cup or 5 servings

Hint
Adding jalapeno peppers makes this a hot salsa recipe. Use whatever amount you want.

Nutritional Analysis

Per Serving
Energy	19 calories
Protein	0.5 gm
Fat	0.1 gm
Carbohydrate	5.5 gm
Fiber	1.2 gm
Cholesterol	0 mg
Iron	0.2 mg
Sodium	1 mg
Calcium	19 mg
Sugar	2.5 gm

Recipe Cost: $0.63

Diet Tip
Avoid overeating. Don't overeat just because there's too much food on your plate.

Lifestyle Tips
Medical science has taught us that the healthiest and happiest people are actively involved with life. Engage in as many productive activities as you can. Seek and enjoy the company of other interesting people with whom you enjoy spending time. Don't let your age or arthritis discourage you from being active and socializing.

Chapter 14 Appetizers 185

Nutritional Analysis

Per Serving
Energy	*25 calories*
Protein	*0.5gm*
Fat	*0.2 gm*
Carbohydrate	*6.5 gm*
Fiber	*1.3 gm*
Cholesterol	*0 mg*
Iron	*0.3 mg*
Sodium	*3 mg*
Calcium	*17 mg*
Sugar	*4.3 gm*

Recipe Cost: $1.43 (approximate, depending on fruits and season)

Lifestyle Tip
If you have trouble turning pages, get a rubber finger tip from an office supply store.

Health Tip
A free radical is a single oxygen molecule that has become excited by picking up an electron. The excited oxygen can damage tissues in the same way that oxygen makes iron rust. Scientists are looking to free radicals as the factors causing degenerative diseases and aging.

FRUIT SALSA WITH RED ONION

This makes such a flavorful salsa that I often see my fellow employees eating it by the spoonful all by itself.

1/2 cup	Orange Sections
1/2 cup	Lime Sections
1/2 cup	Red Onion, diced small
1/4 cup	Fresh Chopped Cilantro
	Jalapeno Peppers

Choose three of the following:

1/2 cup	Pineapple, diced bite size
1/2 cup	Papaya, diced bite size
1/2 cup	Peaches, diced bite size
1/2 cup	Mango, diced bite size
1/2 cup	Cantaloupe, diced bite size
1/2 cup	Seedless Red Grapes, cut in half
1/2 cup	California Green Seedless Grapes, cut in half
1/2 cup	Honeydew Melon, diced bite size

Method of Preparation
Mix all ingredients well. Use whatever combination you prefer that is in season.

Yield
Approximately 3+ cups, or 8 servings

GUACAMOLE

In this recipe we won't use any jalapeno peppers or hot sauce because these products are in the forbidden nightshade family. If you are able to tolerate them, go ahead and enjoy yourself!

2	Fresh Avocados, flesh only
1/2	Small Red Onion, minced and mashed
1 Tbsp.	Fresh Lime Juice
1/2 tsp.	Garlic Paste
1 tsp.	Honey

Method of Preparation
Combine all ingredients in a glass bowl and mash them well so you have a relatively smooth paste. Serve the guacamole after one hour of refrigeration.

Yield
About one pound, or 8 servings

Hints
This is a great dip for vegetables, some good crackers from the health food store, or whatever you enjoy dipping.

Nutritional Analysis

Per Serving

Energy	88 calories
Protein	1.1 gm
Fat	7.7 gm
Carbohydrate	5.4 gm
Fiber	1.2 gm
Cholesterol	0 mg
Iron	0.5 mg
Sodium	6 mg
Calcium	8 mg
Sugar	1.7 gm

Recipe Cost: $0.88

Diet Tip
Salmon oil or fish oil is a very good anti-inflammatory. Look for a standardized brand. Take 3 to 6 grams a day in a divided dosage with meals to be effective.

Diet Tip
Carotenoids provide most of their benefits by protecting body cells from free radicals. The recommended intake of fruits and vegetables is a minimum of five servings per day. Only about one person in ten consumes five servings of fruits and vegetables per day.

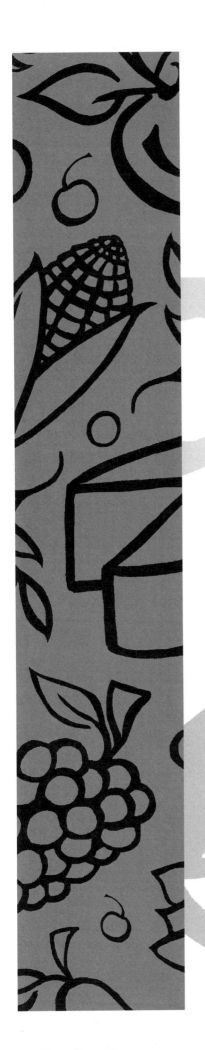

CHAPTER 15

SOUPS

Lifestyle Tip
When possible, use long-handled mops, brooms, and dusters to help reduce strain on your joints.

SOUPS

The French word *soupe* was once used to describe the various ingredients put into bouillon or broth made of meat or fish. How times have changed—now we can put just about anything grown into any liquid and call it soup. There are now so many combinations and flavors out there that I just want to burst with pride for being a chef.

On a cold, gray, blustery day, is there anything better than a bowl of some kind of good, tasty, steaming hot soup? If there is, let me know.

Soups fall into three different classifications: clear, thick, and specialty. All three are included in this section.

America is known for its chowders, gumbos, oyster stews, and the Philadelphia pepper pot, just to name a few. These are the specialty soups.

Here in America we also enjoy topping soups. We use fresh herbs, toasted nuts, toasted coconut, croutons, cheese, bacon bits, egg whites, and yolks, just to name a few.

Once again, go to the library and read, or join a community college cooking class. You'll be surprised to see people of all ages who are learning how to cook. Learn, learn, learn! And enjoy making all of these soups!!

CHILLED YOGURT SOUP WITH FRUITS

This is a great summertime soup. It's cool, refreshing, and healthy for you. My mouth started to water when I wrote down this recipe.

1 pt.	Plain Yogurt
2	Fresh Bananas, ripe, peeled, and sliced
2	Fresh Peaches, ripe, peeled, and sliced
1-1/2 pt.	Apple Juice
	Juice from 1 Fresh Orange or Tangerine
2 Tbsp.	Honey
1/2 tsp.	Ground Nutmeg
1/8 tsp.	Ground Allspice

Method of Preparation
In your blender, puree all of the ingredients until they are smooth. If necessary, you can do this in 3 or 4 batches, adding each to a large bowl. Chill the mixture for 2 hours in the refrigerator.

Garnish with a thin slice of peach. Lay it in the middle of the soup with a sprig of fresh mint on top.

Yield
About 8 servings at one cup each (2+ quarts)

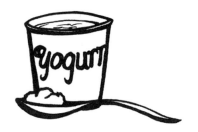

Nutritional Analysis

Per Serving
Energy	122 calories
Protein	3.4 gm
Fat	1.1 gm
Carbohydrate	25.8 gm
Fiber	1 gm
Cholesterol	3 mg
Iron	0.5 mg
Sodium	43 mg
Calcium	114 mg
Sugar	21.1 gm

Recipe Cost: $3.21

Diet Tip
Apples contain 84% pure water, carbohydrates, proteins, minerals, and vitamins A, B, and C. They are also high in iron, potassium, and many other nutrients.

Diet Tip
Quercetin has remarkable anti-inflammatory properties. Red and yellow onions are an excellent source of quercetin.

Nutritional Analysis

Per Serving
Energy	*152 calories*
Protein	*8.4 gm*
Fat	*4.5 gm*
Carbohydrate	*19.8 gm*
Fiber	*4.5 gm*
Cholesterol	*16 mg*
Iron	*1.2 mg*
Sodium	*75 mg*
Calcium	*17 mg*
Sugar	*1.2 gm*

Recipe Cost: $5.53

Diet Tip
Avoid eating iceberg or head lettuce. It's almost worthless nutritionally. There is 100 times more iron and potassium in leaf lettuce than in head lettuce.

Diet Tip
Things that are absorbed through the gut that shouldn't be (leaky gut syndrome) can cause allergic responses or inflammation of joints. Foods high in lectins, such as the nightshade family, milk, and grains, can contribute to increased gut permeability.

CREAM OF BROCCOLI SOUP

Soup is a favorite all over the world. This one is probably one of the real favorites, and its great hot or cold.

2 lbs.	Broccoli Stems, chopped small
8 oz.	Onion, diced small
4 oz.	Celery, diced small
4 oz.	Leeks, diced small
4 oz.	Butter, health food kind
3 qts.	Chicken Velouté, hot (see page 168)
1 qt.	Heavy Cream, health food kind, scalded
	Broccoli Florets from the 2 lbs. of broccoli stems, boiled and shocked in cold water
	Salt Substitute to taste
1/2 tsp.	Ground White Pepper

Method of Preparation
Sweat the broccoli stems, onions, celery, and leeks in the butter for about 5-6 minutes, then add one quart of the veloute and simmer over low heat for 30-35 minutes.

Now mash all the cooked ingredients very well with a potato masher. Add the rest of the veloute and continue cooking for 30 minutes. Add the scalded cream and stir well. Strain through a fine strainer or through a cheesecloth, returning the liquid to your pot. Add the florets, salt substitute, and white pepper. Stir well and serve.

Yield
Approximately one gallon

Cooking Method
Simmer

CREAM OF CRAB CURRY SOUP

Here's a treat for lovers of crabmeat and curry. This is also a great soup when chilled for a hot summer's day.

3/4 cup	Butter, health food kind
2 tsp.	Curry Powder
3-4 Tbsp.	Brown Rice Flour
9 cups	Milk or Half and Half, health food kind (equal to 2 quarts + 1 cup)
1	Celery Stalk, peeled and grated
1	Medium Onion, grated
1 lb.	Crabmeat
1/4 cup	Parsley, chopped

Method of Preparation
In a soup pot, melt the butter, then add the curry powder and stir for a few minutes. Add the flour and simmer over low heat for a few minutes more, taking care that the flour doesn't brown. Slowly add the milk until incorporated. Add the celery and onion and continue simmering for 1/2 hour.

Add the crabmeat and cook 40-50 more minutes. When the soup is done, add the parsley.

Yield
Serves 10-12

Hint
Add half a pound of fresh mushrooms if you like mushroom and crab together. Just sauté the mushrooms in 2 Tbsp. butter (health food kind), over very low heat for 8-10 minutes, and add to the finished soup. Stir well.

Cooking Method
Simmer

Nutritional Analysis

Per Serving	
Energy	157 calories
Protein	12.4 gm
Fat	9.4 gm
Carbohydrate	6.6 gm
Fiber	2.5 gm
Cholesterol	16 mg
Iron	1.5 mg
Sodium	481 mg
Calcium	35 mg
Sugar	0.8 gm

Recipe Cost: $11.47

Diet Tip
Berries are high in fiber, potassium, and vitamin C.

Diet Tip
Weight management is a must to help control the pain of arthritic joints. Ideally, each meal should be nutritious and balanced with approximately 30% protein, 40% carbohydrate, and 30% fat. A balanced meal will result in better hunger management, improved energy levels, improved health, and weight loss.

Nutritional Analysis

Per Serving
Energy	306 calories
Protein	2.9 gm
Fat	26.7 gm
Carbohydrate	14.5 gm
Fiber	1.4 gm
Cholesterol	66 mg
Iron	0.6 mg
Sodium	51 mg
Calcium	127 mg
Sugar	6.9 gm

Recipe Cost: $4.37

Diet Tip
The cure for ignorance is knowledge. Read all you can about your disease, including what foods cause an arthritis flare-up.

Health Tip
Exercise is essential to good health and vitality. People who exercise regularly live longer, have less chronic disease, and have a better quality of life. Everyone has a different capacity for exercise, depending on age and current health status. However, everyone can do some form of exercise. Regular moderate physical exercise strengthens the heart, reduces body fat, and boosts the immune system that helps to control the symptoms of inflammation.

AVOCADO SOUP

Cold avocado soup is a great refresher on a hot summer day.

2	Avocados, ripe, skin and seed removed
1	Medium Onion, sliced
1 pt.	Heavy Cream, health food kind
1 pt.	Rice Milk
1/4 cup	Sherry
	Tabasco Sauce to taste (if you can eat nightshade foods)
1 cup	Chicken Stock (see Chapter 12)
	Salt Substitute to taste
2 oz.	Fresh Orange Juice

Method of Preparation
In a blender, blend the avocado and onion until smooth. Add the rest of the ingredients and blend for a couple of minutes. Chill.

Yield
Serves 6-8

Hint
Add some honey if you want a little sweetness.

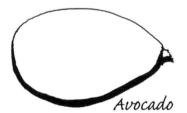
Avocado

BROCCOLI SOUP WITH DICED CHICKEN

This is a great fall and wintertime soup. It is very healthy and can be enjoyed often.

6 cups	Chicken Stock (see Chapter 12)
2 cups	Water
1 lb.	Broccoli, separated into florets and stems, chopped small
1 cup	Onions, diced small
1 Tbsp.	Soy Margarine
3 cups	Cooked Chicken, diced bite size
	Salt Substitute to taste
	White Pepper to taste
	Croutons (see Chapter 16)

Method of Preparation
In a soup pot, heat the chicken broth, water, and broccoli stems till they boil, then turn the heat down and simmer for 1 hour. This will give the broth a good broccoli flavor.

Sauté the onion in the margarine until transparent.

Strain the broth, then add broccoli florets, onion, and diced chicken, cooking over a slow fire until the florets are tender. Season to taste. Serve with croutons on top.

Yield
6-8 servings

Hint
The benefits of parsley are many. You can add 1/2 cup finely chopped parsley to this wonderful soup if you enjoy it as I do.

Cooking Methods
Boil, sauté, simmer

Nutritional Analysis

Per Serving	
Energy	175 calories
Protein	18.4 gm
Fat	6.7 gm
Carbohydrate	10 gm
Fiber	2.2 gm
Cholesterol	47 mg
Iron	1.2 mg
Sodium	178 mg
Calcium	50 mg
Sugar	1.3 gm

Recipe Cost: $3.37

Diet Tip
Meal frequency is important for weight loss. The body is designed to have a meal approximately every four hours. After four hours, the body begins to store fat to protect itself from what it perceives as starvation.

Chapter 15 Soups 195

Nutritional Analysis

Per Serving
Energy	*396 calories*
Protein	*29.5 gm*
Fat	*22.3 gm*
Carbohydrate	*18.8 gm*
Fiber	*2.5 gm*
Cholesterol	*166 mg*
Iron	*2.2 mg*
Sodium	*124 mg*
Calcium	*33 mg*
Sugar	*3 gm*

Recipe Cost: $5.72

Lifestyle Tip
Store out of season clothes in boxes under your bed. It saves trips to the attic and cellar.

Diet Tip
When you eat a lot of starchy foods such as pasta, rice, potato chips, crackers, pastries, and bread, you are setting yourself up to crave more of the same. These foods cause an elevation of insulin that causes a drop in glucose, resulting in increased hunger for more fattening foods.

CHICKEN CORN SOUP WITH NOODLES

When I was a student at Pennsylvania State University, I worked at a great Pennsylvania Dutch restaurant called The Skillington Restaurant, in Skillington, Pennsylvania. This is my adaptation of their recipe.

1	Stewing Chicken (about 3-4 lbs.), disjointed
2	Celery Stalks, cut bite size
1	Medium Onion, cut bite size
	Salt Substitute to taste
3 qts.	Ice Cold Water
1/4 tsp.	Saffron Strands
3 cups	Corn Kernels
3 cups	Noodles, cooked
1/8 tsp.	White Pepper
1/4 cup	Chopped Parsley
3	Hard-Boiled Eggs, chopped

Method of Preparation
Place the chicken and the next five ingredients on the list in a sauce pot or soup pot. Bring to a boil, cook 15 minutes, and remove the white scum. Turn down the heat and simmer until chicken is done, about 45 minutes more.

Remove chicken from the pot, cool, and remove the meat from the bones. Turn the heat back on and return the meat to the pot. Bring to a boil, add the rest of the ingredients from the corn on down, and serve.

Yield
Serves 10-12

Hint
Wouldn't some garlic bread taste great with this?

Cooking Methods
Boil, simmer

196 The Executive Chef's Arthritis Cookbook and Health Guide

CHICKEN NOODLE SOUP

This is a recipe from my great-grandmother, passed down through the family. My mom sent it to me as a Christmas gift, and it turned out to be the best present I have ever eaten.

1	Stewing Chicken (about 4-1/2 lbs.), disjointed
4 qts.	Ice Cold Water
1	Medium Onion, sliced
1	Large Carrot, sliced 1/2" thick
2	Celery Stalks with leaves, sliced 1/2" thick
2	Bay Leaves
1/2 tsp.	Thyme Leaf
1/2 tsp.	Whole Black Peppercorns
3	Parsley Stems
3 cups	Cooked Noodles
1/4 cup	Chopped Parsley

Method of Preparation
In a large soup pot, place all the ingredients except the noodles and the parsley. Cover, bring to a boil, cook 15 minutes, then skim the scum. Turn down the heat and simmer about 1-1/2 hours more, or until the chicken is tender and broth has a good chicken flavor.

Strain the broth and reserve. Let the chicken cool, and remove the meat from the bones. Cut it bite size.

Put the broth back into the pot, return to a boil, then turn down to a simmer. Add the meat, cooked noodles, and chopped parsley.

Yield
Serves 10-12

Cooking Methods
Boil, simmer

Nutritional Analysis

Per Serving

Energy	434 calories
Protein	34.1 gm
Fat	26.3 gm
Carbohydrate	13.4 gm
Fiber	1.8 gm
Cholesterol	141 mg
Iron	2.8 mg
Sodium	133 mg
Calcium	42 mg
Sugar	1.4 gm

Recipe Cost: $4.31

Diet Tip
Fill your salt shaker with the salt substitute in this book (Chapter 4).

Lifestyle Tip
Meal preparation can be made easier by planning rest breaks during meal preparation time. Use good posture to avoid fatigue or strain while performing kitchen tasks. Arrange your kitchen for maximum convenience. Buy presliced or chopped vegetables and use labor-saving kitchen gadgets and appliances to make cooking tasks easier.

Chapter 15 Soups 197

Nutritional Analysis

Per Serving
Energy   *270 calories*
Protein   *33.9 gm*
Fat   *8 gm*
Carbohydrate   *12.7 gm*
Fiber   *1.4 gm*
Cholesterol   *117 mg*
Iron   *5.3 mg*
Sodium   *268 mg*
Calcium   *91 mg*
Sugar   *3.1 gm*

Recipe Cost: $21.60

Health Tip
Watch out for sodium in over-the-counter medications. Some antacids contain more than 25% of the daily recommended amount of sodium in each dose.

Health Tip
Basic communication, relaxation, emotional management, and mind-body skills can prevent a great deal of unnecessary suffering associated with arthritis.

HAWAIIAN STYLE SEAFOOD CHOWDER

Get four of your best friends together with five quart jars, and everyone goes home with soup. Keep one for yourself.

3 qts.	Fish Velouté, heavily thickened
4 oz.	Soy Margarine
1 cup	Carrots, diced small
1 cup	Celery, diced small
2 cups	Onions, diced small
2 cups	Clam Juice
3 oz.	Fresh Lemon Juice
1/4 cup	Fresh Chopped Parsley
	Salt Substitute to taste
1/2 tsp.	Ground White Pepper
2 cups	Non-Dairy Soy Milk, heated
4	Large Potatoes, diced bite size, skin left on
2 lbs.	Mahi Mahi, or whatever white fish you have, cut bite size
1 lb.	Medium Scallops, cut in half
1 lb.	21-25 Shrimp, cut in half the long way
1 lb.	Chopped Clams, fresh if possible, but rinsed canned ones will work fine

Method of Preparation
Prepare the fish velouté, following roux recipe in Chapter 8. Set aside.

In a 2-gallon soup pot, melt the soy margarine over low heat, then add the carrots, celery, onions, and a lid and cook for 5 minutes. Add the fish velouté and clam juice and bring to a boil, then turn down to a simmer and cook till veggies are just about tender.

Add the lemon juice, parsley, salt substitute, white pepper and milk. Return to a boil and add the potatoes; cook over medium heat for 10 minutes.

Turn off the heat, add all the fish products, and stir well. The fish products are cut small enough that the heat from the soup will sufficiently and safely cook them.

This is a thick and creamy soup. Cool it properly, and split it up among the other cooks.

Yield
5+ quarts

Cooking Methods
Sauté, boil, simmer

CHICKEN BARLEY SOUP

Barley was probably the first cereal cultivated by man. Cooked barley has a mild flavor and a chewy texture. It is very good steamed, buttered, or in soups and casseroles.

3 oz.	Soy Margarine
1 cup	Onion, diced small
1 cup	Carrots, diced small
2 cups	Barley
8 cups	Chicken Stock
2 cups	Cooked Chicken, cut bite size
	Salt Substitute to taste
1/4 tsp.	White Pepper
1/4 cup	Chopped Parsley

Method of Preparation
Melt the soy margarine in a soup pot, add the veggies, and cook for a few minutes. Add the barley and stir until coated. Now add the chicken stock, bring to a good rapid boil, and stir well.

Turn down to a simmer and cook about 25-30 minutes, or until the barley is soft. Add the chicken, salt substitute, pepper, and parsley. Stir well and serve.

Yield
Serves 8-10

Cooking Methods
Sauté, boil, simmer

Nutritional Analysis

Per Serving

Energy	*243 calories*
Protein	*13.5 gm*
Fat	*7.2 gm*
Carbohydrate	*31.6 gm*
Fiber	*7.2 gm*
Cholesterol	*25 mg*
Iron	*1.9 mg*
Sodium	*120 mg*
Calcium	*27 mg*
Sugar	*2 gm*

Recipe Cost: $3.33

Diet Tip
Never keep spices close to the stovetop; they'll lose their color and flavor.

Diet Tip
Good nutrition is essential for optimal wellness. Healthy cells make a healthy body, and high quality nutrients help maintain healthy cells. Eat foods that protect you. Fresh fruits and vegetables (broccoli, cabbage, brussels sprouts, and cauliflower) are loaded with phytochemicals that help to protect the joints from the damaging effects of free radicals.

Nutritional Analysis

Per Serving
Energy   *264 calories*
Protein   *11.6 gm*
Fat   *16.3 gm*
Carbohydrate   *18 gm*
Fiber   *2.4 gm*
Cholesterol   *26 mg*
Iron   *0.7 mg*
Sodium   *253 mg*
Calcium   *309 mg*
Sugar   *7 gm*

Recipe Cost: $4.11

Diet Tip
Grow fresh herbs on your window sill.

Diet Tip
Pay attention to trans-fatty acids (french fries, peanut butter, margarine, etc.) and saturated fats (animal fat) because both elevate LDL (bad cholesterol) that contributes to development of coronary heart disease. Your combined intake of saturated fat and trans-fatty acids should be 10% of total calories. These bad fats may be a factor in increased inflammation and joint destruction.

ONION SOUP WITH CHEESE AND CROUTONS

Here is a true classic. Onion soup is healthy, hearty, and flavorful. Great for a cold, or on a cold day.

4	Large Onions, sliced 1/4" thick
4 oz.	Soy Margarine
1 Tbsp.	Chopped Garlic
1 Tbsp.	Soy Flour (approximately)
3 qts.	Chicken Stock, hot (see recipe in Chapter 12)
1 pinch	Thyme Leaf
2	Bay Leaves
2	Parsley Stalks
1/2 tsp.	Salt Substitute
1/4 tsp.	Ground Black Pepper
	Croutons
	Grated Swiss Cheese

Method of Preparation
Preheat the oven to 350°F. In a 4-quart saucepan or soup pot, place the onions, margarine, and garlic. Cover and place in the oven for 45 minutes, stirring occasionally. Cook till onions are golden brown, then add the flour, enough to soak up any remaining margarine.

Now add the stock, herbs, and spices, and return to oven for one hour. Stir once in a while.

To serve, fill a soup crock with hot soup, top it with a handful of croutons and then some cheese, and place under broiler till cheese melts.

Yield
Makes about eight 10-oz. crocks

Hint
This is a great recipe for an appetizer or a full meal.

Cooking Methods
Simmer, bake, broil

200 The Executive Chef's Arthritis Cookbook and Health Guide

SPLIT PEA SOUP WITH CHICKEN:
GREEN OR YELLOW SPLIT PEAS

Since we aren't eating ham or bacon, we'll use chicken in our soup.

2 cups	Dried Split Peas, green or yellow
2 oz.	Butter, health food kind
1 cup	Onion, diced small
2 qts.	Chicken Stock (see recipe in Chapter 12)
1 tsp.	Salt Substitute
1/2 tsp.	Fresh Ground Black Pepper
2 cups	Cooked Chicken, cut bite size

Method of Preparation
Soak the peas overnight in enough water to cover.

In a soup pot, melt the butter, add the onions and sauté over low heat until they are transparent. Add the peas with their water, chicken stock, and seasonings.

Simmer for one hour and 15 minutes, or until peas are mushy. Add the chicken meat and cook ten more minutes. Stir frequently while this is cooking. Garnish with croutons (recipe in Chapter 16).

Yield
8-10 cups

Cooking Methods
Sauté, simmer

Nutritional Analysis

Per Serving

Energy	231 calories
Protein	8.4 gm
Fat	5.7 gm
Carbohydrate	26.9 gm
Fiber	2.5 gm
Cholesterol	25 mg
Iron	2.1 mg
Sodium	89 mg
Calcium	31 mg
Sugar	4.2 gm

Recipe Cost: $3.09

Diet Tip
Fresh herbs can be chopped and frozen for future use in cooked dishes.

Health Tip
The benefits of healthful eating and physical activity are so intertwined that they deserve equal consideration. Exercise 30 minutes a day for health, 45 minutes daily for weight maintenance.

Chapter 15 Soups 201

Nutritional Analysis

Per Serving
Energy	*115 calories*
Protein	*2.5 gm*
Fat	*6.1 gm*
Carbohydrate	*13.7 gm*
Fiber	*1.5 gm*
Cholesterol	*0 mg*
Iron	*0.9 mg*
Sodium	*133 mg*
Calcium	*70 mg*
Sugar	*2.8 gm*

Recipe Cost: $4.81

Lifestyle Tip
Turntables, also known as lazy Susans, make a variety of items easier to reach.

Health Tip
Osteoporosis begins in youth and can occur in people of all genders, races, and ethnic backgrounds. White, post-menopausal women have the highest incidence of osteoporotic fractures. Individuals with the highest peak bone mass after adolescence have the greatest protective advantage when the declines in bone density associated with increasing age, illnesses, and hormonal changes take their toll.

CREAM OF MUSHROOM SOUP

Mushroom soup is a favorite soup all over the globe. Enjoy this easy, basic recipe.

1 lb.	Fresh Mushrooms, sliced 1/8" thick
2	Bay Leaves
1/2 cup	Onion, finely chopped
2 qts.	Chicken Stock (see recipe in Chapter 12)
4 oz.	Butter, health food variety
2 oz.	Whole Wheat Flour
2 cups	Rice Milk
	Salt Substitute to taste
1/2 tsp.	Coarse Ground Black Pepper

Method of Preparation
In a soup pot, place mushrooms, bay leaves, onion, and 2 cups of chicken stock. Cover with a lid and cook over low heat for 20 minutes.

In another pot, place the butter and flour. Cook them over low heat, stirring well for 4-5 minutes. Add the remaining chicken stock slowly, stirring constantly.

Add the rice milk and heat till hot. Now add the very flavorful mushrooms, bay leaves, onions, and liquid from the first pot. Stir well, and cook over low heat for 10 more minutes.

Season with salt substitute and black pepper.

Yield
8-10 servings

Hint
Put a few croutons on top, using crouton recipe in Chapter 16.

Cooking Method
Simmer

202 The Executive Chef's Arthritis Cookbook and Health Guide

VEGETABLE SOUP WITH CHICKEN BROTH

Is there anyone out there who doesn't enjoy a serving of good, hot vegetable soup?

4 oz.	Soy Margarine
2 tsp.	Chopped Garlic
8 oz.	Turnips, diced medium
8 oz.	Carrots, diced medium
1	Medium Onion, diced medium
8 oz.	Celery, diced medium
3 qts.	Chicken Stock (see recipe in Chapter 12)
3	Bay Leaves
8 oz.	Cabbage, cut bite-size
10 oz.	Frozen Peas
12 oz.	Canned Corn, drained
2	Medium Potatoes, cut bite size, optional (remember about the nightshade family)
2	Medium Tomatoes, chopped small (optional: nightshade)
1/4 cup	Chopped Parsley

Method of Preparation

In a soup pot, place the margarine, garlic, turnips, carrots, onions, and celery over medium heat. Cover the pot with a lid and sweat until an aroma is apparent (about 5-7 minutes).

Add the chicken stock and bay leaves. Bring liquid to a boil, then turn the heat down to a simmer and cook for 10 minutes.

Now add the cabbage, peas, corn, potatoes, and tomatoes. Simmer till all vegetables are tender. Add parsley and stir. Season with salt substitute if necessary

Yield

Over one gallon, or ten to twelve 14-ounce portions

Hint

This recipe also works great if you replace the chicken stock with fish stock. You can also add chicken or fish pieces if you want meat in the soup. Either way, make them bite size and simmer till tender.

Cooking Method

Boil, simmer

Nutritional Analysis

Per Serving

Energy	*145 calories*
Protein	*4.1 gm*
Fat	*5.4 gm*
Carbohydrate	*22.1 gm*
Fiber	*4 gm*
Cholesterol	*0 mg*
Iron	*1.4 mg*
Sodium	*167 mg*
Calcium	*47 mg*
Sugar	*5.4 gm*

Recipe Cost: $5.67

Lifestyle Tip

Wearing rubber gloves makes it easier for weak hands to grasp objects and protect hands from cleaning chemicals.

Diet Tip

Avoid refined and processed foods—which strip natural food of their fiber, vitamins and minerals.

SWEET POTATO SOUP

A great, unique-tasting soup, hot or cold.

2	Large Sweet Potatoes (about 1 lb.)
1 qt.	Chicken Stock (see recipe in Chapter 12)
1 cup	Heavy Cream, from health food store
	Salt Substitute to taste
	Coarse Ground Black Pepper to taste
1 cup	Grated Swiss Cheese, from health food store

Method of Preparation

Preheat oven till it reaches 350°F. Wash and dry the sweet potatoes. Bake potatoes on a small sheet pan for 1 to 1-1/2 hours, or until very soft.

When the potatoes are cool enough to handle, peel the skin off. Place potatoes in a soup pot and mash very well.

Add the chicken stock and cream, and simmer over medium heat for 20 minutes. Add the salt substitute and pepper to taste.

Just before serving, whisk the grated cheese into the hot soup until it melts. Don't cook the soup too long after you've added the cheese or it will become stringy.

Yield
Serves 4-6

Cooking Methods
Bake, simmer

Nutritional Analysis

Per Serving
Energy	351 calories
Protein	13.2 gm
Fat	23.5 gm
Carbohydrate	22.1 gm
Fiber	2.3 gm
Cholesterol	79 mg
Iron	0.4 mg
Sodium	35 mg
Calcium	412 mg
Sugar	9.9 gm

Recipe Cost: $4.98

Lifestyle Tip

If you enjoy playing cards but have a hard time shuffling, get a battery powered card shuffler.

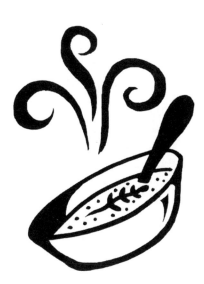

204

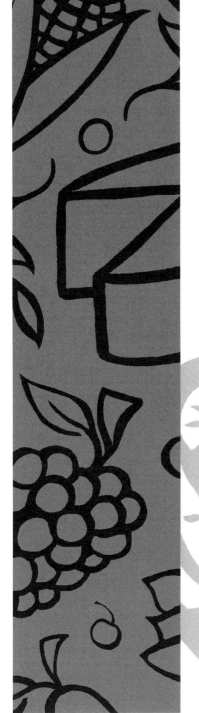

SALADS & DRESSINGS

CHAPTER 16

206

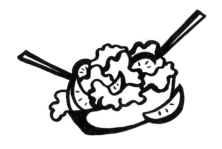

SALADS AND SALAD DRESSINGS

In today's world we need to give thanks to the Pennsylvania Dutch, who are primarily responsible for the many traditional salads that we Americans enjoy today. Salads in America are classified into three main categories: main-dish salads, side-dish salads, and fruit salads. This cookbook includes some of each.

People on the West Coast make salads out of just about anything. They range from a simply dressed green salad to an elaborate salad dish that could contain meats, poultry, seafood, or fruits. They have been very innovative in recent years. The many preparations, styles, and variations have led to what's been called the California Cuisine. Thank God the chefs of the world will always be experimenting with foods. This cuisine is proof of all the hard work that goes into the many new and wonderful recipes of today. Thank you, chefs.

LETTUCE

Here is a list of some of the many kinds of lettuce available to you:

Treviso radicchio, tango, tat-soi, red perella, watercress, Nagoya red kale, Nagoya white kale, chervil, mustard greens, red romaine, green romaine, mizuna, arugula, red chard, green chard, white flowering kale, red flowering kale, red oak, green oak, red Asian mustard, lollo rosso, sorrel, escarole, dandelion greens, Belgian endive, radicchio, spinach, red beet tops, red Russian kale, mache

Lettuces have many different uses and many different flavors. You can learn more about them at your local library.

208 The Executive Chef's Arthritis Cookbook and Health Guide

SPINACH, TURKEY BACON, AND MUSHROOM SALAD

A wonderful alternative: plenty of taste without all the sodium. Very healthy for you.

1/2 lb.	Young Spinach, fresh
16	Turkey Bacon Strips
8	Medium Mushrooms, fresh
1 oz.	Olive Oil
2 Tbsp.	Lemon Juice
	Salt Substitute to taste
	Fresh Ground Black Pepper to taste

Method of Preparation

Wash spinach leaves thoroughly in cold water, remove any tough stems, and shake dry in a towel.

Fry bacon till it's crisp. Drain on a paper towel and crumble.

Slice mushrooms thinly. Tear spinach leaves into bite-size pieces.

In a bowl, toss spinach, bacon, and mushrooms; add oil and lemon juice. Season with salt substitute and fresh ground black pepper.

Yield

Serves four—immediately!

Hint

Add 2 chopped hardboiled eggs and 1/2 tsp. of fresh chopped garlic (for all you garlic lovers). Now you have another healthy variation of this recipe.

Nutritional Analysis

Per Serving

Energy	*120 calories*
Protein	*7.9 gm*
Fat	*8.6 gm*
Carbohydrate	*4.6 gm*
Fiber	*2.7 gm*
Cholesterol	*19 mg*
Iron	*2.4 mg*
Sodium	*332 mg*
Calcium	*61 mg*
Sugar	*0.4 gm*

Recipe Cost: $5.25

Diet Tip

Omit white flour from your diet. Instead use whole wheat, rye, corn, oat, or whole wheat pastry flour.

Diet Tip

Water helps the body get rid of wastes and toxins, tones up the circulation, and enhances the body's immune system, while many beverages such as coffee, tea, and alcohol do just the opposite.

Chapter 16 Salads & Dressings 209

Nutritional Analysis

Per Serving
Energy	*200 calories*
Protein	*2.5 gm*
Fat	*220.4 gm*
Carbohydrate	*11 gm*
Fiber	*0.4 gm*
Cholesterol	*70 mg*
Iron	*0.7 mg*
Sodium	*92 mg*
Calcium	*34 mg*
Sugar	*0.1 gm*

Recipe Cost: $0.96

Lifestyle Tip
Store your grains in a cool, dry place.

Nutritional Analysis

Per Serving
Energy	*89 calories*
Protein	*0.1 gm*
Fat	*8.2 gm*
Carbohydrate	*4.7 gm*
Fiber	*0 gm*
Cholesterol	*0 mg*
Iron	*0.2 mg*
Sodium	*21 mg*
Calcium	*4 mg*
Sugar	*3.2 gm*

Recipe Cost: $4.21

Lifestyle Tip
Buy a big lamp switch. They are easy to see, grip, and turn.

TANGERINE MAYONNAISE

This recipe goes very well with any hot or cold vegetable you enjoy. It also goes well with broiled, steamed, or baked fish. The old standard, tartar sauce, is just that: an old standard. Be adventurous! Try something new.

1 cup	**Soy Mayonnaise**
3 oz.	**Fresh Tangerine or Orange Juice**
1 tsp.	**Grated Tangerine Zest**
1 tsp.	**Chopped Shallots**
1/2 tsp.	**Dijon Mustard**

Method of Preparation
Mix all ingredients well in a small bowl.

Yield
Approximately one cup

Hint
For you garlic lovers out there, add 1 tsp. chopped garlic.

MUSTARD VINAIGRETTE

This is a great recipe to make with heated beet greens, mustard greens, wilted lettuce, etc. You get the idea. Just use enough to flavor the greens. Serve with the juices.

16 oz.	**Red Wine Vinegar**
8 oz.	**Olive Oil**
4 oz.	**Honey**
3 Tbsp.	**French's Mustard**
2 Tbsp.	**Chopped Garlic**
1 Tbsp.	**Chopped Shallots**
	Salt Substitute to taste
1 tsp.	**Coarse ground Black Pepper**

Method of Preparation
In a large pan, heat all the ingredients till they just start to boil. Stir well. Cool and refrigerate.

Temper (let warm to room temperature) 1/2 hour before using.

Yield
Approximately 3-1/2 cups.

Cooking Method
Boil

CROUTONS FOR YOUR SOUPS AND SALADS

Tasty, crunchy croutons really pep up your salad or soup!

2-3 oz.	Olive Oil
1 Tbsp.	Chopped Garlic
7 slices	Whole Wheat Bread, cut into bite size cubes
2 Tbsp.	Soy Parmesan Cheese
1 Tbsp.	Fresh Chopped Parsley

Method of Preparation
In a large skillet over medium high heat, place the olive oil and garlic and sauté for 1 minute. Add the bread and stir well so the oil soaks up into the bread. When the bread becomes golden brown, add the cheese and parsley, and cook 1 more minute.

Yield
Enough for 6-10 soups or salads, depending on how much you enjoy eating these delicious croutons.

Hint
These can be made in large batches and stored in an airtight container for 4-5 days. You can also mix everything well in a bowl then bake in a 350°F oven on a sheet pan or cookie tray till they are golden brown.

BLEU CHEESE DRESSING WITH FRESH BASIL

This is a new recipe I made since I have been experimenting with a great variety of health food products. Bleu cheese is the most nutritious of all the cheeses.

8 oz.	Soy Mayonnaise (unsalted)
4 oz.	Sour Cream (made from tofu or non-fat)
1 Tbsp.	Fresh Lemon Juice
1/8 tsp.	Coarse ground Black Pepper
2 Tbsp.	Fresh Chopped Basil
	Salt Substitute to taste
1 cup	Bleu Cheese (made from cultured milk)

Method of Preparation
In a large bowl, blend together the mayonnaise and sour cream until smooth. Add everything but the bleu cheese and mix well. Crumble in the bleu cheese and mix a little bit till blended.

Yield
Enough for 6-10 salads, depending on how much you enjoy.

Hint
Add 1 Tbsp. fresh tangerine juice for another unique taste.

Nutritional Analysis

Per Serving

Energy	99 calories
Protein	2.3 gm
Fat	6.5 gm
Carbohydrate	8.7 gm
Fiber	0.6 gm
Cholesterol	1 mg
Iron	0.5 mg
Sodium	111 mg
Calcium	33 mg
Sugar	0.7 gm

Recipe Cost: $1.01

Lifestyle Tip
You can get cutlery that is designed for hands with limited grasping ability. Their handles are soft, rubbery, and non-slip.

Nutritional Analysis

Per Serving

Energy	272 calories
Protein	6.3 gm
Fat	27.3 gm
Carbohydrate	1.3 gm
Fiber	0.1 gm
Cholesterol	24 mg
Iron	0.2 mg
Sodium	324 mg
Calcium	134 mg
Sugar	0 gm

Recipe Cost: $3.91

Lifestyle Tip
Use a terry cloth wash mitt with a palm pocket to hold soap.

Nutritional Analysis

Per Serving

Energy	*475 calories*
Protein	*3.5 gm*
Fat	*41.8 gm*
Carbohydrate	*26.3 gm*
Fiber	*5.7 gm*
Cholesterol	*13 mg*
Iron	*2 mg*
Sodium	*51 mg*
Calcium	*107 mg*
Sugar	*18.2 gm*

Recipe Cost: $2.43

Diet Tip
Tooth decay is largely the result of eating refined sugar.

Health Tip
Our bodies and minds function much better when we are more physically active. Get moving a bit more each day. For the most part, that means walking, swimming, gardening, cycling, or generally moving your body around a little more regularly.

COLESLAW

This is a very tasty dish. The horseradish makes it tangy. If you enjoy horseradish, you can add a little more. Remember that a recipe is a foundation, so you can change the structure a little bit to suit your tastebuds.

1	Small Head Cabbage, shredded
1	Small Onion, chopped small
1	Green Pepper, chopped small (optional)*
1	Red Pepper, chopped small (optional)*
2 Tbsp.	Chopped Parsley

Dressing:

3/4 cup	Soy Mayonnaise
2 Tbsp.	Honey
2 oz.	Horseradish
4 tsp.	Cider Vinegar
	Salt Substitute to taste
1/4 tsp.	Ground Black Pepper

* Remember these are nightshade plants. Your doctor can help you determine if you're affected by them.

Method of Preparation
Combine cabbage, onion, green and red peppers, and parsley. Mix them well in a bowl. Combine the dressing ingredients in another bowl and mix well. Pour dressing over the slaw and mix well again. Cover and chill.

Yield
Serves 4

Hint
So often people use way too much mayonnaise. It just seems to spoil the taste by overpowering everything else.

SPINACH AND ROMAINE SALAD
WITH CREAMY HORSERADISH DRESSING

I created this recipe because I enjoy horseradish and English mustard together.

1 lb.	Fresh Spinach, washed and dried, with stems discarded
1	Romaine Lettuce, large head, washed and dried

Dressing:

4 oz.	Sour Cream, health food store or non-fat kind
2 Tbsp.	Horseradish
1 Tbsp.	White Vinegar
3/4 tsp.	English Mustard
	Salt Substitute to taste
	Coarse Ground Black Pepper to taste
4 oz.	Salad Oil

Method of Preparation
Cut the romaine into 2" pieces lengthwise.

In a bowl, whisk together all the dressing ingredients except the oil. When they're well mixed, continue whisking while you add the salad oil; whisk until smooth.

Now add the spinach and romaine, and toss lightly till coated. Enjoy!

Yield
Serves 6-8

Hint
You can also add any garnishes you enjoy; for example, sliced onions, celery, carrots, cukes, and so on.

Nutritional Analysis

Per Serving

Energy	157 calories
Protein	4.1 gm
Fat	14.6 gm
Carbohydrate	4.4 gm
Fiber	3.3 gm
Cholesterol	0 mg
Iron	2.2 mg
Sodium	62 mg
Calcium	90 mg
Sugar	1.4 gm

Recipe Cost: $3.21

Lifestyle Tip
Buy extenders for your comb, hair brush, bath brush, nail file, etc. They are made to help with limited hand and arm mobility.

Health Tip
Expose yourself to the beauties of nature, to the fresh air, sunlight, the scents of the flowers, the songs of the birds, and the wonders of the world. This releases hormones, chemicals, and enzymes that promote healing. Sunlight aids in osteoporosis prevention. Enjoying the wonders of the world boosts your immune system and helps to control your disease.

Chapter 16 Salads & Dressings   213

Nutritional Analysis

Per Serving
Energy	*429 calories*
Protein	*1.5 gm*
Fat	*40.2 gm*
Carbohydrate	*19.3 gm*
Fiber	*2.8 gm*
Cholesterol	*23 mg*
Iron	*0.5 mg*
Sodium	*11 mg*
Calcium	*29 mg*
Sugar	*13.7 gm*

Recipe Cost: $4.84

Health Tip
The following herbs can be very beneficial for rheumatism and arthritis: bitterroot, buckthorn bark, burdock, wintergreen, yellow dock, sassafras, and bearsfoot. Look up their descriptions and take those best suited to your case. Use singly or in combination.

Diet Tip
So-called COX-2 inhibitors, such as the reservatrol in red grapes and the curcumin in turmeric, may suppress production of inflammation.

SIX FRUIT SALAD MAUI STYLE

This recipe tastes soooo gooood, it almost melts in your mouth. I made up this recipe when I had a bunch of fruit leftover from our Sunday brunch. Here in Alohaville it disappears very rapidly when we place it on the salad bar. You can use whatever fresh fruits are ripe. Use what is in season, on sale, or available in your area.

1 cup	Each, cut bite size: Fresh Peaches, Pineapple, Papaya, Grapes, Melon, and Strawberries Juice from 1/2 Lemon
1/2 cup	Heavy Whipping Cream, whipped stiff; substitute health food variety
1 cup	Soy Mayonnaise
2 Tbsp.	Fresh Lemon Juice
1 tsp.	Grated Lemon Peel
1 tsp.	Curry Powder

Method of Preparation
Place all the fruit in a large bowl. To keep fruit from browning, squeeze juice from half the lemon over the fruit and mix well. Chill for 1 hour.

Fold the heavy cream substitute into the soy mayonnaise, blend in the lemon juice, lemon peel, and curry powder. Pour the mixture over the chilled fruit and mix well.

Serve on a bed of Boston lettuce or whatever delicate lettuce is available in your area. Garnish with a sprig of fresh mint.

Yield
Serves 4-6 for a lunchtime meal

STUFFED PAPAYAS OR AVOCADOS

Is there anything more attractive than a fresh stuffed papaya? Yes: two of them!

2	Fresh Papayas, cut in half lengthwise, seeds removed, and soaked in cold water for 2-3 minutes

or

2	Avocados, cut in half, seed removed
	Chopped Lettuce
1	Turkey Salad Recipe, chilled (in Chapter 20)
1 tsp.	Chopped Parsley

Method of Preparation

Place one papaya half or one avocado half on a cold plate with a bed of chopped lettuce. Do this four times. Fill with turkey salad and sprinkle a little chopped parsley on top. Garnish with 6-8 crackers from the health food store.

Yield
Serves 4

Hint
You can also stuff the papayas or avocados with shrimp salad, chicken salad, or Kula crab salad (they're all in this book).

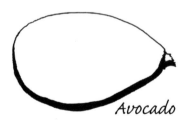
Avocado

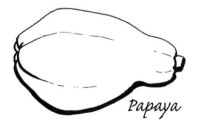
Papaya

Nutritional Analysis

Per Serving
Energy	935 calories
Protein	68 gm
Fat	66.5 gm
Carbohydrate	15.2 gm
Fiber	2.5 gm
Cholesterol	190 mg
Iron	4.4 mg
Sodium	182 mg
Calcium	100 mg
Sugar	8.5 gm

Recipe Cost: $3.47

Diet Tip
Eat more whole grain bread and cereal. This will also add vitamins, minerals, and fiber to your diet.

Diet Tip
Fiber and lignans in fresh produce help move toxins and chemicals through the gut. Certain bacteria in the gut can react with chemicals and toxins and cause a flare-up of arthritis. Fiber helps to clear the bowel of toxins. Eat lots of fibrous foods.

Chapter 16 Salads & Dressings 215

Nutritional Analysis

Per Serving
Energy	*701 calories*
Protein	*34.3 gm*
Fat	*58.3 gm*
Carbohydrate	*19.1 gm*
Fiber	*2.2 gm*
Cholesterol	*76 mg*
Iron	*4 mg*
Sodium	*197 mg*
Calcium	*426 mg*
Sugar	*13.3 gm*

Recipe Cost: $3.98

Diet Tip
Cut down on processed foods. Nearly 70% of the sugar we eat is hidden in these foods.

Health Tip
High stress and pressures of life can cause digestive problems, impaired body defenses against disease, lower productivity, ulcers, headaches, burn-out, and lead to substance abuse. These are the consequences of inadequate rest and recreation. Take a break and enjoy life. Set aside some time for relaxing and rebalancing. This will lower stress hormones and will decrease pain and stiffness.

CHICKEN AND FRUIT SALAD

I really have a great liking for this recipe. It has many of my culinary favorites in it.

2 cups	Chicken, white meat, cooked and diced
1/2 cup	Crushed Pineapple, strained
1 cup	Cheddar Cheese, health food kind, diced small
1/2 cup	Celery, diced small
	Juice from 1/4 Fresh Lemon
1/2 cup	Macadamia Nuts, diced
1 cup	Seedless Green Grapes, halved
2	Bananas, diced
1 cup	Soy Mayonnaise
	Salt Substitute to taste
	Paprika, to sprinkle on top

Method of Preparation
In a large bowl, mix all ingredients well. You may choose to add a little more mayonnaise if you like.

Serve on a bed of whatever lettuce is available in your area. Garnish with sliced oranges.

Yield
Serves 4-6

Hint
This goes ideally with homemade corn bread or muffins.

216   The Executive Chef's Arthritis Cookbook and Health Guide

CHUTNEY DRESSING

Gene, my Army cook friend, gave me this recipe when he was
my sous chef. Thanks, Gene!

1-1/2 cups	Salad Oil
5/8 cup	Wine Vinegar
2	Garlic Cloves, chopped fine
	Salt Substitute to taste
1 tsp.	Fresh Lemon Juice
1-2/3 cup	Chutney, chopped fine

Method of Preparation
Mix all the ingredients in a bowl. Store in a jar in the refrigerator. Stir well before using.

Yield
Makes about 12 servings

Hint
This dressing goes well with both green salads and fruit salads.

Nutritional Analysis

Per Serving
Energy	334 calories
Protein	0.5 gm
Fat	27.3 gm
Carbohydrate	24.2 gm
Fiber	0 gm
Cholesterol	0 mg
Iron	0.5 mg
Sodium	76 mg
Calcium	12 mg
Sugar	0 gm

Recipe Cost: $4.17

Diet Tip
Pay attention to food
labels. Any word ending in
-ose is a form of sugar.

PINEAPPLE-LEMON DRESSING

Here is a recipe for a dressing to put on all kinds of summer
salads.

1 cup	Salad Oil
1/2 cup	Pineapple Juice, unsweetened
3 Tbsp.	Fresh Lemon Juice
	Salt Substitute to taste
3/4 tsp.	English Mustard

Method of Preparation
In a container with a lid, combine all the ingredients. Close the
top and shake thoroughly. Refrigerate till you need it. Shake
before using.

Yield
Seven 2-oz. servings

Hint
Adding two teaspoons of fresh mint will make another kind of
dressing.

Nutritional Analysis

Per Serving
Energy	288 calories
Protein	0.2 gm
Fat	31.2 gm
Carbohydrate	3.1 gm
Fiber	0 gm
Cholesterol	0 mg
Iron	0 mg
Sodium	2 mg
Calcium	5 mg
Sugar	2.4 gm

Recipe Cost: $1.07

Diet Tip
The closer any sugar is to
the beginning of the list of
ingredients on a nutritional
label, the greater its percentage in the product.

Nutritional Analysis

Per Serving
Energy	298 calories
Protein	2.7 gm
Fat	24.6 gm
Carbohydrate	21.6 gm
Fiber	4.6 gm
Cholesterol	0 mg
Iron	1.2 mg
Sodium	10 mg
Calcium	29 mg
Sugar	9.3 gm

Recipe Cost: $6.22

Diet Tip
Every American consumes about 135 pounds of sugar each year. Any way you can cut down on this amount will be a health benefit to you.

Lifestyle Tip
Living well with arthritis depends on your attitude. We are what we think, feel, and believe. Our attitude can stimulate or suppress cells in our bodies that are responsible for some of the signs and symptoms of arthritis.

AMBROSIA SALAD HAWAIIAN STYLE

When you read this recipe, I'll bet your mouth starts to water!

1 can	Pineapple Chunks
1 can	Fruit Cocktail
1 sm. can	Sliced Pears
1 sm. can	Mandarin Oranges
1 sm. can	Shredded Coconut
5 oz.	Macadamia Nuts or Walnuts, crushed
1-1/2 cup	Whipping Cream, health food kind, whipped stiff, or Non-Dairy Whipped Topping

Method of Preparation
Drain the juice from all the cans. In a large cold stainless steel bowl, combine the fruits, coconut, and nuts; mix well. Pour the whipping cream over this mixture and fold well. Serve immediately on a bed of delicate lettuce, like butter lettuce.

Yield
Serves 6-8

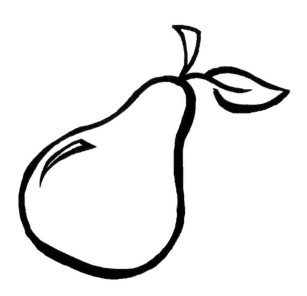

218 The Executive Chef's Arthritis Cookbook and Health Guide

ORANGE CREAM DRESSING

This dressing makes a nice sweet topping for all fresh berry recipes.

1 cup	Soy Mayonnaise
1/2 cup	Light Corn Syrup
2Tbsp.	Orange Rind, cut as fine as possible
3 Tbsp.	Fresh Orange Juice
1 tsp.	Fresh Lemon Juice
1/2 tsp.	Nutmeg
1 cup	Heavy Whipping Cream (health food kind), whipped to a stiff peak

Method of Preparation
Blend mayonnaise and corn syrup until smooth. Add rind, juices, and nutmeg. Fold in whipped cream.

Yield
Serves 10

Hint
For more orange flavor, add one orange cut into small segments.

TOASTED COCONUT CHIPS

I once trained three young Tongan men how to cook. In turn, they taught me how to prepare and enjoy one of their favorite *pupus* ("appetizers").

1	Fresh Coconut
	Salt Substitute to taste

Method of Preparation
This is a very easy recipe to prepare, once you get the coconut open.

Scoop out the fresh meat, and with a knife or potato peeler, cut all the meat as thin as possible. Spread on a cookie sheet and sprinkle with salt substitute. In a pre-heated oven, bake at 325°F until golden brown. Stir a few times to ensure even baking. Cool before serving.

Store in an air-tight container.

Nutritional Analysis

Per Serving

Energy	269 calories
Protein	0.3 gm
Fat	24 gm
Carbohydrate	15.4 gm
Fiber	0 gm
Cholesterol	7 mg
Iron	0.1 mg
Sodium	24 mg
Calcium	6 mg
Sugar	8.9 gm

Recipe Cost: $2.31

Diet Tip
Drink plenty of water: 6-8 ten-ounce glasses every day.

Nutritional Analysis

Per Serving

Energy	389 calories
Protein	3.7 gm
Fat	36.8 gm
Carbohydrate	16.7 gm
Fiber	9.9 gm
Cholesterol	0 mg
Iron	2.7 mg
Sodium	22 mg
Calcium	15 mg
Sugar	0 gm

Recipe Cost: $2.00

Lifestyle Tip
Carrying items in a backpack will reduce the stress on your shoulders and the joints in your hands.

Chapter 16 Salads & Dressings 219

Nutritional Analysis

Per Serving
Energy	*332 calories*
Protein	*3.7 gm*
Fat	*31.6 gm*
Carbohydrate	*12.7 gm*
Fiber	*4.4 gm*
Cholesterol	*0 mg*
Iron	*2.6 mg*
Sodium	*240 mg*
Calcium	*72 mg*
Sugar	*4.7 gm*

Recipe Cost: $4.16

Diet Tip
Salt is added to food by commercial processors. Limit the amount of salt you add to processed food.

Lifestyle Tip
People who get involved in meaningful loving relationships, travel, and social events have a tendency to live longer and have less pain and suffering associated with their arthritis.

MARINATED BROCCOLI SALAD

This salad should be served in your nicest clear glass bowl so people can see the beauty of what the Almighty puts on earth for us to enjoy.

1	Bunch Fresh Broccoli (about 1 lb.)
2 qts.	Boiling Water
1/2 lb.	Fresh Mushrooms, stems trimmed and quartered
3/4 cup	Pitted Black Olives, no juice, sliced in thirds
1	Cucumber, sliced thin, leave skin on
1	Medium Red Onion, sliced thin

Marinade:

4 oz.	Olive Oil
1 Tbsp.	White Wine Vinegar
1 Tbsp.	Fresh Lime Juice
3 Tbsp.	Fresh Parsley, chopped
2	Green Onions, cut in 1/4" slices
1 tsp.	Minced Garlic
1/2 tsp.	Salt Substitute
1/4 tsp.	Ground Black Pepper

Method of Preparation
Trim off broccoli florets; save the stems for another use. Cook broccoli in boiling water for 2 minutes; remove and shock in ice water until cold. Remove to a large bowl.

Trim stems from mushrooms and quarter the mushroom tops. Combine broccoli, mushrooms, olives, cucumbers, and red onion.

Mix the marinade well and pour over the vegetables. Toss lightly. Refrigerate 2 hours, mix well, and serve in your clear bowl.

Yield
Serves 4

Cooking Method
Boil

HOMEMADE YOGURT

From *Prescription for Cooking*, p. 85.

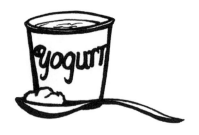

Once you taste homemade yogurt you will never buy yogurt again. It is creamier, lighter, and is not tart. I love my homemade yogurt and make a gallon weekly. I eat mine plain because I love the cool creamy taste. If using for a health reason, consume first in the morning on an empty stomach and a couple hours after dinner. It works best on an empty stomach.

1 quart	Raw, Skim, Goat, Cow, or 2% Homogenized Milk
4 Tbsp.	Unflavored, Unpasteurized Yogurt *(or a yogurt culture, and follow instructions on the package).*
3-4 Tbsp.	Non-Instant, Non-Fat Dried Milk Powder for a firmer yogurt *(optional),* I prefer just to use milk.

Method of Preparation

Make a paste from a small amount of milk and the milk powder, add to rest of milk. Put in a heavy pan over low heat. Scald the milk to the boiling point. **It should be steaming and bubbles on top, but not boiling.** *(Your health food store carries yogurt thermometers and automatic yogurt makers. It would help to get the thermometer.)*

Keep milk at 140-150 degrees for 10 minutes to destroy any unwanted organisms present. Remove from heat and let cool to 110 degrees (lukewarm) or warm to the touch. Mix your yogurt or culture into the milk. Make sure it is smooth and without lumps, but do not beat, mix gently. Put into clean jars (scald them first) and cover. Keep the jars at a steady 110 degrees. *If kept too hot or too cold it will not thicken.*

It will thicken more after it is refrigerated. 1 tablespoon unsweetened gelatin can be added in place of dry milk for thicker yogurt and added protein.

Add fresh fruit or preserves, honey or sweetener of your choice before serving, or eat it plain.

Chapter 16 Salads & Dressings 221

HOMEMADE YOGURT
(Continued)

Hints on Places to Keep Yogurt at 110 Degrees

In a heavy skillet with a few inches of water over a pilot light.

In a pretested oven of 110 degrees (use an oven thermometer).

Electric frying pan with water and insert yogurt jars, keep on lowest heat. Test with a thermometer.

Note
Always keep 4 tablespoons back for the next batch. Made with yogurt culture, it takes 8-10 hours, with fresh yogurt from the last batch, 3-5 hours.

LOW-FAT WHIPPING CREAM

From *Prescription for Cooking*, p. 115.

Make before serving because this cannot be stored, it will separate in about 15-25 minutes, but it is great on desserts and fruit.

Place 1/2 cup skim milk into a stainless steel bowl (this is best because it holds in the cold). Place in the freezer for 20 minutes or just until ice crystals begin to form on top.

Use a hand-held electric mixer and beat in 1/4 cup of non-fat dry milk solids slowly until the mixture thickens and soft peaks form. Add 1/2 teaspoon barley malt sweetener or 1 tablespoon of honey. Continue to beat for about 3 minutes.

222 The Executive Chef's Arthritis Cookbook and Health Guide

LOW-FAT MIRACLE SPREAD

From *Prescription for Cooking*, p. 116.

1 tub	Hain's Soft Safflower Margarine (found in health food stores)
1/2 cup	Unrefined Canola Oil

Optional:

1/2 cup	Homemade Lowfat Yogurt

Method of Preparation
Using a hand mixer or food processor, blend all the ingredients at low speed.

Spoon into a tub and refrigerate. Use in place of butter or margarine for all recipes and for spreading on top of all vegetables, potatoes, etc.

LOW-FAT SOUR CREAM

From *Prescription for Cooking*, p. 116.

1/2 lb.	Tofu
2 Tbsp.	Lemon Juice
3 Tbsp.	Canola Oil

Method of Preparation
Place tofu and lemon juice in blender or food processor, blend until creamy. While still mixing, add oil through feeder tube and continue to process until mixture is thick. If too thick, blend in a little water as needed.

Yield
Makes one cup serving with only 3 grams of fat.

INSTANT NON-FAT DRY MILK

From *Prescription for Cooking*. P 167.

If you use milk in cooking, this is the product to use. It costs less, does not spoil and has a natural sweetness. It can be used in make-ahead recipes for biscuit mix, pancake mix, or any recipe that calls for milk.

Chapter 16 Salads & Dressings 223

EASY SOY MILK

From *Prescription for Cooking,* p. 187.

This can be used in all cooking recipes in place of cow's milk, it's good on cereals and any place calling for milk.

> 1 cup   Soy Powder (from health food store)
> 3-1/2 cups Distilled Water

Method of Preparation
Soak soy powder in distilled water for three hours. Place in a double boiler and simmer for fifteen minutes. You can strain this or use as is.

Keep refrigerated.

Hints
The following ingredients will improve the flavor and texture:

> 1 tsp.   Pure Vanilla Extract
> 8 oz.   R.W. Knudsen's Papaya Juice or
>   Fresh Papaya
> 1 cup   Fresh White Grape Juice

TOFU

From *Prescription for Cooking,* p. 167.

Derived from the soybean, it is known as a soybean curd. It is white, cheese-like in texture and very high in protein and the B-vitamins. It is bland in taste, but takes on the flavor of any food that is combined with it. It is a gourmet item. It will keep approximately two weeks under refrigeration. Store covered with water in a bowl or jar. After opening, drain off the water and cover with fresh water. Before using tofu in recipes like cream cheese frosting or tofu cheesecake, always drain and pat dry. Tofu is also excellent sliced, patted dry, dipped in tamari sauce, and soaked a few minutes, then dipped in sesame seeds and sautéed. It will take the place of a burger, it is a good meat substitute with any meal.

224 The Executive Chef's Arthritis Cookbook and Health Guide

CARROT AND RAISIN SALAD WITH PINEAPPLE

When many people travel to the South Pacific, they expect this item on a menu or salad bar. I ate it growing up in the South Pacific island of Pennsylvania.

Dressing:

4 oz.	Soy Mayonnaise
4 oz.	Sour Cream, health food kind or non-fat
4 oz.	Rice Milk
4 oz.	Pineapple Juice
2-1/2 lbs.	Carrots, grated on large holes
1 cup	Raisins
1 cup	Crushed Pineapple, drained
	Salt Substitute to taste

Method of Preparation
Mix dressing ingredients well, then pour over the carrots and fruit, and mix again. Chill well.

This is a fine recipe for a buffet style party. It will last 3-4 days properly chilled.

Yield
Serves 10-12 as an appetizer salad

Hints
When serving on a buffet, put some kiwi fruit slices on top. This makes it exceptionally attractive.

You can make half the recipe without any problem.

Nutritional Analysis

Per Serving

Energy	175 calories
Protein	2.5 gm
Fat	9 gm
Carbohydrate	23.4 gm
Fiber	3.9 gm
Cholesterol	3 mg
Iron	0.8 mg
Sodium	44 mg
Calcium	53 mg
Sugar	17.2 gm

Recipe Cost: $4.47

Lifestyle Tip
A vegetable brush with suction-cup feet is a great kitchen item for cleaning vegetables.

Diet Tip
Hydrogenated oils can worsen your arthritis as well as other ailments. Hydrogenated oils to avoid include fast foods, deep fried foods, margarine, cheese, peanut butter, and TV dinners because they contain toxic trans-fatty acids and stiffen cell membranes. They can lead to early cell death. Other oils to avoid are saturated fats such as animal fats which are high in cholesterol.

Nutritional Analysis

Per Serving
Energy   *604 calories*
Protein   *6.1 gm*
Fat   *55.5 gm*
Carbohydrate   *25 gm*
Fiber   *3.7 gm*
Cholesterol   *17 mg*
Iron   *1 mg*
Sodium   *69 mg*
Calcium   *144 mg*
Sugar   *19.2 gm*

Recipe Cost: $3.12

Diet Tip
Eat a variety of good, fresh, wholesome food.

Diet Tip
Many adults with arthritis have high blood pressure or heart disease. Reducing fats and cholesterol in your diet will help control or prevent these diseases.

COLESLAW AND PINEAPPLE SALAD

I created this recipe just to fill up some space on the salad bar. It became so popular we only served it on weekdays, because we got too busy to make enough of it on weekends.

16 oz.	**Crushed Pineapple, drained**
1 head	**Cabbage (about 2 lbs.)**

Dressing:

2 cup	**Sour Cream, health food kind**
2 cup	**Soy Mayonnaise**
1/4 cup	**Fresh Lemon Juice**
2 Tbsp.	**White Vinegar**
2 Tbsp.	**Honey**
2 Tbsp.	**Horseradish**

Method of Preparation
Blend all dressing ingredients well. This will make about 1 quart. Properly stored in the refrigerator, it will last about 3 weeks.

Cut the amount of cabbage you wish to serve. Add to this the amount of crushed pineapple you would like.

Pour enough of the dressing over the cabbage and pineapple to moisten it as you would coleslaw.

Yield
Serves 8-12 if you make this recipe all at once.

Hints
If you want less dressing, you can make half the recipe with good results.

If you are serving this in a bowl, red cherries around the edge with a circle of crushed pineapple in the middle and a sprinkle of paprika on the top makes a nice garnish.

FRUIT SALAD DRESSING WITH HONEY

This is one of my own creations—a honey lover to the max. This dressing goes well with just about any fruit salad.

1-1/4 cup	Salad Oil
3/8 cup	Fresh Lemon Juice
	Salt Substitute to taste
1 cup	Sage Honey (here in Hawaii we use macadamia nut honey)
1/4 cup	Parsley

Method of Preparation
In a bowl, whisk together salad oil, lemon juice, and salt substitute. Slowly whisk in the honey, add the parsley, and whisk well. Chill.

Take out of the refrigerator half an hour before serving.

Yield
Serves 10

Nutritional Analysis

Per Serving

Energy	*347 calories*
Protein	*0.2 gm*
Fat	*27.3 gm*
Carbohydrate	*28.8 gm*
Fiber	*0.1 gm*
Cholesterol	*0 mg*
Iron	*0.2 mg*
Sodium	*2 mg*
Calcium	*5 mg*
Sugar	*27.2 gm*

Recipe Cost: $1.91

Health Tip
Plan your days according to your stamina. Do your harder chores first, rest, then do your easier ones.

CREAMY COCONUT DRESSING

This recipe comes from French Master Chef Eugene Bernard, my mentor. He was a great fresh fruit eater, and he always put something sweet on top.

2 cup	Sour Cream, health food kind
1/2 cup	Soy Mayonnaise
1-2/3 cup	Flaked Coconut
1/4 tsp.	Mace
1 Tbsp.	Fresh Lemon Juice
3 oz.	Honey

Method of Preparation
Blend sour cream and mayonnaise until smooth. Add the rest of the ingredients and mix well.

This goes well on all fruit salads.

Yield
Dressing for 8-10 salads

Nutritional Analysis

Per Serving

Energy	*236 calories*
Protein	*5.8 gm*
Fat	*19.6 gm*
Carbohydrate	*11.9 gm*
Fiber	*0.7 gm*
Cholesterol	*3 mg*
Iron	*0.5 mg*
Sodium	*30 mg*
Calcium	*37 mg*
Sugar	*6.8 gm*

Recipe Cost: $3.17

Health Tip
A balanced multivitamin and mineral supplement is a good foundation to which to add all other supplements. Taking some individual supplements (like beta-carotene) alone can actually be harmful.

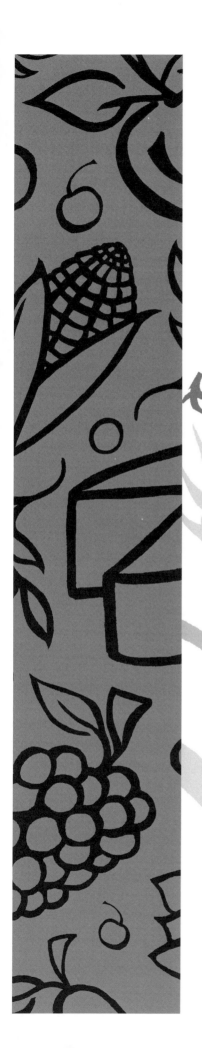

RICE & GRAINS

CHAPTER 17

228

RICE

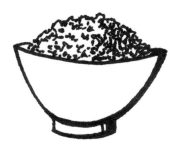

Rice is perhaps the most important crop in the world. It provides over half the world's total population with a palatable and nutritious food source at a low cost.

Rice is classified by the length of the grain. Here in the United States varieties include short grain, medium grain, and long grain types.

Long grain rice separates and looks light and fluffy when cooked. Short grain rice is fatter and more tender, moister, and sticky when cooked. Medium grain rice falls between the two. It is a good all-purpose rice. Most rice consumed in America is white or polished rice.

Commercial rice is cleaned before packaging, so it isn't necessary to wash it before cooking. Washing the rice increases the loss of soluble nutrients. Also, never use too much water when cooking any rice.

Rice yields are as follows:

1 cup white rice yields 3 cups cooked
1 cup uncooked parboiled rice (e.g., Uncle Ben's) yields 4 cups cooked
1 cup uncooked brown rice yields 4 cups cooked

> From *Prescription for Cooking*, p. 166

RICE - ANOTHER OPINION

Rice should be consumed in its brown form. Never eat white rice. There are three types of brown grain rice. Short grain is higher in nutritional value and lower in calories than the long grain, but it clumps together more than the long grain variety. Use long grain when having company and short grain for yourself. There is also sweet rice, which is slightly softer, sweeter, and stickier than the other varieties. Sweet rice has been used traditionally in Japan to make special holiday cakes. When toasted, sweet rice puffs up like popcorn. Rice malt syrup is a good natural sweetener, found in a health food store. Try substituting brown rice for potatoes with meals. Brown rice is by far one of the most nutritious foods that can be found. It is especially high in the B-complex vitamins.

From *Prescription for Cooking,* p. 121

GRAINS

Grains have particular attributes which make them unique. Rice is non-allergenic and gluten-free, except for sweet glutinous rice. While oats are relatively high in fat for a grain, they contain an antioxidant which delays rancidity. Wheat contains gluten and is the only grain suitable for baking leavened breads without the addition of any other grains. Quinoa is the only grain to contain a complete protein source.

Whole grains are high fiber, complex carbohydrate foods, they are rich in both fat in sodium. They are a good source of minerals and the B-complex vitamins. Grains have been a staple food throughout the world's history. Grains are a complex carbohydrate that promotes energy, which is vital to the body. All whole grains, except wheat, help reduce fat in the body. Grains are an excellent source of complex carbohydrates needed by body builders to ensure a steady blood sugar level. Grains are good for all blood sugar disorders.

A whole grain is made up of these basic parts: the bran, the germ, and the endosperm and exosperm. When grains are refined they are stripped of the bran, and sometimes the germ. The bran is the outermost part of the grain, and a good source of roughage, as well as B vitamins, proteins, fats, and minerals. Each part of a whole grain has nutritional value. The exosperm, which is rich in bran; the endosperm, which is principally starch; the husk, which is primarily fiber; and the germ, which is rich in protein, polyunsaturated fatty acids, vitamins, and minerals.

Whole grains, like corn, oats, rice, and wheat account for some of the most sought-after foods found in a natural foods outlet.

Whole grains provide complete nourishment when complemented with legumes, beans, or vegetables. These foods eaten together will form a complete protein.

Chapter 17 Rice & Grains 231

Nutritional Analysis
(1 cup cooked wild rice)

Energy	*166 calories*
Protein	*6.5 gm*
Fat	*0.6 gm*
Carbohydrate	*35 gm*
Fiber	*? gm*
Cholesterol	*0 mg*
Iron	*1 mg*
Sodium	*5 mg*
Calcium	*5 mg*
Sugar	*1.1 gm*

Recipe Cost: $0.41

Health Tip
Keeping close to your ideal body weight helps decrease the pressure on knees and hips, which bear much of the weight of the body.

Health Tip
Potential risks of alternative therapies include immune system stimulation, interactions with prescribed drugs, financial considerations, and perceived strain on doctor-patient relationship. It's good to consult with your physician before and during the use of alternative therapies.

WILD RICE

Wild rice is not really a rice, it's a wild grass. This strain of wild grass is very susceptible to drought and wind. It is a crop which is harvested by hand. Native American Indians still harvest most wild rice today.

The value of this grain is its unique nutty flavor and its nutritional value. Wild rice is a great addition to meals of wild game, such as elk, deer, pheasant, goose, duck, or porcupine. (To catch a porcupine, shine a very bright light in its eyes at night. Roll it over on its back and grab it by its belly. When I was a young mountain man back in rural Pennsylvania, people used to get very excited when I walked into our hunting cabin carrying a porcupine. Incidently, we never ate them—the quills were too hard to swallow.)

Wild rice should always be washed before cooking. It is best when simmered by using 1 part rice to 3 parts water, and cooking for about 45 minutes or until all the water is absorbed.

ELECTRIC RICE COOKER

It's really simple to cook rice in an electric rice cooker: put the rice and water in the pot, and switch it on. (Use the amount of water in the instructions that come with the cooker.) Don't add any salt.

When the rice is done, the cooker will switch off automatically. Let the rice stand for 10-15 minutes, and it will be ready to serve.

The electric cooker will also cook brown rice and glutinous rice correctly; it takes a little longer but the machine will look after this.

BROWN RICE

Brown rice usually has a special nutty flavor and slightly chewy texture. The following recipe is the stove top method.

3 cups	Water
1 cup	Brown Rice
1 Tbsp.	Soy Margarine
	Salt Substitute to taste

Method of Preparation
Bring water to a boil. Stir in rice, margarine, and salt substitute. Bring to a boil. Reduce heat to low, cover, and simmer until all liquid is absorbed, about 45 minutes.

Remove from heat and let stand, covered, for 5 minutes. Fluff with a fork.

Yield
3 cups, or 4-6 servings

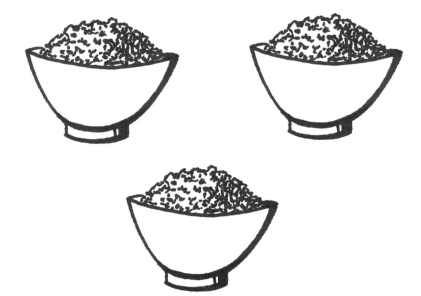

Nutritional Analysis
(1 cup cooked brown rice)

Energy	216 calories
Protein	5 gm
Fat	1.8 gm
Carbohydrate	44.8 gm
Fiber	3.3 gm
Cholesterol	0 mg
Iron	0.8 mg
Sodium	10 mg
Calcium	20 mg
Sugar	0 gm

Recipe Cost: $0.21

Diet Tip
For people with arthritis, it is important to keep trim by reducing fat, cholesterol, and sugar in diets.

Diet Tip
Whole grains are nutritional powerhouses, chockfull of B vitamins, magnesium, fiber, phytochemicals, and the antioxidants vitamin E and selenium. They're also a wonderful source of the complex carbohydrates that patients with arthritis need for energy.

Chapter 17 Rice & Grains 233

Nutritional Analysis

Per Serving
Energy   *477 calories*
Protein   *7.9 gm*
Fat   *23.9 gm*
Carbohydrate   *57.8 gm*
Fiber   *3.1 gm*
Cholesterol   *91 mg*
Iron   *3.3 mg*
Sodium   *296 mg*
Calcium   *51 mg*
Sugar   *9.5 gm*

Recipe Cost: $1.03

Diet Tip
Eat foods with enough starch and fiber.

Diet Tip
Nightshade foods are defined as foods derived from plants from the genus solanaceae which include tomatoes, potatoes, peppers, and eggplants. These substances are believed to promote inflammation in a small percentage of people. There has been no valid research to substantiate this claim. I still advise patients to do an elimination diet, refraining from eating these foods for six weeks and then reintroducing them one by to one to see whether there is a change in their symptoms.

FRIED RICE

Fried rice is nothing more than white rice with whatever you like fried added to it. Here is a recipe we enjoy.

3 oz.	Olive Oil
2	Garlic Cloves, chopped fine
1	Medium Onion, chopped small
2	Celery Stalks, chopped small
2	Carrots, chopped small
3 cups	White Rice, cooked, cold
1 oz.	Soy Sauce, low sodium kind
1 Tbsp.	Honey
2	Eggs, beaten
3	Green Onions, minced
	Salt Substitute to taste

Method of Preparation
In a large, deep skillet with 1 oz. of the olive oil, saute the garlic, onions, celery, and carrots till tender. Remove to a side dish.

Break up the cold white rice so there are no lumps. In the skillet, heat another ounce of oil and add the rice. Stir so it doesn't stick. Add back the vegetables and, over low heat, heat till hot. Add the soy sauce and honey. Stir well.

With the last ounce of olive oil, cook the egg like you would scrambled eggs, except don't stir it. When it is done, chop it up with a wooden spoon. Add to rice and stir in well. Sprinkle the green onion over the rice and serve.

Yield
Serves 4

Hint
Add some of the following for flavor, for more servings, or just for looks. Remember, food is beautiful!

1 cup	Chicken, bite size, or
1 cup	Turkey, bite size, or
1/4 cup	Macadamia Nuts, diced, or
1 cup	Shrimp, bite size, or
1 cup	Crabmeat, or
1 cup	Cooked Fish, bite size, or
1 cup	Mushrooms, sliced, or
1 cup	Whatever you enjoy

You can make whatever amount you want, let it cool, and refrigerate. Reheat for two minutes in the microwave, or until hot in a non-stick skillet.

234 The Executive Chef's Arthritis Cookbook and Health Guide

LUNDBERG WILD BLEND™
WILD AND BROWN RICE RECIPE

To me this gourmet blend of wild and premium brown rices is the best there is to offer. I have used this for many years as a healthy alternative wherever I have been the Executive Chef.

1 cup	Lundberg Wild Blend™
3-1/2 cups	Chicken Stock (see recipe in Chapter 12)
1 Tbsp.	Olive Oil
	Salt Substitute to taste

Method of Preparation
Rinse rice. Put all ingredients in a pot with a tightly fitting lid. Bring to a boil, reduce heat, then cover and simmer for 45 minutes. DO NOT REMOVE THE LID.

Remove from heat and let sit, covered, for 10 minutes. Fluff with a fork.

Yield
Serves 4-6

Hint
A rice cooker may be used with the same rice to chicken stock ratio.

Nutritional Analysis

Per Serving

Energy	124 calories
Protein	2.7 gm
Fat	3.5 gm
Carbohydrate	23.7 gm
Fiber	2 gm
Cholesterol	0 mg
Iron	0 mg
Sodium	1 mg
Calcium	0 mg
Sugar	0 gm

Recipe Cost: $1.06

Lifestyle Tip
Join the Arthritis Foundation and get *Arthritis Today* magazine. It has all the latest news about your disease.

Diet Tip
Brown rice helps keep blood sugar stabilized so you don't feel hungry for longer periods of time.

Chapter 17 Rice & Grains 235

Nutritional Analysis
(1 cup cooked white rice)

Per Serving
Energy	205 calories
Protein	4.3 gm
Fat	0.4 gm
Carbohydrate	44.5 gm
Fiber	0 gm
Cholesterol	0 mg
Iron	1.9 mg
Sodium	2 mg
Calcium	16 mg
Sugar	0.3 gm

Recipe Cost: Depends on how much rice you cook. Whatever amount you use, it is affordable, unless it is a boxcar full.

WHITE RICE

White rice must never be rinsed thoroughly. All this does is wash away the nutrients. It used to be a good idea to thoroughly wash rice, but new laws and harvesting methods have greatly reduced the dirt in rice.

White rice is very simple to cook in any size container. Place the rice in a saucepan with enough water to rise 1/2 inch above the rice. Usually you can measure this by the length to the first knuckle of your middle finger. See how simple it is!

Turn the heat on high until it boils, then turn it down to medium and cook for 12-15 minutes. The rice will look like this: small holes begin to form on the surface of the rice, and most of the water has been absorbed.

Now, cover the rice and cook over very low heat for 10-15 minutes longer. Leave covered and remove from heat. Let it sit for about 10 minutes more.

Any remaining water will be absorbed and the cooking is done. The rice will remain hot for about half an hour if covered.

236

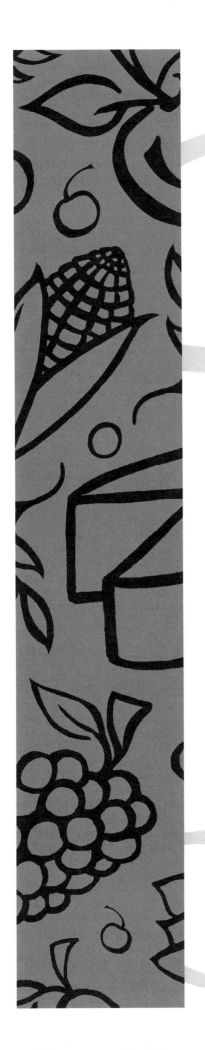
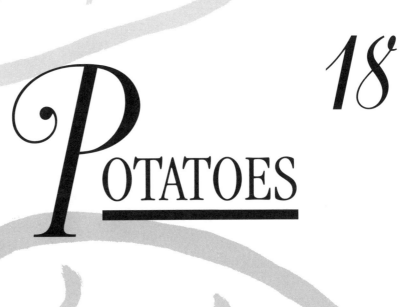

POTATOES

CHAPTER 18

238

POTATOES

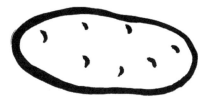

The potato is the edible, starchy tuber of the common plant *Solanum tuberosum*, a perennial of the nightshade family. The potato is related to the deadly nightshade, but that does not make the potato harmful. It just means that all the green parts of the plant are poisonous. Other members of the family are the tomato, tomatillo, and eggplant.

We include potatoes in this book because they taste good and are good for you in many instances. If you have any questions about eating food from the nightshade family, go to your doctor and get an opinion from him or her. Some people who suffer from arthritis are affected by nightshade family members, while others are not.

Potatoes have been cultivated by the Native Americans since 3000 B.C. The potatoes grown by the Indians ranged in size from a peanut to a plum. The first Europeans introduced to potatoes were Spanish Conquistadors, Pizarro's men, in about 1353.

There are about 2,000 varieties of potatoes grown around the world. Varieties of potatoes have been developed to fit into the various growing climates and the different cuisines throughout the world. Potatoes may be round, oval, irregular, oblong, or even kidney shaped. They can weigh up to one pound, and their colors vary from whitish brown to purple.

There are many labels and classifications of potatoes: Pennsylvania, Idaho, Maine, California, Washington red ones, long red ones, white ones, long white ones, new potatoes, fall potatoes, young potatoes, baking potatoes, and on and on and on: potatoes, potatoes, potatoes.

When a potato is cooked, it develops either a fine, waxy texture, or a starchy mealy consistency.

The waxy textured ones are better for steaming whole, or boiling, or making potato salad. The mealy textured ones are great for baking, mashing, or frying. The round white thick-skinned potatoes are marked all-purpose. These are good for potato chips.

Look for potatoes with shallow eyes. Avoid those with split skin, or ones that are spongy. A good potato will smell like freshly turned earth.

Do not refrigerate potatoes. Store them between 40°F and 50°F when possible. The starch in potatoes stored at too high or low a temperature turns to natural sugar.

Potatoes are best enjoyed with their skin on. The vitamins and minerals of the potato are stored in or just below the skin, so removing the skin removes the vitamins and minerals.

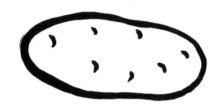

Potatoes are enjoyed when cooked in just about all of the cooking methods. Here in America we all love the baked potato—that's why I included the recipe for the Perfect Baked Potato.

REMEMBER: Only 4-5% of arthritis sufferers can't eat potatoes. This means 95-96% of you can enjoy the recipes in this chapter.

Health Tip
Do not exercise if joints are hot or inflamed. If they are inflamed, just slowly move them through gentle range of motion several times a day to maintain mobility. Inflamed joints can cause shortening and tightening of surrounding tissues. Do not move the joint past the point of pain. Do all movements slowly and smoothly one to five times daily.

Chapter 18 Potatoes 241

Nutritional Analysis

Per Serving

Energy	*310 calories*
Protein	*5.5 gm*
Fat	*14.4 gm*
Carbohydrate	*41.5 gm*
Fiber	*4 gm*
Cholesterol	*0 mg*
Iron	*3.1 mg*
Sodium	*18 mg*
Calcium	*33 mg*
Sugar	*0 gm*

Recipe Cost: very affordable

Health Tip
Exercise will make your heart stronger, giving you more energy for daily tasks.

Nutritional Analysis

Per Serving

Energy	*388 calories*
Protein	*5.9 gm*
Fat	*22.1 gm*
Carbohydrate	*44 gm*
Fiber	*4.9 gm*
Cholesterol	*0 mg*
Iron	*3 mg*
Sodium	*30 mg*
Calcium	*45 mg*
Sugar	*4.4 gm*

Recipe Cost: $1.38

Health Tip
For osteoporosis, increase your calcium intake. It influences bone density.

THE PERFECT BAKED POTATO

Select a smooth, medium-size potato, wash it thoroughly, and prick all over with a fork to let moisture escape.

Now rub the potato all over with some type of healthy oil. Bake on a rack in a hot 375°F oven for 45 minutes to 1 hour. Serve immediately.

Hint
Many people think that wrapping a potato in aluminum foil and putting it in the oven is a baked potato. Wrong! You actually have a steamed potato. The aluminum foil does not allow the steam to escape, so the cooking process becomes a steaming process and not the proper baking process. DON'T USE FOIL.

Cooking Method
Bake

POTATOES FRIED IN GARLIC OIL WITH ONIONS AND GARLIC

Here is a healthy alternative for making fried potatoes. No unhealthy saturated fats, just a lot of good flavor.

3 oz.	Garlic Oil (see Chapter 19)
1 tsp.	Soy Margarine
2 lbs.	Idaho Potatoes, boiled, chilled, sliced, with skin on
1	Large Onion, sliced 1/4" thick, boiled, and drained
1 tsp.	Chopped Garlic
1/4 tsp.	Salt Substitute
1/8 tsp.	White Pepper

Method of Preparation
In a large skillet, heat the garlic oil till hot. When hot, add the margarine; when it has melted add the potatoes and pan fry 5 minutes. Next, add the onions, cook 5 minutes more, then add the garlic and cook till the potatoes and onions are nice and brown. Add the seasonings.

Yield
Serves 4

242 The Executive Chef's Arthritis Cookbook and Health Guide

PARSLEY BUTTERED POTATOES

For many years now, this has been a very popular item to serve with any white fish. We used to make this at our hunting cabin in Pennsylvania to go along with a batch of freshly caught native brook trout.

12	New Potatoes (about 2-1/2" long), skin on, steamed till tender, cooled, and cut bite size
2-3 oz.	Olive Oil
1 tsp.	Lemon Juice
1/3 cup	Chopped Parsley
	Salt Substitute to taste
	Coarse Ground Black Pepper to taste

Method of Preparation
In a bowl, place all of the ingredients and toss well. Place ingredients on a sheet pan and bake in a 375°F oven for 20 minutes. Then turn on the broiler and place the pan under it for a few minutes so the potatoes get golden brown. Stir when necessary.

Yield
Serves 4

Hint
You can add 1 tablespoon of chopped shallots and 1 tablespoon of chopped garlic to this recipe. Saute them first in a little olive oil till you can smell the garlic in your kitchen. Then add to the bowl and mix well.

Cooking Methods
Steam, bake, broil

Nutritional Analysis

Per Serving

Energy	463 calories
Protein	10.1 gm
Fat	14.7 gm
Carbohydrate	75.8 gm
Fiber	8.4 gm
Cholesterol	0 mg
Iron	6.3 mg
Sodium	35 mg
Calcium	66 mg
Sugar	0.1 gm

Recipe Cost: $1.65

Health Tip
Exercise is beneficial because it can help you keep your joints moving.

Diet Tip
Suppression of the inflammation of arthritis can be manipulated through dietary fats. The alpha-linolenic oils such as fish oil, grapeseed oil, flaxseed oil, evening primrose oil, and borage oil suppress inflammation and reduce the symptoms of arthritis.

Chapter 18 Potatoes 243

Nutritional Analysis

Per Serving
Energy	*369 calories*
Protein	*10.3 gm*
Fat	*15.4 gm*
Carbohydrate	*51.9 gm*
Fiber	*3.7 gm*
Cholesterol	*78 mg*
Iron	*4.2 mg*
Sodium	*155 mg*
Calcium	*240 mg*
Sugar	*3.8 gm*

Recipe Cost: $1.67

Health Tip
After exercising, try gentle stretching the next day to avoid stiff or sore muscles.

Diet Tip
A small percentage of arthritis can be attributable to hypersensitivities to food such as dairy products, corn, and cereal as evidenced by reduced disease activity on withdrawal of offending food and flare-up upon eating them again.

BAKED STUFFED POTATOES

Almost everyone really enjoys this truly great American dish.

4	Idaho Potatoes, baked until tender and cooled
1 oz.	Butter, use 94% saturated fat free
3 oz.	Cream, from health food store
1	Egg Yolk
	Salt Substitute to taste
	White Pepper to taste
1/3 cup	Parmesan Cheese (organic tofu kind)
2 Tbsp.	Chives, chopped

Method of Preparation
When the potatoes have cooled, cut them in half lengthwise, scoop the potato pulp into a bowl. Mash the pulp the best way you can. Heat the butter and cream till the butter melts; add this and the rest of the ingredients to the pulp and mix well. Spoon the mixture back into the potato skins and bake in a 350°F oven for 15-20 minutes. Serve immediately.

Yield
Serves 4

Hints
You can also add your favorite grated cheese to the top. Just remember to use the kind from the health food store.

Use your imagination: you can chop bite-size a great number of culinary delights and add 1 cup to this recipe. For example, use leftover corn, broccoli, onions, spinach, and so forth—whatever you enjoy.

Cooking Method
Bake

MASHED POTATOES

Where I was born in Pennsylvania, we call these "mountain potatoes." You'll probably like this so much, you'll always eat your potatoes this way. When you cook a small amount of onion with potatoes, the flavor isn't overpowering.

2 lbs.	Potatoes (about 6 medium ones), cut bite-size, skin on
1	Medium Onion, diced small
4 oz.	Soy Milk
1 oz.	Soy Margarine
	Salt Substitute to taste
	White Pepper to taste

Method of Preparation

In a sauce pan, place the potatoes and onions, cover with cold water, and bring to a boil over high heat. Turn heat to medium and continue simmering until potatoes are tender. When done, strain and pour out on a sheet pan. Leave for 10 minutes so the potatoes will start to dry.

Put the potatoes back in the sauce pan and mash them, or place in a mixing bowl and mix on low.

In a separate pan, heat the milk and margarine till hot. Pour this into the potatoes, half at a time. (You might not need it all.) Mash and blend until smooth. Add the seasonings to taste.

Yield
Serves 6-8

Hint
Homemade mashed potatoes with a lump or two always taste better than the smooth no-lump ones.

Cooking Method
Boil, simmer

Nutritional Analysis

Per Serving

Energy	*110 calories*
Protein	*2.8 gm*
Fat	*1.6 gm*
Carbohydrate	*21.9 gm*
Fiber	*2.4 gm*
Cholesterol	*0 mg*
Iron	*1.5 mg*
Sodium	*48 mg*
Calcium	*37 mg*
Sugar	*1.8 gm*

Recipe Cost: $1.82

Diet Tip

For gout, drink 10-12 eight ounce glasses of non-alcoholic fluids daily. This will help wash the uric acid crystals out of your body.

Diet Tip

Fasting appears to reduce disease activity in rheumatoid arthritis by impairment of immune function, increased levels of cortisol, and decreased intestinal permeability. You should see a dietitian to learn the proper way of fasting or see a minister to learn about spiritual fasting.

Nutritional Analysis

Per Serving
Energy	*110 calories*
Protein	*2.8 gm*
Fat	*1.6 gm*
Carbohydrate	*21.9 gm*
Fiber	*2.4 gm*
Cholesterol	*0 mg*
Iron	*1.5 mg*
Sodium	*48 mg*
Calcium	*37 mg*
Sugar	*1.8 gm*

Recipe Cost: $2.14

Diet Tip
Eat foods that are high in fiber, such as fruits and vegetables. This will cause a softer stool and a rapid elimination of waste.

Health Tip
Nutritional supplements should not take the place of appropriate dietary habits or proper medical care. Nutritional supplementation helps to assure that you are getting the levels of essential nutrients that your body needs. Diseases and medications can deplete your body of essential nutrients that might not be replaced by your diet.

CANDIED SWEET POTATOES

This is a great healthful recipe to add to your Thanksgiving dinner. Remember everyday should be a day of thanksgiving. We truly have so much to be grateful for.

6 oz.	Honey
3 oz.	Fresh Tangerine, Lemon, or Orange Juice
2 oz.	Butter (health food store kind)
	Salt Substitute to taste
6	Fresh Sweet Potatoes, steamed, cooled, and sliced

Method of Preparation
As usual, we won't peel the potatoes. In a skillet, place everything except the potatoes, and simmer over medium heat till it starts to become syrupy. Now add the cooked potatoes and stir well, so all potatoes are coated.

In a preheated 400°F oven, place the skillet and cook for 15 minutes, or until potatoes are piping hot.

Yield
Serves 4-6

Hint
This recipe is easily doubled.

Cooking Methods
Steam, simmer, bake

GERMAN POTATO SALAD

Here's a very rich recipe that doesn't follow our guidelines. I included it here because the flavor and taste are so good. Make it for your family and friends and have a taste, but be careful if you're sensitive to this kind of food.

8	Medium New Potatoes, boiled, cooled, and sliced, with skin on
8	Slices of Bacon, fried, cooled, and crumbled
1/4 cup	Bacon Fat (from the fried bacon)
3 Tbsp.	Brown Rice Flour
1-3/4	Hot Water
3 oz.	Cider Vinegar
1 oz.	Honey
	Salt Substitute to taste
1/2 tsp.	Ground Black Pepper
1-1/2 tsp.	English Mustard

Method of Preparation

In a frying pan, place the bacon fat, heat, stir in the flour, cook slowly over low heat, stirring constantly. Take off the heat and add the cups hot water and vinegar; mix well, return to low heat and cook, stirring till smooth and thick.

Add honey, salt substitute, mustard, and pepper, then cook 3 more minutes. In a bowl, put the sliced potatoes and crumbled bacon. Pour the bacon mixture over these and mix well.

Yield
Serves 6-8

Cooking Methods
Boil, fry

Nutritional Analysis

Per Serving	
Energy	251 calories
Protein	4.9 gm
Fat	11.1 gm
Carbohydrate	33.6 gm
Fiber	2.2 gm
Cholesterol	13 mg
Iron	0.7 mg
Sodium	128 mg
Calcium	15 mg
Sugar	2.9 gm

Recipe Cost: $1.91

Health Tip
Being very overweight or obese increases your risk of developing osteoarthritis in the knee.

Health Tip
Glucosamine sulfate is used to treat osteoarthritis. It is a protective agent that may stop the progression of cartilage degradation and stimulate production of new cartilage. It is easily absorbed with minimal to no side effects. Chondroitin sulfate is a component of joint cartilage. It is a very large molecule that is not easily absorbed into the joint.

Chapter 18 Potatoes **247**

Nutritional Analysis

Per Serving
Energy	*368 calories*
Protein	*4.2 gm*
Fat	*9.2 gm*
Carbohydrate	*46.8 gm*
Fiber	*3.8 gm*
Cholesterol	*0 mg*
Iron	*1.7 mg*
Sodium	*12 mg*
Calcium	*65 mg*
Sugar	*0 gm*

Recipe Cost: $2.69

Health Tip
Avoid smoking. Tobacco is a plant from the nightshade family, all of which potentially cause an arthritis flare-up.

Health Tip
When shopping for an herbal or natural preparation, look for a standardized product that should be stamped on the bottle. Standardized herbal extract means that the product is guaranteed to contain a minimum level of the major active ingredient. With the traditional method of herbal extraction there is no guarantee that the active ingredient is present.

OVEN ROASTED POTATOES IN GARLIC OIL AND FRESH BASIL

Here is a trick learned in my classical French training. For many years I have served these potatoes with various fish products. People ask how they have such a wonderful garlic flavor without seeing any garlic.

Oil infusions have been used for many years, and are now popular again. You can read about them in many old French cookbooks.

3 lbs.	Idaho Potatoes, boiled then chilled and sliced; leave skin on
4 oz.	Garlic Oil (recipe in Chapter 19)
1/2 cup	Fresh Chopped Basil
	Salt Substitute to taste
1/8 tsp.	White Pepper

Method of Preparation
In a bowl, place all the ingredients except the potatoes, and mix well. Now add the potatoes and mix so they are coated.

Preheat oven to 450°F (yes, 450°F). Put the potatoes on a sheet pan and bake 20-30 minutes, or until they get nice and golden. Serve immediately.

Yield
Serves 4-6

Hint

For you onion lovers, add 1 pound of sliced, boiled, and cooled onion to this recipe.

Cooking Methods
Boil, bake

248

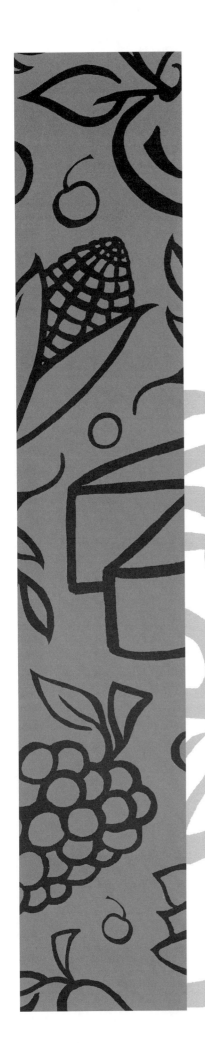

FACTS ABOUT Veggies & GARLIC

CHAPTER 19

250

Chapter 19 Facts About Veggies & Garlic 251

LEAFY AND GREEN

Green and leafy vegetables are an important part of the daily diet. They add variety and are excellent sources of chlorophyll, iron, magnesium, calcium, manganese, vitamin C, potassium, vitamin A, essential fatty acids and other minerals, vitamins, and fiber needed for your immune system and to ward off diseases. Most of them are very low in fat and calories. Leafy greens are good for the gall bladder, spleen, heart, blood, and brain. You can cook greens in many ways to make them appetizing. The tasty and nourishing recipes in this chapter will encourage you to make vegetables a part of every meal.

To taste really good, vegetables have to be fresh and properly prepared. Buy the freshest and best looking vegetables you can find. The vegetables with the darkest, most intense colors tend to contain the highest levels of nutrients. Clean them by soaking in the sink for a few minutes, then swirl them around and drain. Tear the leaves up and chop the stems. Greens can be added to soups, stews, or cooked in broth with a little chopped onion, carrots, and celery. They are also good when steamed and seasoned before serving.

Make it a point to eat at least one serving of lightly cooked greens each day: spinach, beet greens, chard, kale, collards, or mustard greens. Onions can help lower cholesterol and garlic can help fight germs if you eat them raw. For vegetarians, cooked greens are an important source of iron. Make sure to have both raw and cooked vegetables in your diet. Make a salad of different kinds of lettuce, radishes, carrots, cucumbers, onions, and tomatoes to get some raw vegetables in your diet.

Some vegetables contain natural toxins. For example, the sprouts and green skins of potatoes are poisonous, so remove them before cooking. Most of the natural toxins in vegetables are easily destroyed by the heat of cooking. Cabbage and cauliflower, Brussels sprouts, kale, collards, mustard greens, and broccoli are better for you when lightly cooked. They may offer some protection against colon cancer.

Try making a broth to use in cooking. Cook a finely chopped onion, a couple of cloves of minced garlic, 1 finely chopped carrot with 1/2 cup reduced-sodium chicken or turkey broth (vegetarians use miso) in a large covered skillet until the onion is completely wilted, about 10 to 15 minutes. You do not need to add salt.

Get on the vegetable bandwagon—it's headed for good health!

ASPARAGUS

Asparagus is one of the very first plants harvested in the spring —a sign of spring finally arriving. Asparagus is a good source of vitamins A and C and of potassium. It is best cooked immediately after picking.

Asparagus should be vibrant green, and the stems should snap easily between your fingers. Thick or thin asparagus usually tastes the same; the cooking time is the only difference. Trim off the stem ends by about one inch, and wash in cold water. Then boil, steam, bake or stir-fry.

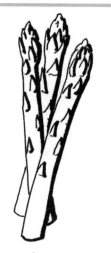

Asparagus

STIR-FRIED ASPARAGUS WITH CHICKEN AND NUTS

Every spring I've made this as a Chef's Special to celebrate the fresh bounty of American foods which will be available for the next six to seven months. Thank you, Lord, for the springtime.

2 oz.	Olive Oil
4	Boneless, Skinless Chicken Breasts (about 6 oz. each), cut in 1/2" strips
1 Tbsp.	Chopped Garlic
1 tsp.	Chopped Ginger
2 oz.	Orange or Tangerine Juice
1 lb.	Asparagus, cut off stems leaving 3" tips
1 Tbsp.	Honey
4 oz.	Low or No Sodium Soy Sauce
	Cornstarch and Water to thicken
1/4 cup	Toasted Pine Nuts, Macadamia Nuts, or your favorite

Method of Preparation
In a large skillet, frying pan, or wok, pour the olive oil. Heat until HOT. Add the chicken and cook over medium heat about 4-5 minutes. Add the garlic and ginger; cook 1 minute more.

Add tangerine or orange juice, asparagus, honey, and soy sauce. Cook until asparagus is as tender as you like.

Remove everything but the juice in the bottom of the pan. Thicken it with a slurry of cornstarch and water. Add the nuts, and cook 2-3 minutes. Dish out on a separate platter and add sauce and nuts over the top.

Yield
Serves 4-8

Cooking Methods
Pan fry, simmer

Nutritional Analysis

Per Serving
Energy   296 calories
Protein   30.7 gm
Fat   14.4 gm
Carbohydrate   12.5 gm
Fiber   1.9 gm
Cholesterol   66 mg
Iron   2.5 mg
Sodium   706 mg
Calcium   38 mg
Sugar   5.1 gm

Recipe Cost: $5.25

Health Tip
After menopause, women lose bone mass when their menstrual cycles stop and their bodies produce less of the hormone estrogen. Consider taking estrogen, which must be prescribed by your doctor.

Chapter 19 Facts About Veggies & Garlic 253

Nutritional Analysis

Per Serving
Energy	*32 calories*
Protein	*2.6 gm*
Fat	*0.2 gm*
Carbohydrate	*6.7 gm*
Fiber	*2.4 gm*
Cholesterol	*0 mg*
Iron	*1 mg*
Sodium	*2 mg*
Calcium	*24 mg*
Sugar	*3.8 gm*

Recipe Cost: $1.23

Health Tip
As you get older, you can reduce your risk of falling and breaking a bone by exercising. This will make you more flexible and stable.

Health Tip
I advise patients with arthritis to first focus on positive changes in the mind, body, and spirit, optimal nutrition, and water intake. Identify and eliminate food allergens, reduce animal fats in the diet. Take high potency multivitamins with minerals and fish oil/omega fatty acids. Depending on the type of arthritis, severity, and acuteness of the arthritis, I will then help the patient decide whether to add traditional therapies, alternatives, or a combination of both.

STEAMED ASPARAGUS

Asparagus is a great springtime vegetable. When it is in full season it is usually quite affordable. One pound is usually enough for four servings.

	Water
1 tsp.	**Honey**
1 tsp.	**Fresh Lemon Juice**
1 lb.	**Fresh Asparagus, cut off growing end about 2"**

Method of Preparation

In your vegetable steaming pot, place the water, honey and lemon juice. Then put the steamer in and place the asparagus on top. Turn the heat on high and steam till tender.

Yield
Serves 4

Cooking Method
Steam

BEANS: GREEN AND YELLOW

Green beans and yellow wax beans are commonly called snap beans. Both of them are usually available year round, but are at their best from June to September. Both beans are just about equal in nutritional value, except the green ones contain about twice as much vitamin A. One pound usually feeds 4 people.

Look for green and yellow beans that are about as thin as a pencil. They should have smooth pods. If they are sold loose, pick ones that have the same size for even cooking. Avoid beans that are limp or spotted with brown. Green beans should have a very intense color; yellow ones should have a shiny Manila color, possibly tinged with light green.

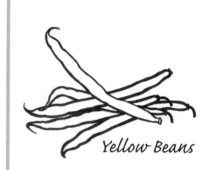
Yellow Beans

GREEN BEANS SAUTÉED WITH SLICED ALMONDS

Here in Maui we have exceptionally sweet fruit. I use their juices often in cooking. If your juice needs a little sweetener, just add a little bit of honey.

2-3 oz.	Shallot Oil (recipe in book)
1 lb.	Fresh Green Beans, cleaned and blanched
1/4 cup	Finely Chopped Parsley
1/2 cup	Sliced or Slivered Almonds
1 oz.	Fresh Orange or Tangerine Juice
	Salt Substitute to taste
	Coarse Ground Black Pepper to taste

Method of Preparation
In a large sauté pan, over medium heat, place the shallot oil and heat till hot. Add the green beans and sauté for 2-3 minutes. Add the parsley, almonds, and tangerine or orange juice, and continue cooking for 2 more minutes, or until the beans are piping hot. Season to taste. Serve immediately.

Yield
Serves 4

Cooking Method
Sauté

Nutritional Analysis

Per Serving
Energy	*241 calories*
Protein	*4.7 gm*
Fat	*20.7 gm*
Carbohydrate	*12.6 gm*
Fiber	*3.6 gm*
Cholesterol	*0 mg*
Iron	*2.2 mg*
Sodium	*7 mg*
Calcium	*91 mg*
Sugar	*2.9 gm*

Recipe Cost: $1.61

Lifestyle Tip
To avoid falling, keep hallways, stairs, and rooms well lit.

Diet Tip
Do not use soda when cooking vegetables. It destroys the vitamins you are after.

Chapter 19 Facts About Veggies & Garlic   255

Nutritional Analysis

Per Serving
Energy   *197 calories*
Protein   *6.2 gm*
Fat   *14.1 gm*
Carbohydrate   *15.6 gm*
Fiber   *3.7 gm*
Cholesterol   *0 mg*
Iron   *2.6 mg*
Sodium   *11 mg*
Calcium   *74 mg*
Sugar   *3.5 gm*

Recipe Cost: $3.92

Lifestyle Tip
To avoid falls, keep a flashlight beside your bed and use it if you get up during the night.

Diet Tip
Carotenoids obtained from pigments of colorful fruits and leafy vegetables such as apricot, peach, strawberry, cantaloupe, mango, papaya, carrot, spinach, squash, greens, broccoli, pink grapefruit, sweet potato, kale, red bell pepper, watercress, and onions have been shown to decrease the free radicals which contribute to joint inflammation.

GREEN BEAN SALAD WITH MUSHROOMS AND SPROUTS

Beans, mushrooms, sprouts: healthy, healthy, healthy, and healthy for you.

1	**Recipe of Green Beans Sautéed with Sliced Almonds, cooled and refrigerated 2 hours**
1 lb.	**Sprouts, your favorite kind**
1/2 lb.	**Sliced Mushrooms, your favorite kind**
2 oz.	**Fresh Orange or Tangerine Juice**

Method of Preparation
In a large bowl, toss everything together and mix well. Refrigerate 1 hour.

Serve on a bed of your favorite lettuce and garnish with a few pieces of fresh tangerine.

Yield
Serves 6 for a healthy, hearty lunch

Cooking Method
Sauté

GREEN BEANS IN OLIVE OIL WITH GARLIC AND NUTS

This is such a wonderful combination of flavors, that just about melts in your mouth.

2 oz.	Olive Oil
1 Tbsp.	Chopped Garlic
1 oz.	Tangerine, Lemon, or Orange Juice
1 lb.	Whole Green Beans, stems removed and blanched until tender
1/4 cup	Your Favorite Nuts, chopped fine or crushed with a rolling pin to desired consistency
	Salt Substitute to taste
	Fresh Ground Black Pepper to taste

Method of Preparation
Heat olive oil till hot. Add garlic and sauté 2 minutes. Add juice and green beans. Cook till green beans are hot, then add the nuts and cook 1 more minute. Add salt substitute and pepper to taste.

Yield
Serves 4

Hint
With all the types of beans, nuts, and juice available, just think of all the different ways you can make this simple recipe. The combination of flavors is simply too great to even consider trying to list. Yum! Yum!! Yum!!!

Cooking Method
Blanch, sauté

Nutritional Analysis

Per Serving

Energy	*222 calories*
Protein	*3.8 gm*
Fat	*18.9 gm*
Carbohydrate	*12.6 gm*
Fiber	*2.9 gm*
Cholesterol	*0 mg*
Iron	*1.8 mg*
Sodium	*5 mg*
Calcium	*64 mg*
Sugar	*2.2 gm*

Recipe Cost: $2.33

Lifestyle Tip
Avoid throw rugs. They make a dangerous slippery surface.

Health Tip
Always inform your doctor of all supplements that you are taking. If you have a serious illness, a history of liver or kidney disease, are pregnant, or are taking anticoagulant medications (Coumadin, Ticlid, Plavix, heparin, etc.) always check with your doctor before starting any supplements or herbs.

Chapter 19 Facts About Veggies & Garlic 257

Nutritional Analysis

Per Serving
Energy	*265 calories*
Protein	*5.3 gm*
Fat	*22.7 gm*
Carbohydrate	*14 gm*
Fiber	*3.9 gm*
Cholesterol	*0 mg*
Iron	*2.4 mg*
Sodium	*8 mg*
Calcium	*7 mg*
Sugar	*0.1 gm*

Recipe Cost: $2.94

Lifestyle Tip
Use non-skid wax on floors to prevent slips.

Health Tip
Rheumatoid arthritis is a crippling and disabling disease. New therapeutic options have been developed over the past five years. These new drugs have the potential to change the downward spiral of rheumatoid arthritis. Methotrexate is considered the gold standard in the pharmacological treatment of rheumatoid arthritis. Since 1998, several new innovative treatments have entered the market such as Arava (leflunomide), Enbrel (etanercept), and Remicade (infliximab).

YELLOW BEANS WITH NUTS AND GARLIC CHIVES

In using most beans from the string or pod families, you can plan on using one pound for four people.

2 oz.	Garlic Oil (see page 266)
1 lb.	Fresh Yellow Beans, cleaned and blanched
1/2 cup	Crushed Nuts, use your favorite kind
1/4 cup	Finely Chopped Parsley
1/4 cup	Finely Chopped Garlic Chives
	Salt Substitute to taste

Method of Preparation
In a large sauté pan over medium high heat, place the garlic oil; when hot, add the yellow beans and sauté for 2-3 minutes. Add the nuts, parsley, and garlic chives, and continue to sauté for 2 more minutes, or until the beans are piping hot. Serve immediately.

Yield
Serves 4

Hint
If you're a mushroom lover, add 1/2 pound of sliced mushrooms to extend the recipe and make it tastier.

Cooking Method
Sauté

SAUTÉED BEET GREENS

People usually throw beet greens away, but they are a great bonus that comes with fresh beets. Beets are usually fresh year-round, and are an excellent source of potassium.

1 oz.	Olive Oil
1 Tbsp.	Chopped Garlic
1 Tbsp.	Honey
1 oz.	Lemon Juice
	Salt Substitute to taste
	Fresh Ground Black Pepper to taste
2 lb.	Beet Greens, cooked till limp, then cooled, dried, and coarsely chopped

Method of Preparation
In a large skillet, heat the olive oil, add the garlic, and sauté over medium heat till you have a good garlic aroma.

Add all the remaining ingredients except the greens and cook till hot. Then add the beet greens and heat through. Serve immediately.

Yield
Serves 4

Hint
The beet greens are excellent with Orange Mustard Sauce (see Chapter 13).

Cooking Methods
Steam or boil, sauté

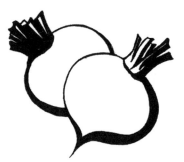

Nutritional Analysis

Per Serving

Energy	145 calories
Protein	6 gm
Fat	7.6 gm
Carbohydrate	18.1 gm
Fiber	2.4 gm
Cholesterol	0 mg
Iron	4.4 mg
Sodium	547 mg
Calcium	264 mg
Sugar	4.4 gm

Recipe Cost: $3.06

Lifestyle Tip
Install and use sturdy handrails.

Health Tip
There is sufficient circumstantial evidence to support the notion that rheumatoid arthritis is infectious in origin. At present, viruses are the leading candidates, particularly retroviruses. It is likely, however, that several viruses may trigger rheumatoid arthritis in a genetically predisposed subject or in someone who has a dysfunctional immune system caused by stress, sleep deprivation, lack of adequate water, and poor nutrition.

Chapter 19 Facts About Veggies & Garlic 259

BROCCOLI

Broccoli is an excellent source of vitamins A and C, and a source of potassium. One large bunch will usually provide enough florets to serve four people. The leftover stalks can be stir fried or steamed—just peel them with a paring knife or vegetable peeler first.

Broccoli should be a deep, rich, green color with tightly closed buds on a firm head. Avoid heads with yellow flowers. They will taste somewhat like cabbage because they are overly mature.

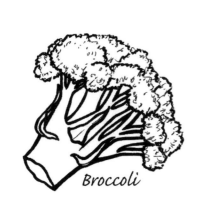

STEAMED BROCCOLI

Steamed broccoli...soooooo gooood for you!

1 lb.	Broccoli
	Water
1 oz.	Lemon Juice

Nutritional Analysis

Per Serving
Energy	4 calories
Protein	3.4 gm
Fat	0.4 gm
Carbohydrate	6.5 gm
Fiber	3.5 gm
Cholesterol	0 mg
Iron	1 mg
Sodium	31 mg
Calcium	55 mg
Sugar	2.4 gm

Recipe Cost: $1.09

Method of Preparation
In a pot with water and the lemon juice in the bottom and your stainless steel steamer, place the broccoli. Steam till tender.

Yield
Serves 4

Cooking Method
Steam

Lifestyle Tip
In the kitchen, make sure all items are within your easy reach.

BRUSSELS SPROUTS

Brussels sprouts are an excellent source of vitamin C and potassium. One pound will serve four people. Choose only the ones that are vibrant green. Pull off any loose or damaged leaves, and trim the stem end with a paring knife, then cut an X in the bottom.

They are excellent boiled, steamed, stir-fried, or microwaved. Bring water to a boil, then add Brussels sprouts and cook for about 12 minutes or until tender.

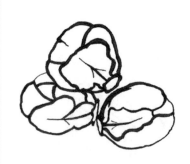

BRUSSELS SPROUT SALAD

This recipe comes from an old Army cook I had the pleasure of working with for a year or so here on Maui. Aloha, Gene!

1 box	Brussels Sprouts, frozen, or 1 lb. fresh
3 oz.	Red Wine Vinegar
3 oz.	White Wine Vinegar
	Salt Substitute to taste
1 Tbsp.	Caraway Seeds
1 Tbsp.	White Pepper
1 cup	Sweet Onion, diced small
2 Tbsp.	Honey

Method of Preparation
Cook the Brussels sprouts in boiling water till tender. Shock in ice cold water. Drain and place in a large bowl.

Heat the rest of the ingredients till they come to a boil. Simmer a few minutes, then pour over Brussels sprouts. Chill 2-3 hours.

Yield
Serves 4-6

Cooking Methods
Boil, simmer

Nutritional Analysis

Per Serving
Energy	77 calories
Protein	3.3 gm
Fat	0.5 gm
Carbohydrate	18.1 gm
Fiber	4 gm
Cholesterol	0 mg
Iron	1.6 mg
Sodium	21 mg
Calcium	51 mg
Sugar	9 gm

Recipe Cost: $2.23

Lifestyle Tip
Use a rubber mat or rubberized decals in the bathtub to prevent falling.

CARROTS

Carrots are native to Afghanistan. They spread under cultivation to the Mediterranean area around 500 B.C. They are a common garden vegetable which is grown for its thick, fleshy root. Carrots can be eaten raw or cooked. They seem to taste best when cooked in stews.

A carrot contains 10-15% natural sugar, and is also rich in vitamins B, C, and E. Carrots are also a great source of carotene, which converts to vitamin A when eaten. The darker the carrot, the greater the amount of carotene inside. The longer a carrot is stored after harvest, the darker it becomes, and the source of carotene is greater. It also takes on a more assertive, carroty flavor.

HONEY GLAZED CARROTS

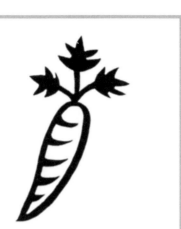

Heres a healthy choice for all of you carrot lovers out there.

1 lb.	Carrots, peeled and sliced thin on the bias
2 oz.	Soy Margarine
1 tsp.	Fresh Lemon Juice
4 oz.	Honey
2 Tbsp.	Chopped Parsley

Method of Preparation
Peel and slice the carrots; cook them in boiling water till tender. In a non-stick frying pan, melt the margarine, then add the lemon juice and honey. Cook over medium heat till the mixture bubbles.

Put the drained carrots into the pan and sauté, stirring with a wooden spoon till hot. Sprinkle parsley over the top of the carrots and stir again. Serve right away.

Yield
Serves 4

Cooking Methods
Boil, sauté

Nutritional Analysis

Per Serving
Energy   *185 calories*
Protein   *1.4 gm*
Fat   *5.7 gm*
Carbohydrate   *35.1 gm*
Fiber   *3.7 gm*
Cholesterol   *0 mg*
Iron   *0.8 mg*
Sodium   *178 mg*
Calcium   *38 mg*
Sugar   *30.1 gm*

Recipe Cost: $1.57

Lifestyle Tip
To avoid falls, keep electrical cords out of high traffic areas.

SAUTÉED RED CABBAGE

I used to make this in very large batches. I would cool it down, refrigerate it, and use it as a cold buffet item. It's great in the fall, and very inexpensive.

1	Medium Onion, diced small
2 oz.	Olive Oil
1	Small head of Red Cabbage, chopped bite size
1 oz.	Honey
1 oz.	Apple Cider Vinegar, unfiltered if possible
4	Granny Smith Apples, cored, skin on, chopped bite size
3 oz.	Chicken Stock (use recipe in Chapter 12)
	Salt Substitute to taste

Method of Preparation

Sauté onion in olive oil till transparent. Add the rest of the ingredients and cook over low heat for 20-25 minutes or till tender.

Yield
Serves 4-6

Cooking Method
Sauté

Nutritional Analysis

Per Serving

Energy	*183 calories*
Protein	*.5 gm*
Fat	*10.1 gm*
Carbohydrate	*24.8 gm*
Fiber	*4.8 gm*
Cholesterol	*0 mg*
Iron	*0.6 mg*
Sodium	*9 mg*
Calcium	*50 mg*
Sugar	*21.5 gm*

Recipe Cost: $2.61

Lifestyle Tip
For your feet's sake, wear comfortable shoes that provide the proper support.

Health Tip
Recent research has suggested that natural isoflavones, estrogen-like compounds found in soy, may be a boon to bones. Ipriflavone has been shown to prevent bone breakdown and help increase bone density. Ipriflavone is sold as Ostivone. Recommended dose is 1200mg a day plus Calcium Citrate 1500mg a day and Vitamin D 800 units. A bone density study should be obtained before you start this approach if you are postmenopausal. Repeat the bone density study approximately two years later. If there is bone loss, you need to consider traditional treatments for osteoporosis.

GARLIC

Garlic has been a valued food and medicine for thousands of years. Garlic is mentioned in the writings of the ancient Hebrews, Greeks, Babylonians, Romans, and Egyptians who celebrated its uses in food and medicine. An undisturbed head of garlic has little odor. The flavor and smell of garlic are due to water and oil soluble sulfur compounds that are created and released when the clove is crushed. These sulfur compounds are believed to have the medicinal properties.

Garlic is not only a strong-flavored seasoning for food, it's a powerful natural medicine. Garlic has the ability to lower cholesterol and reduce the clotting tendency of the blood. It can help lower high blood pressure, relieve arthritis, and boost the immune system. Raw garlic is a powerful antibiotic that is especially active against fungal infections. Eating several cloves of raw garlic at the first onset of cold symptoms is a home remedy worth trying. A clove, incidentally is just one segment of the head or bulb. Since garlic reduces the blood's ability to clot, people taking aspirin or blood thinners should talk to their doctor before eating more than one or two cloves of garlic on a regular basis.

Not everyone is up for eating raw garlic, but garlic loses its antibiotic properties when you cook or dry it. Commercial garlic capsules do not preserve the full activity of the fresh bulb. Try chopping garlic fine, mixing it with food, and eating it with a meal. Or you might cut a clove into chunks and swallow them whole like pills. To minimize the odor, chew some fresh parsley after eating garlic.

GARLIC: SOME FACTS

Garlic flesh contains the same sulphur compounds responsible for the pungency of onions, which can be controlled by preparing it properly. "Garlic oils" don't exist in whole, undisturbed garlic flesh. Only when garlic is crushed do the cells produce the oil, in an enzymatic reaction.

Take a whole bulb of garlic and roast it in some olive oil in an oven dish at 350°F for 25-35 minutes. Baste it frequently. The garlic is ready to eat when the flesh is tender when pierced.

Remove from oven and place it on a cutting board. Now tenderly mash it. It will be a paste, which you can use in many culinary dishes. For people who don't like the strong taste of garlic, this is the way to prepare it.

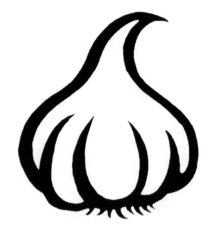

Health Tip
Garlic, ginger, and turmeric (the main ingredient in curry) have powerful immunity stimulating effects. Each day consume three cloves of garlic (or four 500mg garlic pills), one teaspoon of ginger (or four 500mg pills), and one-quarter teaspoon of turmeric (or two 500mg turmeric pills). These spices have been shown to decrease the inflammation of arthritis.

Chapter 19 Facts About Veggies & Garlic

Nutritional Analysis

Per Serving
Energy   *423 calories*
Protein   *23.1 gm*
Fat   *29 gm*
Carbohydrate   *17.4 gm*
Fiber   *0.3 gm*
Cholesterol   *67 mg*
Iron   *1.4 mg*
Sodium   *134 mg*
Calcium   *54 mg*
Sugar   *0.2 gm*

Recipe Cost: $4.16

Lifestyle Tip
Keep fire extinguishers in places throughout your home where fires may occur—especially in the kitchen and workshop areas—and make sure you know how to use them.

CREAM OF ROASTED GARLIC SOUP WITH CHICKEN

8	Cloves of Fresh Garlic
2 oz.	Olive Oil
1-1/2 qt.	Chicken Stock (use recipe in Chapter 12)
2 cups	Heavy Cream, health food store substitute
2 cups	Cooked Chicken, sliced bite size
	Salt Substitute to taste
	White Pepper to taste
2 Tbsp.	Fresh Chopped Parsley

Method of Preparation
In a shallow oven dish, place the garlic and olive oil. Roast at 350°F for 25-35 minutes, or until tender. Baste every 15 minutes with the hot olive oil. When done, remove from oven, cool, and mash so you have a paste.

In a pot, place the garlic paste and chicken broth. Bring to a boil, stirring constantly. Heat the cream substitute to just below a boil and add to the pot.

Then add chicken, salt substitute, and white pepper. Stir well. Finally, add chopped fresh parsley and stir well. Serve immediately.

Yield
Serves 4-6 for a very healthy meal

Cooking Methods
Roast, boil

266 The Executive Chef's Arthritis Cookbook and Health Guide

GARLIC OIL

This recipe makes a wonderful oil in which to sauté all your favorite foods for a garlic flavor.

20	Garlic Cloves, peeled, smashed and cut in half lengthwise, or chopped in food processor
1 cup	Olive Oil
1 cup	Canola Oil

Method of Preparation

Place the garlic in a 1 quart jar, then fill it up with the oils. Close the lid and refrigerate for 1 week before using.

The oil will last up to 4 weeks when properly refrigerated. When finished, throw away the garlic.

Nutritional Analysis
(1 ounce garlic oil)

Energy	243 calories
Protein	0.1 gm
Fat	27.1 gm
Carbohydrate	0.6 gm
Fiber	0 gm
Cholesterol	0 mg
Iron	0.1 mg
Sodium	0 mg
Calcium	3 mg
Sugar	0 gm

Recipe Cost: $2.80

Lifestyle Tip
Today scientists are looking at four broad areas of arthritis research: causes, treatments, education, and prevention. Get more information from the Arthritis Foundation.

Diet Tip
Researchers have observed powerful anti-inflammatory properties in chives, leeks, shallots, scallions, garlic, and onions that are beneficial for reducing the symptoms of arthritis. Garlic also has powerful effects on free radicals.

Chapter 19 Facts About Veggies & Garlic 267

LEEKS

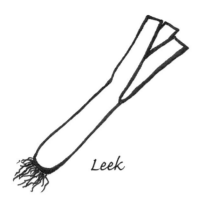
Leek

Leeks contain calcium, potassium, and vitamin C. They are a good source of fiber. Select leeks which are unwrapped and untrimmed, have a clean white base, and are firm with fresh leaves.

For use, cut off leaves about three inches above the white part (you can use the leaves in a vegetable broth), cut in half lengthwise, and clean out any dust by running under cold tap water till clean.

MUSHROOMS

Mushrooms are an edible fungus. There are over 38,000 kinds of mushrooms throughout the world. They come in all shapes and sizes. About 3/4 of them are edible, but only 2,000 or so varieties are palatable. Even fewer varieties are deadly—about 1 to 2 percent. Mushrooms are found wild in all temperate parts of the world.

Mushrooms

The stem and cap of the mushroom are the fruit, not the fungus. The fungus grows underground and consists of a mass of thin, thread-like roots or stems called spawn. Mushrooms that are commercially grown are started from the spawn, not the seeds, which are called spores.

The mushroom industry started in the United States in southwest Pennsylvania, and now Kennet Square is called the mushroom capital of the world. The famous limestone caves of Pennsylvania are ideal growing areas. Many other areas around the United States also grow mushrooms. The particular and delicate flavor of the mushroom is present in fresh and dried forms only.

When preparing mushrooms, remember that they are very absorbent. If necessary, gently wipe with a damp cloth and trim the ends of the stems. If you feel you need to rinse them, do so by holding each mushroom under running cold water. Never allow them to sit in water; they will become soggy.

SAUTÉED MUSHROOMS WITH ORANGE MUSTARD SAUCE

Here is a flavorful dish for all of you mushroom lovers out there. You'll need one pound of mushrooms, sliced bite size. Shiitake, button, oyster, porcini, morels, chantarelles—use your favorite kind, or a combination.

1 lb.	Mushrooms
1 oz.	Olive Oil
4 oz.	Soybean Margarine
3 oz.	Orange Juice
1 Tbsp.	Dijon Mustard
2 Tbsp.	Fresh Chopped Garlic Chives
	Salt Substitute to taste

Method of Preparation
In a bowl, toss the mushrooms in a little olive oil, just enough to coat them.

Melt margarine over medium heat, add the orange juice and Dijon mustard, then stir well. Add the mushrooms. Turn heat on high and sauté till they're hot.

Add fresh chopped garlic chives and the salt substitute. Stir well.

Yield
Serves 4-6

Cooking Method
Sauté

Nutritional Analysis

Per Serving

Energy	*136 calories*
Protein	*1.8 gm*
Fat	*12.5 gm*
Carbohydrate	*5.3 gm*
Fiber	*1 gm*
Cholesterol	*0 mg*
Iron	*1 mg*
Sodium	*259 mg*
Calcium	*10 mg*
Sugar	*1.5 gm*

Recipe Cost: $2.00 - $6.00 depending on the variety of mushroom used

Lifestyle Tip
Educate yourself! Read all you can about your disease. Get Arthritis Foundation materials and booklets. Go to the library. Get on the Internet. Read, read, read.

Diet Tip
Some sources have reported that eating almonds might be beneficial for arthritis. This is because almonds are a good source of copper. Most Americans' diets don't supply the recommended daily allowance for copper of two milligrams. Most multivitamins contain a copper compound (cupric oxide) that your body can't absorb. Choose multivitamins with easy to absorb copper sulfate or age-proof your diet with copper-rich nuts, whole grains, leafy green vegetables, and beans.

Chapter 19 Facts About Veggies & Garlic

ONIONS

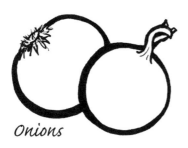
Onions

Onions are a source of vitamins A and C and folic acid. Sweet onions include the famous Maui onion, Walla Walla onion and the Vidalia onion. These varieties are grown in low-sulfur soil, which produces exceptionally sweet onions.

Other onion varieties include the red Italian onion, white Bermuda onion, yellow all-purpose onion, pearl onion and green onion. There are many other varieties throughout the world, but these are the most common here in America.

Onions and Tears

One school of thought for preventing tears is to thoroughly chill an onion before cutting. This seems to help somewhat. All of the other ways I have heard and tried don't seem to work for me.

There is only one true way to not have yourself bothered when an onion is sliced, diced, chopped, or whatever: ask someone else to do it.

270 The Executive Chef's Arthritis Cookbook and Health Guide

MAUI ONIONS AND MUSHROOMS

I created this recipe while here on Maui. It has been very well received over the years. The alcohol cooks out and you have a very mild brandy taste which is very enjoyable.

4	Cloves of Garlic, chopped fine
1 oz.	Olive Oil
3/8 cup	Heavy Cream, use health food store variety made with no animal products or preservatives
1 Tbsp.	Fresh Lemon Juice
2 oz.	White Wine
1 oz.	Brandy
2 Tbsp.	Parsley, chopped fine
	Salt Substitute to taste
3	Large Maui Onions, or another sweet onion, quartered twice
1 lb.	Medium Mushrooms, quartered

Method of Preparation
Over medium heat, sauté garlic in olive oil for 2-3 minutes. Add the rest of the ingredients except the onions and mushrooms, and heat for 2 minutes.

Add onions and heat for 6 minutes. Now add mushrooms and cook till just tender.

Dish out into small casserole dishes, and pour the sauce over top.

Yield
Serves 6-8

Hint
You had better make some garlic bread with this recipe! The sauce tastes sooo good you'll want to sop it all up.

Cooking Method
Sauté

Nutritional Analysis

Per Serving

Energy	103 calories
Protein	1.5 gm
Fat	4.8 gm
Carbohydrate	11.4 gm
Fiber	2 gm
Cholesterol	0 mg
Iron	0.4 mg
Sodium	14 mg
Calcium	27 mg
Sugar	6.7 gm

Recipe Cost: $4.93

Lifestyle Tip
By joining the Arthritis Foundation you get their wonderful magazine, *Arthritis Today*. It contains the latest up-to-date stories to help you with your disease.

Diet Tip
For optimal immunity you need a minimum of two servings of fruit and a minimum of five servings of vegetables each day. Fruits and vegetables contain hundred of phytochemicals. These natural substances protect cells against damaging effects of free radicals and boost the synthesis of neutralizing enzymes. Eat a variety of colorful fruits and vegetables for optimal benefit. Half the vegetables you eat should be orange or red and half should be dark green. Focus on fruits that are colorful all the way through--blueberries, cherries, oranges, etc.

Nutritional Analysis

Per Serving
Energy	120 calories
Protein	11.4 gm
Fat	3.2 gm
Carbohydrate	10.8 gm
Fiber	1.5 gm
Cholesterol	74 mg
Iron	2.1 mg
Sodium	123 mg
Calcium	49 mg
Sugar	4.6 gm

Recipe Cost: $12.16

Lifestyle Tip
Stop clutter before it accumulates.

Health Tip
Do your homework before you go shopping for herbs. The name of an herb can mean many different things and be very confusing because of the various species, some of which have no value. Know the scientific (Latin) name of the herb and which part is used for medicine (root, leaves, flowers, or whole plant). Read the labels carefully. Make sure that the product contains the right plant part, otherwise you could be wasting your money.

STIR FRIED PEA PODS WITH SHRIMP AND WATER CHESTNUTS

Get out your stir-fry pan and try to keep your mouth from watering in anticipation of these great tastes!

1/2 lb.	Fresh Pea Pods, snow, Chinese, etc., (whatever kind you enjoy), make sure they're stringed
24	Medium Raw Shrimp, peeled and deveined
1	Small Sweet Onion, sliced
2 Tbsp.	Soybean Margarine
2 oz.	Orange Juice
1 cup	Sliced Water Chestnuts
1/4 tsp.	Sesame Seed Oil
	Salt Substitute to taste

Method of Preparation
String the pea pods, clean the shrimp, and slice the onion.

In a large non-stick frying pan, melt the margarine. When melted, add the orange juice.

Add the onion and sauté 2 minutes. Add the water chestnuts, pea pods, and shrimp. Cook until shrimp is done over high heat.

One minute before it's done, add sesame seed oil and salt substitute. Stir well. Serve your desired way.

Yield
Serves 4-6

Hint
This is a fine recipe for a luncheon or light supper. You can chill this and serve it over your favorite lettuce for a summer salad. Also, you could mix in your favorite sprouts.

Cooking Method
Sauté

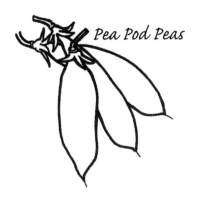
Pea Pod Peas

SHALLOTS

Shallots are technically a member of the onion family, but they possess a mild taste, totally unlike the strong flavors of the onion. Their scent is delicate, and almost never irritates your eyes.

Shallots are small and bulb-like, sometimes consisting of two or three separate cloves attached to the root end. The skin is reddish brown.

Shallots should be firm and heavy for their size. Smaller shallots have a more delicate flavor, but the larger ones are easier to peel. They will usually last two months or more if stored in a cool, dry place with air circulation. I keep mine in a wicker basket.

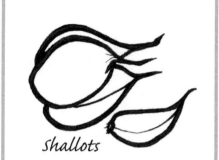
shallots

ROASTED SHALLOTS AND NEW POTATOES

A different twist of flavor. Roasted shallots are mild, and make this a great tasting dish.

2 oz.	Olive Oil
6	Large Shallots, cleaned
8	White Potatoes, washed and cut in half
1 Tbsp.	Chopped Basil
1 Tbsp.	Lemon Juice
	Salt Substitute to taste
	Fresh Ground Black Pepper to taste

Method of Preparation
Preheat oven to 400°F. In a large baking dish place half of the oil and all of the shallots. Add the potatoes and toss so they are coated with oil. Bake in oven, uncovered, for 12 minutes.

While baking, mix the remaining ingredients together. After 12 minutes, pour over the potatoes. Bake 15-18 minutes more, or until done. Remove and serve.

Yield
Serves 2

Cooking Method
Bake or roast

Nutritional Analysis

Per Serving
Energy	723 calories
Protein	14.2 gm
Fat	29 gm
Carbohydrate	106.4 gm
Fiber	11.2 gm
Cholesterol	0 mg
Iron	8.7 mg
Sodium	46 mg
Calcium	107 mg
Sugar	1.1 gm

Recipe Cost: $1.17

Lifestyle Tip
Work with a rhythm. Playing music helps.

Lifestyle Tip
The Arthritis Foundation has a toll-free information hotline at 1-800-283-7800. It has automated information on arthritis available 24 hours a day.

Chapter 19 Facts About Veggies & Garlic 273

Nutritional Analysis
(1 ounce shallot oil)

Energy	242.calories
Protein	0.1.gm
Fat	27.1 gm
Carbohydrate	0.4.gm
Fiber	0.gm
Cholesterol	0.mg
Iron	0.1 mg
Sodium	0 mg
Calcium	1 mg
Sugar	0.1gm

Recipe Cost: $2.97

Lifestyle Tip
Pulling weeds is much easier after a rain when the ground is still moist.

Health Tip
The Arthritis Foundation website is located at www.arthritis.org with information available 24 hours a day.

SHALLOT OIL

10	Medium Shallot Bulbs, peeled, smashed and cut in half engthwise, or chopped in food processor (most of the time shallots grow 3 bulbs per head)
1 cup	Olive Oil
1 cup	Canola Oil

Method of Preparation
Place the shallots in a 1 quart jar, then fill it up with the oils. Close the lid and refrigerate for 1 week before using.

The oil will last up to 4 weeks when properly refrigerated. When finished, throw away the shallots.

SPROUTS

Soybean sprouts, alfalfa sprouts, radish sprouts, mung bean sprouts...sprouts, sprouts, sprouts.

Bean sprouts have a subtle, nutty flavor, possess a high water content, and are usually available all year long. Bean sprouts are a good source of protein and vitamin C.

One pound as a side dish or salad is enough to serve 4-6 people. Soybean sprouts are slightly toxic and should be cooked so you don't get an upset stomach.

When purchasing bean sprouts, look for white shoots. Use them as soon as possible. Rinse sprouts thoroughly by running cold tap water over them. Place them in a sieve if necessary. Pick out the ones with dark green hulls and ones not crisp and fine. Pat them dry with a towel before use.

Sprouts can be added to many recipes, depending on individual taste.

ZUCCHINI

Zucchini are a good source of vitamins A and C. They have a mild, delicate flavor and are great simply sliced and sautéed; or stuffed and baked; or stir-fried, deep-fried, or many other ways.

There are three kinds of zucchini—the familiar green cylinder type, a milder golden variety, and round zucchini.

When cooking, leave the skin on. Wash well under cold water and dry. You can steam, deep-fry, stir-fry, bread or fry it. My favorite is sautéed with a little garlic and olive oil.

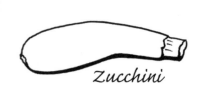

GRILLED ZUCCHINI

Here in Hawaii, we use fresh Kula zucchini when it's in season. Kula is a region of Upcountry Maui where the famous Kula Onion comes from. All the foods grown in this area are exceptionally sweet because of the soil.

3	Large Zucchinis, cut 1/4" on a bias
1/2 cup	Olive Oil
1 tsp.	Chopped Parsley
1/2 tsp.	Chopped Chives
1/2 tsp.	Chopped Basil
1 tsp.	Fresh Tangerine, Lemon, or Orange Juice
	Salt Substitute to taste

Method of Preparation
In a large bowl, place the zucchini. In a small bowl, mix the rest of the ingredients well, pour over the zucchini, and mix well. Refrigerate for 1 hour.

Heat your grill to 350°F and grill 2 minutes on each side, or place under a broiler for 1-2 minutes each side. Serve immediately.

Yield
Serves 6

Hint
This recipe can also be used as a cool vegetable salad for a summer lunch. Just cut the zucchini bite size, and chill, don't grill.

Cooking Method
Grill

Nutritional Analysis

Per Serving
Energy	173 calories
Protein	1.1 gm
Fat	18.1 gm
Carbohydrate	2.9 gm
Fiber	0.5 gm
Cholesterol	0 mg
Iron	0.5 mg
Sodium	3 mg
Calcium	16 mg
Sugar	2 gm

Recipe Cost: $1.88

Lifestyle Tip
Sitting on a garden stool could make your gardening easier.

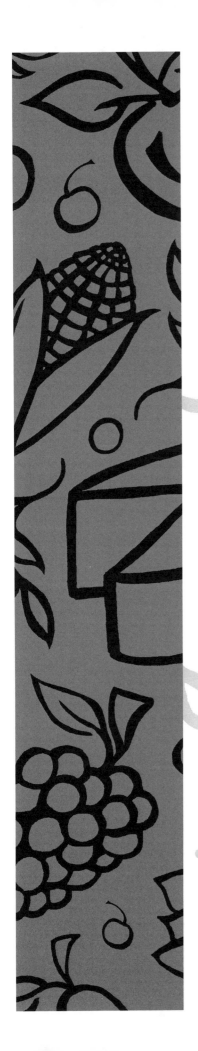
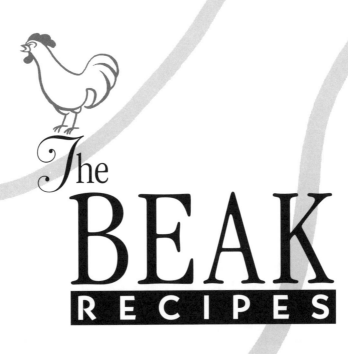

The BEAK RECIPES

CHAPTER 20

POULTRY

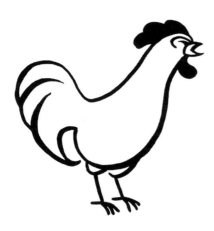

Chicken wasn't always as available as it is in today's market. It used to be a special treat, usually served for Sunday dinner or a special occasion. Chickens were so special because they also gave eggs, and you didn't want to eat the bird that feeds you. Only the young roosters were chosen to eat. What could be better than a heaping platter of fresh, tender, young, crispy fried chicken? Don't ask me!

Turkey was originally an American native game bird about the size of a pheasant. Long before the white man arrived, Native Americans had domesticated the turkey. Many years later, after cross-breeding superior strains of turkey, we now eat a much tender, juicier bird which requires less cooking time than its tough ancestors.

Here in America we enjoy a stuffed turkey, roasted and served with traditional giblet gravy, as a Thanksgiving or Christmas meal. The leftovers are used for sandwiches, soups, salads, and much, much more. Don't forget to check out Carl's Perfect Way to Roast a Turkey recipe.

There are many other types of poultry: game hens, ducks, geese, and capons, just to name a few. The library is a good source of books or cookbooks where you can learn about these great creatures that the Good Lord put on the earth.

BUYING, STORING, AND HANDLING POULTRY

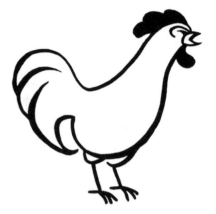

Buying Poultry
When you buy fresh poultry, make sure it has been refrigerated, and choose packages with little or no water in them.

Good quality chickens and turkeys have smooth, tight skin, with plump breasts and drumsticks. Skin color ranges from yellow to bluish white, depending on what the bird fed on. A chicken's skin color is no indication of quality.

Storing and Freezing Poultry
Fresh poultry is very perishable and should be cooked within three days of buying. You can freeze poultry just as it comes from the market. Add a layer of insulation, such as freezer wrap or aluminum foil, to prevent freezer burn. Squeeze the excess air out of the package before freezing. Use within 4 to 6 months. When you bone poultry, save and freeze the trimmings for your stocks and sauces.

Thawing Frozen Poultry
Thaw in the refrigerator to prevent bacterial growth. Allow 24 hours for a whole chicken, 4 to 8 hours for the parts. Whole turkeys will take up to three days to defrost, depending on their size. Thawing under cold water usually takes 6 to 8 hours. This method keeps all the parts cooled until the entire bird is thawed.

Never thaw poultry at room temperature! That can cause rapid bacterial growth, and that bacteria can make you very ill or even kill you. The danger zone for all foods is 45°F to 140°F.

Testing Poultry for Doneness
The cooking method you use determines how you test for the doneness of poultry. You can roast, bake, broil, fry, simmer, steam, poach, or barbecue poultry. You can also *imu* it ("cook in a hot underground pit") as we do here in Hawaii.

A meat thermometer is the most accurate way to check doneness for a roasted turkey or chicken. Insert the thermometer into the thickest part of the thigh, but not touching the bone. When done, it should read 185°F. Stuffing should be cooked to an internal temperature of 165°F.

A test that seems to work well for all types of poultry is to make a slash in the thickest part of the meat. It should not look pink. Also, inserting a fork into the thickest part of the thigh will let you know it's done, if the juices run clear.

Chapter 20 Beak Recipes

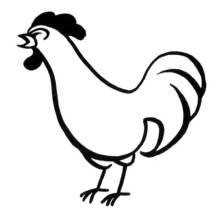

POULTRY CLASSIFICATION AND POINTERS

Rock Cornish Game Hen
Very tender, suitable for all cooking techniques. Delicately flavored, a hybrid developed from the Cornish breed of chicken.
Small birds yield   1 serving
Large birds   2 servings
Age: 4 - 6 weeks   Weight: 1 - 1-1/2 pounds

Fryer, Broiler
Very tender, suitable for all cooking techniques. These are the perfect all-purpose birds. They are sold whole, cut up, and in parts, boned or bone-in.
Age: 8 - 12 weeks   Weight: 3 - 4 pounds

Roaster
Very tender, suitable for all cooking techniques. They are a good choice when serving dinner for six.
Yield: approximately 7 servings
Age: 2-1/2 - 5 months   Weight: 5 - 6 pounds

Stewing Hen
Old female birds; they require slow, moist cooking. Used in soups or stews, a long, slow simmering brings out their flavor.
Age: Over 10 months   Weight: 3 - 5 pounds

Capon (castrated male)
Very tender. Usually roasted.
Age: Under 8 months   Weight: 5 - 8 pounds

Young Hen or Tom Turkey
Tender, suitable for all cooking techniques.
Age: 5 - 7 months   Weight: 8 - 22 pounds

Yearling Turkey
Fully mature birds, tender, usually roasted. Size has no bearing on flavor or tenderness. Heavier birds have more meat.
Age: Under 15 months   Weight: 10 - 35 pounds

Duck
Tender, usually roasted. Usually sold frozen, but some stores offer them fresh.
Age: 4 months   Weight: 5 - 6 pounds

Young Goose or Gosling
Tender, usually roasted. Usually sold frozen; often a special order item.
Age: Under 6 months   Weight: 8 - 14 pounds

TURKEY NOODLE SOUP
OR
TURKEY RICE SOUP

Here are two great recipes to make with leftover turkey. You can freeze the soup and use it a few months later, so you won't get tired of eating all the turkey at once.

1/2 lb.	Cooked Noodles
	or
4 cups	Cooked Rice
2-3 oz.	Soy Margarine
2	Large Carrots, chopped small
1	Large Onion, diced small
3	Celery Stalks, chopped small
2 qts.	Turkey Stock (see Chapter 12)
4 cups	Cooked Turkey Meat, cut bite size
1/4 cup	Finely Chopped Parsley
	Salt Substitute to taste
	White Pepper to taste

Method of Preparation
In a soup pot, place the margarine and melt over low heat. Turn heat up to medium, and add carrots, onions, and celery. Cook for 2 minutes. Add 1 pint turkey stock and cook until carrots are almost tender.

Add the rest of the ingredients, except seasonings, and bring to a rapid boil. Turn off heat and season to taste. Serve while hot.

Yield
10-12 servings

Hint
For you garlic lovers, use 2-3 ounces of garlic oil (recipe in book), instead of soy margarine. This will give the soup a slight garlic accent.

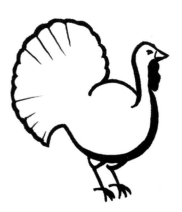

Nutritional Analysis

(Turkey Noodle Soup)

Per Serving
Energy	201 calories
Protein	23.9 gm
Fat	6.6 gm
Carbohydrate	10.1 gm
Fiber	1.3 gm
Cholesterol	57 mg
Iron	1.8 mg
Sodium	115 mg
Calcium	34 mg
Sugar	2.4 gm

(Turkey Rice Soup)

Per Serving
Energy	243 calories
Protein	24.4 gm
Fat	6.6 gm
Carbohydrate	19.6 gm
Fiber	1 gm
Cholesterol	57 mg
Iron	2.2 mg
Sodium	115 mg
Calcium	38 mg
Sugar	2.3 gm

Recipe Cost: $3.37 - $3.12

Chapter 20 Beak Recipes 281

Nutritional Analysis

Per Serving
Energy	*121 calories*
Protein	*17.9 gm*
Fat	*3.9 gm*
Carbohydrate	*2.7 gm*
Fiber	*1.1 gm*
Cholesterol	*43 mg*
Iron	*1.1 mg*
Sodium	*70 mg*
Calcium	*63 mg*
Sugar	*1 gm*

Recipe Cost: $3.14

Diet Tip
Cherries and strawberries seem to offer some relief to people who suffer from gout.

Health Tip
Cat's Claw has been reported to be beneficial in arthritis because of its immunostimulant effects. The problem is choosing the right Cat's Claw. The Cat's Claw plant (*Uticaria tomentosa*) exists in two types that are identical in appearance but contain different active ingredients. When shopping for Cat's Claw, look for a product that is certified to be entirely free of tetracyclic alkaloids.

WATERCRESS SOUP WiTH TURKEY

Here is another great fall and winter soup. So healthy and flavorful, it is great to enjoy.

1 cup	Onions, diced small
1 Tbsp.	Soy Margarine
6 cups	Chicken Broth (recipe in book)
2 cups	Water
1 lb.	Watercress, separated into tops and chopped up stems
3 cups	Cooked Turkey, diced bite size
	Salt Substitute to taste
	White Pepper to taste
	Croutons (recipe in Chapter 16)

Method of Preparation
Sauté the onions in the margarine until they're transparent.

In a soup pot, heat the chicken broth, water, and watercress stems until they boil. Turn down the heat and simmer steadily for 45 minutes. The stems will give the broth a light watercress flavor.

Strain the liquid and replace it back in the pot. Add turkey, watercress tops and onion; simmer for 30 minutes. Season to taste. Serve with croutons on top.

Yield
10-12 cups for lunch; or will feed 6-8 for dinner

Cooking Methods
Sauté, boil, simmer

282 The Executive Chef's Arthritis Cookbook and Health Guide

TURKEY SALAD/SANDWICH

Here's a tasty salad for you to make the first day after
Thanksgiving. I usually like to use only the dark meat, but use
whatever you enjoy.

4 cups	Turkey, cut bite size
1/2 cup	Celery, finely chopped
1 cup	Soy (or other health food store) Mayonnaise
2 oz.	Fresh Orange or Tangerine Juice
1 tsp.	Honey
1 Tbsp.	Finely chopped Parsley
	Salt Substitute to taste
1/8 tsp.	White Pepper

Method of Preparation
In a large mixing bowl, place all the ingredients and mix well.
Chill for 2 hours or until very cold. This gives the turkey
enough time to soak up the other flavors in the recipe.

To serve, place a bed of lettuce on a chilled plate and spoon
your desired amount of salad on top. Garnish with 6-8 health
food store crackers.

Yield
Serves 4-6

Hint
With 8-12 slices of cracked wheat bread, some chopped lettuce,
and 4-6 pickles, you have 4-6 sandwiches and garnish.

Nutritional Analysis

Per Serving

Energy	*593.calories*
Protein	*44.8.gm*
Fat	*44.2.gm*
Carbohydrate	*2.6.gm*
Fiber	*0.2.gm*
Cholesterol	*127.mg*
Iron	*2.9.mg*
Sodium	*118.mg*
Calcium	*47.mg*
Sugar	*1.gm*

Recipe Cost: $2.46 - $3.04
per sandwich

Diet Tip
Herbs can play such an
important role in flavoring
foods that you should feel
free to adjust the amounts
in any recipe to suit your
tastebuds.

Chapter 20 Beak Recipes

Nutritional Analysis

Per Serving
Energy   383 calories
Protein   33.9 gm
Fat   2.4 gm
Carbohydrate   11 gm
Fiber   2.4 gm
Cholesterol   105 mg
Iron   1.7 mg
Sodium   114 mg
Calcium   41 mg
Sugar   9 gm

Recipe Cost: $3.88

Lifestyle Tip
For grasping small items, use needle-nose pliers or long handled surgical tweezers.

Health Tip
The National Osteoporosis Foundation recommends 30 minutes of walking at least three days a week for stronger bones. Remind yourself that every time your feet hit the pavement, your bone-building cells are stimulated to make new bone. Drink calcium-fortified orange or ruby red grapefruit juice. They have as much calcium as milk. Absorption of calcium pills is better when you take them in divided dosage (500mg twice a day). Broccoli and almonds are loaded with calcium and healthier than dairy products. If you are over fifty, you should take 1500mg of calcium per day. If you are under fifty 1000mg is suggested.

ORANGE CHICKEN SALAD

I enjoy chicken salad at least one day a week. Here is a recipe and a variation that each have a slight orange flavor.

4 cups	Cooked Chicken, diced
1 cup	Celery, chopped small
1/2 lb.	Green Seedless Grapes, cut in half
1-1/2 cups	Fresh Orange Sections, cut in half
	Salt Substitute to taste
2 oz.	Fresh Orange Juice
1/2 cup	Soy Mayonnaise
	Boston or Bibb Lettuce

Method of Preparation
In a bowl, combine all the ingredients except the lettuce, and mix well. Serve on a bed of lettuce with 4-6 crackers as a garnish; also garnish with a sprig of fresh mint.

Yield
Serves 6-8

Variation
Leave out the mayonnaise and orange juice, and use enough Orange Cream Dressing (recipe in Chapter 16) to hold the recipe together.

Hints
Add 1 Tbsp. fresh chopped basil to give it a unique flavor.
Add 1 Tbsp. fresh chopped tarragon for another great tasting recipe.

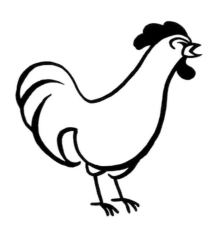

284 The Executive Chef's Arthritis Cookbook and Health Guide

APRICOT AND TANGERINE GLAZED GAME HENS

On a cold winter's day this great dish lifts your spirits and warms your insides so you can shovel the snow.

Herb Sauce:

1/4 lb.	Soy Margarine
1 tsp.	Fresh Basil, chopped
1 tsp.	Fresh Rosemary, chopped
1 tsp.	Fresh Tarragon, chopped
1/8 tsp.	White Pepper
	Salt Substitute to taste

4	Game Hens (1-1/4 to 1-1/2 lb. each)
1	Orange, cut into quarters
	Enough of your favorite stuffing for 4 game hens

1/2 cup	Apricot Jam
2 oz.	Fresh Orange or Tangerine Juice

Method of Preparation

Preheat oven to 425°F.

Melt margarine over low heat, and blend in the herbs and seasonings.

Remove game hen necks and giblets; reserve for other uses or throw them away. Wash the hens under cold running water; pat dry. Squeeze the orange quarters over the outside and inside of the hens and let dry.

Stuff the hens and coat the outside with the herb sauce. In a roasting pan, roast the hens in the preheated oven for 20 minutes.

In a separate pan, melt the apricot jam and orange or tangerine juice together over low heat. This is your basting liquid.

Turn the oven down to 350°F, and baste the hens after 10 minutes. Do it two more times. It should take about 1 hour total cooking time for the hens to be done and the stuffing cooked to 165°F (the proper temperature for doneness of stuffing).

Yield

Serves 4

Hint

With all the other types of jam out there, just think of all the variations you can come up with for this recipe. Just replace the apricot jam with your favorite.

Nutritional Analysis

Per Serving

Energy	1510 calories
Protein	136.3 gm
Fat	38.4 gm
Carbohydrate	152.5 gm
Fiber	3.1 gm
Cholesterol	518 mg
Iron	8.9 mg
Sodium	4023 mg
Calcium	308 mg
Sugar	22.5 gm

Recipe Cost: $10.57

Lifestyle Tip

Buy laundry detergent with a small cup inside so you don't have to lift a heavy box every time you do your laundry.

Diet Tip

Vitamin D allows calcium to enter the bloodstream, and reabsorbs some of it before the kidneys can excrete it. If you are under fifty, 400 international units (IU) are recommended. If you are over fifty, take 800 IU. This amount can be obtained in one to two multivitamins. Vitamin D can be obtained from fortified cereal, eggs, and saltwater fish such as salmon. It is recommended that you take a multivitamin for insurance.

Nutritional Analysis

Per Serving
Energy   *471 calories*
Protein   *53.6 gm*
Fat   *20.9 gm*
Carbohydrate   *15.1 gm*
Fiber   *3 gm*
Cholesterol   *149 mg*
Iron   *2.1 mg*
Sodium   *158 mg*
Calcium   *75 mg*
Sugar   *9 gm*

Recipe Cost: $3.91

Lifestyle Tip

Do all of your shopping at non-peak hours, then if you need special services you may be able to have them done for you.

Diet Tip

While there is no single diet that helps all people with all forms of arthritis, research studies indicate that a proper, healthy diet is extremely important in the management of arthritis. So take advantage of lots of fruits and vegetables. Eating the right foods and maintaining your recommended weight, or losing weight if necessary, will decrease some of the pain and suffering associated with arthritis.

PAPAYA SURPRISE FILLED WITH CHICKEN SALAD

People who travel to Hawaii love to try our papayas. They like the stuffed ones, so on our menus we give them a variety of stuffings.

3 cups	Chicken, white meat, cooked and diced
2	Celery Stalks, diced
1	Medium Onion, diced small (optional)
1/4 tsp.	English Mustard
	Soy Mayonnaise, to bind the salad, however moist you like it
	Salt Substitute to taste
	White Pepper to taste
1/2 tsp.	Fresh Lemon Juice
1 Tbsp.	Fresh Chopped Basil
2	Papayas, cut in half, seeds removed, and soaked in cold water

Method of Preparation

Combine all ingredients except papaya, mix well. Refrigerate 1 hour.

While salad is chilling, cut off the bottom of the papaya so it sits level. Put whatever lettuce is in season on a large plate, and place the papaya in the middle.

Now garnish with whatever you have to make this look attractive, such as cucumber wedges, black and green olives, 1/4 dill pickle, or a slice of orange twisted. Keep this cold until the salad is chilled.

Divide the salad in quarters and fill the papayas. This is a very attractive and impressive dish to serve.

Yield

Serves 4

286 The Executive Chef's Arthritis Cookbook and Health Guide

CHICKEN BREAST TERIYAKI STYLE

I have made this recipe at least a thousand times here in Alohaville.

6	10 oz. Chicken Breasts
	Teriyaki Sauce and Marinade, enough to cover plus 1-1/2 cup for the sauce (recipe in Chapter 13)

Method of Preparation
Place the chicken breasts in a container and cover with Teriyaki Marinade. Refrigerate for 3-4 hours.

You can cook the breasts any of these ways:

1. Bake in a 350°F oven for 15-20 minutes
2. Broil in the oven
3. Sauté them
4. Grill them over charcoal

When they're done, just cover with hot Teriyaki Sauce.

Yield
Serves 4-6

Hint
Fried Rice (recipe in Chapter 17) and a fresh green vegetable, whatever's in season, are excellent accompaniments.

Nutritional Analysis

Per Serving

Energy	398 calories
Protein	70.3 gm
Fat	3.5 gm
Carbohydrate	16.8 gm
Fiber	0 gm
Cholesterol	164 mg
Iron	2 mg
Sodium	224 mg
Calcium	31 mg
Sugar	0 gm

Recipe Cost: $4.69

Lifestyle Tip
Use a plastic drinking bottle with a flexible straw to water plants that are hard to reach.

Lifestyle Tip
Safe-proof your house. Floors seem to cause a great deal of pain and suffering for patients with arthritis. You are more likely to slip and fall on a waxy mirror-like floor. I suggest removing door sills between rooms to keep you from tripping or injuring your toes. Throw rugs could cause you to trip and fall. Install over-sized handles on doors, faucets, and toilets for convenience. No-slip strips in shower and bathtubs and a rubber-backed mat outside the tub or shower will provide firmer footing.

Chapter 20 Beak Recipes

Nutritional Analysis
(1/2 lb. turkey meat)

Energy	*386 calories*
Protein	*66.5 gm*
Fat	*11.2 gm*
Carbohydrate	*0 gm*
Fiber	*0 gm*
Cholesterol	*172 mg*
Iron	*4 mg*
Sodium	*159 mg*
Calcium	*57 mg*
Sugar	*0 gm*

Recipe Cost: $10.00 or so depending on what time of year you roast your turkey

Health Tip
There is no real cure for arthritis. With proper maintenance you are able to become much more comfortable. Read, read, read all you can about your disease.

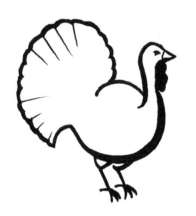

CARL'S PERFECT WAY TO ROAST A TURKEY

Turkey is excellent year round, not just at Thanksgiving and Christmas time. We once took a roasted turkey to a Fourth of July party. People were surprised, but it was the first dish to run out!

Method of Preparation

This recipe is for a 20-25 pound bird. If frozen, thaw the turkey for 48 hours in your refrigerator. It may require more time, so purchase it three days before you are ready to use it.

Now remove the giblet and neck package from the inside. Save the neck. Wash the turkey inside and out with cold water. Dry with a towel.

Cut an orange in half. Squeeze one half over the inside, and the other half over the outside. This will freshen up the turkey. Now fill the cavity with your favorite wheat bread stuffing. Truss the turkey with a large needle and thread. Tie the legs together with string. Tuck the wings under the back of the bird. The bird is now ready to roast. Rub olive oil all over the outside of the bird.

Preheat oven to 350°F. Now place the rack inside your turkey roasting pan, and place the bird on the rack. Roast it breast side up, covering your roasting pan and placing it in the oven.

Roasting time is approximately 5 hours. When the bird has been roasting for 3-1/2 hours, remove the lid. For the next 1-1/2 hours, baste the turkey every 15-20 minutes.

The turkey is ready when the legs move easily in their sockets, or when the juices run clear when a skewer is inserted into the thickest part of the thigh. You can also insert an internal meat thermometer in that same place and it will read 180°F when the bird is done.

Remove the turkey from the oven, replace the lid, and let it rest for 30 minutes. Remove the lid and place the bird on a cutting board. Untie the legs and the trussing thread. Remove the stuffing and keep warm. To reheat the stuffing, place in an oven-safe dish and bake in a preheated 350°F oven for 20-25 minutes. Now carve the turkey and serve.

If you can debone the turkey, do so and save those bones. You can turn them into stock using the recipe in Chapter 12, and you will be able to make soups, salads, and sandwiches from the leftovers.

288

CHAPTER

21

The
FIN
RECIPES

290

Chapter 21 Fin & Seafood Recipes

Diet Tip
Omega-3 oils such as salmon, fish oil, and flaxseed oil are important in the diet because they provide two of the most important fats for building tissue and construction of tissue hormones called prostaglandins. Fish oil can decrease the inflammatory response that causes the pain, swelling, and stiffness of arthritis. Eating salmon three times a week would supply recommended amounts of omega-3.

FISH AND SEAFOOD

The United States is surrounded by vast expanses of water. We also have many rivers, lakes, and streams. When the White Man first came to visit the Native Americans, the waters were teeming with a great abundance of fish and shellfish.

At one time, fish and fresh shellfish were only enjoyed in the limited areas where nature provided them. Today, thanks to air travel, modern refrigeration, and freezing, fish products can be enjoyed all around the nation throughout the year.

Thanks to the culinary influence of the great Chef James Beard, we are now able to enjoy and appreciate nature's bounty of fish and shellfish.

Most people tend to greatly overcook fish and shellfish dishes. Pay attention to the time and details of a recipe. Recipes in a cookbook are tested many times, at great length, for many reasons. Read, read, read.

Fresh fish is one of God's great treasures. There are so many kinds of fish, with so many different flavors for us to enjoy, that all are wonderful if cooked the right way. Don't be afraid to try some different varieties and also try some of the many different ways you can cook fish and other seafood products.

FISH FLAVORS

These lists group together fishes of similar flavor and richness. These different seafoods in each category taste a lot alike and usually can be prepared in the same manner. If a fish called for in a recipe isn't available, use a substitute from these lists. Learn the fish that are available in the different seasons. Whatever is abundant will be more reasonably priced.

Very Light, Delicate Flavor

- Alaska Pollock
- Brook Trout
- Brown Trout
- Cod
- Dover Sole
- Haddock
- Lake Whitefish
- Orange Roughy
- Pacific Halibut
- Pacific Ocean Perch
- Petrale Sole
- Rainbow Trout
- Rock Bass
- Smelt
- Sunfish
- Walleye
- White Sea Bass
- Yellowtail Snapper

Light to Moderate Flavor

- Atlantic Ocean Perch
- Atlantic Salmon
- Black Sea Bass
- Bluefish
- Brown Bullhead
- Burbot
- English Sole
- King (Chinook) Salmon
- Lake Trout
- Lingcod
- Mahi Mahi
- Mullet
- Muskellunge
- Northern Pike
- Ono (or Wahoo)
- Pacific Whiting
- Perch
- Pollock
- Pompano (or Papio)
- Rock Sole
- Rockfish
- Sablefish
- Sand Shark
- Scup/Porgie
- Sheepshead
- Silver (Coho) Salmon
- Sockeye (Red) Salmon
- Striped Bass
- Swordfish
- Tuna
- White Perch
- Yellow Perch

Strong Flavor

- Atlantic Mackerel
- Barracuda
- Freshwater Eels
- King Mackerel

SHELLFISH

Crustaceans (Crab, Lobster, Shrimp)

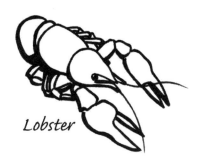
Lobster

- Alaska King Crab
- Blue Crab
- Crawfish
- Dungeness Crab
- Snow Crab
- Soft Shell Crab
- Stone Crab

- American Lobster
- Rock Lobster
- Slipper Lobster
- Spiny Lobster

- Brown Shrimp
- Cold Water Shrimp
- Pink Shrimp
- Red Shrimp
- Rock Shrimp
- Tiger Shrimp
- White Shrimp

Mollusks (Clams, Scallops, Oysters, Mussels)

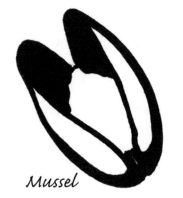
Mussel

- Butter Clam
- Geoduck Clam
- Littleneck Clam
- Pismo Clam
- Quahog Clam
- Razor Clam
- Soft Clam/Steamer

- Bay Scallop
- Sea Scallop

- Eastern/Atlantic Oyster
- Gulf Oyster
- Olympia Oyster
- Pacific Oyster

- Blue Mussel
- California Mussel
- Green Shell Mussel
- New Zealand Mussel

Others

- Octopus
- Squid

294 The Executive Chef's Arthritis Cookbook and Health Guide

HOW TO SELECT QUALITY SEAFOOD

Fresh Whole Fish

Good Quality
- Clear eyes; bright, bulging, black pupils
- Bright red gills, free of slime; clear mucus
- Flesh firm and elastic to touch, tight to the bone
- Ocean fresh odor
- Scales adhere tightly to skin, very few missing, bright color

Poor Quality
- Dull eyes; sunken, cloudy, gray pupils
- Brown to grayish gills, thick yellow mucus
- Flesh soft and flabby, separating from the bone
- Ammonia odor, fishy smell
- Dull scales, large quantities missing

How to store: Refrigerate covered, at 32-38°F. Store 1-2 days. Freeze promptly if you aren't going to cook it immediately.

Fresh Fillets/Fish Steaks

Good Quality
- Color varies with species, but should be consistent throughout meat, and bright

- Ocean fresh odor
- Clean cut flesh, free of skin, firm and moist
- Packaged with tight wrapping, moist appearing

Poor Quality
- Color shows bruising, red spots, yellow or brown edges

- Ammonia smell
- Ragged flesh, traces of bone and skin, soft and mushy, dried out
- Packaged with excessive liquid, dripping, smelly

How to store: Refrigerate covered at 32-38°F. Store 1-2 days.

Canned Seafood

Good Quality
- Cans not dented, full, free from foreign matter, vacuum sealed

Poor Quality
- Cans bulging and leaking, no vacuum seal

Frozen Fish and Shellfish

Good Quality
- Solidly frozen, glossy; when thawed, should pass the same criteria as fresh fish or shellfish
- Tight, moisture resistant wrapping
- Stored in lower part of freezer; temperature at least 0°F

Poor Quality
- Partially thawed, white or dark spots, signs of drying
- Packaging has a hole or shows ice crystal buildup
- Improper storage, excessive glazing

How to store: Tightly wrapped in a freezer of at least 0-20°F. Fat fish can be stored 1-3 months, lean fish 2-3 weeks.

Crabs, Lobsters, Crustaceans

Good Quality
- Legs move when touched, tail curled under, heavy weight

Poor Quality
- No movement, tail hangs limp, light weight, soft shell

How to store: Keep alive in well-ventilated refrigerator in a leak-proof container. Cover with a damp cloth. Store 2-3 days.

Seafood

Most seafood are low calorie sources of high quality protein. The fats in all fish and shellfish are mainly polyunsaturated and monounsaturated, so they have very little unhealthy saturated fats.

In addition, some fish have a unique polyunsaturated fatty acid called omega-3. This fatty acid is believed to help reduce blood clots, prevent heart disease, and lower cholesterol. You can read about this at the library.

New research has shown high amounts of cholesterol in shrimp and squid. Other shellfish have amounts of cholesterol comparable to most fin fish, which have about as much cholesterol as white meat poultry or other well trimmed meat.

Fish are low in sodium, but shellfish contain more than fin fish. All seafood contains some B vitamins, iron, potassium, magnesium, and phosphorous. In addition, saltwater fish contain iodine. Oysters are a rich source of copper, zinc, iron, and iodine.

COOKING FISH AND SEAFOOD

Cooking methods and other preparations used with seafood are: bastes, marinades, baking, barbecuing, curing, deep frying, broiling, smoking, frying, steaming, poaching, simmering, *imu*-ing ("using an underground hot rock pit"), and any other cooking method that strikes your fancy. The many ways of cooking fish and seafood are interchangeable for most dishes.

CRAB SALAD KULA STYLE

Here is a recipe I created one day by adding a little bit of this and a little bit of that to some leftover crabmeat.

1 lb.	Crabmeat, fresh (thawed, if frozen)
1/4	Whole Pimento, chopped fine
1 tsp.	Pimento Juice (remember what you read about the nightshade family)
1/2 tsp.	Dry Mustard
1/2 cup	Soy Mayonnaise
2 Tbsp.	Brandy
2 tsp.	Fresh Lemon Juice
1/2 cup	Crushed Macadamia Nuts or whatever nuts you like
1 cup	Sliced Mushrooms
	Salt Substitute to taste

Method of Preparation
Mix all ingredients well. Chill for 1 hour. Serve on a bed of fresh lettuce with a nice slice of fresh lemon, a slice of fresh pineapple, and fresh tomato slices, or whatever you think tastes good with this and makes it look attractive.

Yield
Serves 4-6 as a meal, or 10-12 as an appetizer

Hints
You can add 1 cup of fresh, seedless grapes (cut in half) to stretch the recipe, since crabmeat is expensive.

You can use this recipe for stuffing avocados, papayas, peaches, tomatoes (if you can eat them), or whatever else you like to stuff that goes well with crab salad.

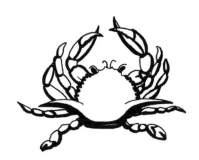

Nutritional Analysis

Per Serving

Energy	283 calories
Protein	15.4 gm
Fat	21.7 gm
Carbohydrate	4.9 gm
Fiber	0.8 gm
Cholesterol	74 mg
Iron	1.3 mg
Sodium	463 mg
Calcium	78 mg
Sugar	0.7 gm

Recipe Cost: $13.62

Lifestyle Tip
Buy a trash compactor to reduce the frequent task of handling your trash and garbage.

Lifestyle Tip
Make your home user friendly. Make sure the sidewalk leading to your house is even. If you have to go up any steps, make sure you have a handrail installed. Touch-sensitive lamps could be used. Make sure you have a couple of good sturdy step stools and high stools for sitting, with good rubber stoppers on the legs. Your back will thank you for a long-handled dustpan. Any convenience item that will make your tasks and living easier should be obtained if you can afford it. The less stress applied to damaged joints means less pain.

Chapter 21 Fin & Seafood Recipes 297

Nutritional Analysis

Per Serving
Energy   *1727 calories*
Protein   *1.7 gm*
Fat   *172.7 gm*
Carbohydrate   *7.2 gm*
Fiber   *0.2 gm*
Cholesterol   *116 mg*
Iron   *0.9 mg*
Sodium   *181 mg*
Calcium   *48 mg*
Sugar   *1.5 gm*

Recipe Cost: $5.-10 depending on the cost of the fish.

Diet Tip
Eat less (or no) red meat.

POACHED COLD FISH WITH OIL, LEMON JUICE, AND FRESH HERB DRESSING

I eat this for my lunch every day at work. It is so full of flavor, I never get tired of the taste.

4   **6 oz. Portions of Poached Cold Fish**

Dressing:
   24 oz.   **Salad Oil (your healthy choice)**
   8 oz.   **Fresh Lemon Juice**
                Salt Substitute to taste
   1/2 tsp.   **Black Pepper**
   1 tsp.   **Each chopped fresh herbs:**
                Basil, Dill, Parsley, and Cilantro
   2 Tbsp.   **Chopped Garlic**
   1 Tbsp.   **Chopped Shallots**

Method of Preparation
Poach your fish with the Fish Poaching Liquid (recipe in Chapter 12). Remove, cool, and refrigerate.

In a glass jar, place the dressing ingredients and shake well. You can keep the dressing refrigerated for 2-3 weeks. If you use olive oil, you'll need to temper it (let it warm up) for 30 minutes before use, because the olive oil solidifies in the refrigerator.

Now take a plateful of your favorite lettuces and mix them together. You can use up to two or three or four kinds if you want. Make sure lettuce is chopped or broken bite size.

Take each portion of fish and cut it bite size. Place the fish on top of the lettuce. Shake the dressing well and ladle 1-1/2 to 2 oz. over each dish.

Impress your friends! A very easy and tasteful culinary delight.

Cooking Method
Poach

298 The Executive Chef's Arthritis Cookbook and Health Guide

BROILED SEAFOOD BROCHETTE
WITH LEMON AND HERBS

Everyone loves making brochettes. They are always so healthy for you. Tasty and pretty, too.

8 pieces	Mahi-Mahi, Halibut, or other firm white fish, cut 1-1/2" thick; 1 lb. will make 8 nice pieces
8	Mushroom Caps
8	Cherry Tomatoes
8	Large Scallops
2 oz.	Olive Oil
2 oz.	Lemon Juice
	Salt Substitute to taste
1/8 tsp.	Coarse Ground Black Pepper
2 Tbsp.	Chopped Parsley
4	10" Skewers

Method of Preparation
Preheat broiler. Always preheat it when you are going to broil something.

Cut fish so you have 8 equal pieces. Start with 1 skewer: put on 1 mushroom cap, 1 piece of fish, 1 cherry tomato, 1 scallop, then another cherry tomato, scallop, fish, and mushroom cap. Do this for each skewer.

Mix olive oil, lemon juice, salt substitute, pepper, and parsley together in a small bowl. Brush the skewers well with this mixture.

Arrange skewers on a broiling pan with no holes, and place 3-4 inches under broiler. Broil 4-6 minutes on each side. Brush on the oil mixture several times while broiling.

Yield
Serves 4

Hints
When done, slide the skewered products over a bed of Fried Rice, and serve with Steamed Broccoli (Chapter 19) and Orange Mustard Sauce (Chapter 13). This is a basic recipe. If you enjoy shrimp, add 8 to the recipe.

Cooking Method
Broil

Nutritional Analysis

Per Serving

Energy	*265 calories*
Protein	*27 gm*
Fat	*15.4 gm*
Carbohydrate	*4.7 gm*
Fiber	*0.8 gm*
Cholesterol	*93 mg*
Iron	*2 mg*
Sodium	*153 mg*
Calcium	*14 mg*
Sugar	*1.1 gm*

Recipe Cost: $7.77

Diet Tip
Eat more fresh fish.

Lifestyle Tip
Never rush to answer the phone. Many fractures and injuries occur while trying to get to the phone. A speakerphone will allow you to converse without trying to hold the handset. Having a phone that you can program all your family, friends, and emergency numbers would be ideal. It is much easier to hit one or two keys than dialing a phone number.

Chapter 21 Fin & Seafood Recipes 299

Nutritional Analysis

Per Serving
Energy	*489 calories*
Protein	*32.1 gm*
Fat	*30.7 gm*
Carbohydrate	*35.5 gm*
Fiber	*13.6 gm*
Cholesterol	*56 mg*
Iron	*9 mg*
Sodium	*736 mg*
Calcium	*773 mg*
Sugar	*5.5 gm*

Recipe Cost: $14.09

Diet Tip
Avoid all dairy products coming from cows' milk.

Diet Tip
Green tea is very beneficial in protecting cells from disease-related injury. Green tea helps to prevent oxidative damage that can cause cancer, arthritis, and many other chronic diseases. It also increases the utilization of energy, giving a healthy boost far greater than caffeine. I recommend three cups a day.

ARTICHOKE BOTTOMS WITH KULA STYLE CRABMEAT

In today's world, canned artichoke bottoms can be found in just about any supermarket's specialty department. Usually there are 7 to 9 in a can. For this recipe, you'll need two cans.

2 cans	Artichoke Bottoms
1 recipe	Crab Salad Kula Style (see page 296)
1 lb.	Cheese. Use the health food store variety, made from cultured milk or organic tofu (which is lactose free and has NO cholesterol). Many types and flavors are available. Choose the one you like best with crabmeat.

Method of Preparation
Preheat oven to 350°F.

Trim off the stem of the artichoke bottom so it sits flat. In an oven dish or pan, place all the artichoke bottoms. Put an equal amount of the crabmeat on each bottom so you use all the crabmeat. Cover with cheese. Bake in the preheated oven for 10-12 minutes.

Yield
Serves 4-8 as an appetizer

Hint
In my experience as a fine dining chef, I have used this recipe as an appetizer for many years. It is a popular dish if you're in the restaurant business. If you have friends in the business, show them this recipe. I'm sure they'll thank you.

Cooking Method
Bake

SHRIMP COCKTAIL ON A PLATE WITH BASIL MAYONNAISE

Is there anyone out there who doesn't enjoy a shrimp cocktail? If so, try this variation and enjoy it.

1-1/2 qts.	Court Bouillon, recipe in Chapter 12
1 lb.	21-25 count Shrimp, thawed, peeled and
or 24 pcs.	deveined

Basil Mayonnaise:

1 cup	Soy Mayonnaise
1 Tbsp.	Fresh Orange or Tangerine Juice
	Salt Substitute to taste
2 Tbsp.	Fresh Chopped Basil
	Lettuce, chopped, for garnish
	Black Olives, for garnish

Method of Preparation

Bring the Court Bouillon to a boil, add the shrimp, and cook for 2-3 minutes only. Turn off the heat and let the shrimp sit inside the liquid for 1 more minute. Shock immediately in ice cold water with ice cubes in it. Let sit for 10-12 minutes. Remove and dry on a towel. Refrigerate.

Mix all the Basil Mayonnaise ingredients together. Stir well.

In each of 4 small dipping dishes, place 1/4 of the mayonnaise. On a 6"-7" plate, place some chopped lettuce. Put a dipping dish in the middle. Put 6 shrimps around the plate with a black olive between each shrimp.

Yield

Serves 4

Hint

You can add garnish of whole wheat crackers and whatever else you enjoy with shrimp.

Cooking Method

Boil

Nutritional Analysis

Per Serving

Energy	628 calories
Protein	24 gm
Fat	57.1 gm
Carbohydrate	6.3 gm
Fiber	0.8 gm
Cholesterol	190 mg
Iron	3.4 mg
Sodium	182 mg
Calcium	79 mg
Sugar	1.5 gm

Recipe Cost: $11.23

Lifestyle Tip

A speakerphone makes using your telephone much easier than gripping the receiver with sore hands.

Diet Tip

Thaw frozen fish in rice milk. This draws out the frozen flavor and makes the fish taste more like freshly caught fish.

Nutritional Analysis

Per Serving
Energy	420 calories
Protein	23.4 gm
Fat	33.6 gm
Carbohydrate	3.8 gm
Fiber	0.1 gm
Cholesterol	199 mg
Iron	2.9 mg
Sodium	899 mg
Calcium	96 mg
Sugar	0.9 gm

Recipe Cost: $13.13

Diet Tip
Eat plenty of garlic. Roasted garlic is very sweet.

Health Tip
Tips to lessen pain: set aside 10 to 15 minutes of privacy without noise; sit or lie in a comfortable position with head supported and eyes closed; breathe deeply for a count of 1 to 4, hold your breath for a count of 1 to 7, exhale slowly on a count of 1 to 8; while you are breathing, visualize all of your muscles relaxing and pain resolving. Relaxing music will greatly add to the experience.

SCAMPI OLOWALU

My long-time chef friend Drew Previti and I created this recipe. It was (and still is) the talk of Maui.

24	16-20 size Shrimp, peeled and deveined
1 cup	Sweet Butter, health food kind
3 tsp.	Capers with Juice
1/4 cup	White Wine
4 Tbsp.	Fresh Lemon Juice
2 tsp.	Chopped Parsley
4 tsp.	Chopped Garlic
1 cup	Heavy Cream, health food kind

Method of Preparation
Combine all ingredients, except shrimp, in a saucepan and bring to a rolling boil. Add the shrimp and cook for 2 minutes only.

Remove shrimp and continue to boil till sauce coats the back of a spoon. Put the shrimp in little casserole dishes, 6 per dish, and pour the sauce over the shrimp. The heat of the sauce will continue cooking the shrimp, and you'll have shrimp that is properly cooked, not rubbery.

Yield
Serves 4

Hints
Get out the French bread for dipping. This is a wonderful sauce.

This recipe is great doubled or even tripled.

Cooking Method
Boil

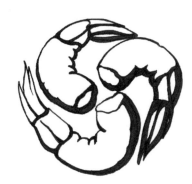

302 The Executive Chef's Arthritis Cookbook and Health Guide

SHRIMP SALAD WITH BASIL MAYONNAISE

For all you seafood lovers out there, here is a salad that's very versatile. You can stuff whatever you enjoy with it.

1-1/2 cups	Soy Mayonnaise (adjust according to taste)
3 Tbsp.	Fresh Lemon Juice
2 tsp.	Fresh Ground Basil
	Salt Substitute to taste
24	Size 16-20 Shrimp, cooked, cooled, and cut in 3 pieces
1/2 lb.	Fresh Mushrooms, sliced

Method of Preparation

In a bowl, whisk the mayonnaise, lemon juice, basil, and salt substitute together. Add the shrimp and mushrooms, and mix well.

On a plate with whatever fresh lettuce is available, place 1/6 of the salad. Garnish with a lemon wedge, sliced cucumbers, and carrot sticks, or whatever goes well and looks attractive. Do this for 6 plates.

Yield

Serves 6

Cooking Method

Boil or poach

Nutritional Analysis

Per Serving

Energy	*558 calories*
Protein	*13.1 gm*
Fat	*55.8 gm*
Carbohydrate	*3 gm*
Fiber	*0.6 gm*
Cholesterol	*127 mg*
Iron	*2.5 mg*
Sodium	*131 mg*
Calcium	*38 mg*
Sugar	*0.2 gm*

Recipe Cost: $11.59

Lifestyle Tip

Use a tablespoon as a doorstop: just turn the spoon upside-down and push the handle under the door.

Lifestyle Tip

If the everyday dressing routine presents some difficulties, try using velcro fastenings, nylon plastic clasps, and snap tape. Knits and stretch fabrics are particularly suited for women with arthritis.

Nutritional Analysis

Per Serving
Energy   254 calories
Protein   13.9 gm
Fat   19.2 gm
Carbohydrate   4.9 gm
Fiber   1 gm
Cholesterol   66 mg
Iron   1.3 mg
Sodium   412 mg
Calcium   74 gm
Sugar   1.2 mg

Recipe Cost: $17.13

Diet Tip
Apple cider vinegar has been shown to be a helpful aid for arthritic conditions.

CRAB LOUIS

This salad goes well with homemade corn bread. Thanks, Louie!

4-5 oz.   Crab Salad Kula Style (recipe in this chapter)
          Fresh Lettuce

Method of Preparation
Place the crab salad on a bed of lettuce. Now use your imagination and garnish the dish with whatever is attractive and in season in your area.

Yield
Serves 4

Hint
In the summer, there's such a variety of grapes to add. Just cut in half and remove the seeds if necessary.

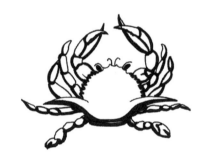

304 The Executive Chef's Arthritis Cookbook and Health Guide

BAKED STUFFED SHRIMP

Here's a recipe for you and your friends to cook and enjoy together. Baked stuffed shrimp goes great with Brown Rice (see Chapter 17) and Honey Glazed Carrots (see Chapter 19). Talk about a tasty, healthful meal!

24	Pieces of 21-25 Count Shrimp, cleaned and deveined
12 oz.	Crabmeat, cleaned
3 oz.	Soy Mayonnaise
1 Tbsp.	Fresh Lemon Juice
2 Tbsp.	Onion, chopped small
2 Tbsp.	Celery, chopped small
1 tsp.	Soy Sauce, low sodium
1 tsp.	Lemon Grass (white part), chopped fine
1/3 cup	Dried Bread Crumbs
1 Tbsp.	Chopped Parsley
	Salt Substitute to taste
1/8 tsp.	White Pepper

Method of Preparation
Preheat oven to 350°F.

Cut the shrimp almost all the way through lengthwise on the bottom side. In a bowl, combine the rest of the ingredients and mix well to make stuffing.

Stuff each shrimp with an equal amount of stuffing. Put them in an oven dish large enough to hold them all.

Bake in the preheated oven for 10-12 minutes or until done.

Hint
If you like cheese, sprinkle the tops with a health food store kind of cheese during the last 3-4 minutes of baking. This gives you another tasty recipe.

Cooking Method
Bake

Nutritional Analysis

Per Serving

Energy	*276 calories*
Protein	*27.9 gm*
Fat	*15.3 gm*
Carbohydrate	*5.6 gm*
Fiber	*0.4 gm*
Cholesterol	*170 mg*
Iron	*2.6 mg*
Sodium	*339 mg*
Calcium	*107 mg*
Sugar	*0.3 gm*

Recipe Cost: $19.46

Diet Tip
Use olive oil whenever possible. It is a monounsaturated oil which almost never causes allergic reactions and has major health-enhancing properties.

Chapter 21 Fin & Seafood Recipes 305

Nutritional Analysis

Per Serving
Energy   *251 calories*
Protein   *19.9 gm*
Fat   *16.3 gm*
Carbohydrate   *3.5 gm*
Fiber   *0.1 gm*
Cholesterol   *65 mg*
Iron   *0.6 mg*
Sodium   *567 mg*
Calcium   *262 mg*
Sugar   *0.3 gm*

Recipe Cost: $16.62

Diet Tip
It is highly recommended to add tofu to your diet.

CRAB DIP

What a great way to start a gathering with friends. Serve the crab dip first, with a seafood dinner to follow.

1 Tbsp.	Olive Oil
1/4 cup	Onion, chopped fine
1 tsp.	Fresh Garlic, chopped
16 oz.	Cream Cheese, health food kind
1 lb.	Crabmeat, cleaned
1/2 cup	Soy Mayonnaise
2 tsp.	Dijon Mustard
2 oz.	Fresh Orange or Tangerine Juice
1 tsp.	Chopped Parsley
	Salt Substitute to taste
	White Pepper to taste

Method of Preparation
In a saucepan, heat the olive oil on medium for 2 minutes. Add the onion and garlic, then sauté for 2-3 minutes, or till onion is transparent. Add the rest of the ingredients and heat till the cheese melts and is smooth. Stir constantly. Season with salt substitute and pepper.

Transfer dip to a serving dish; serve with nice crackers or toast points.

Yield
Serves 6-8

Hint
If you crush the pulp of 1 fresh avocado and add it to the recipe while the cheese is melting, you'll get a new recipe which will feed more people.

Cooking Method
Sauté

306 The Executive Chef's Arthritis Cookbook and Health Guide

OYSTER STEW

In early American days, oysters were very plentiful. Here's an old family recipe from that era that is still being enjoyed.

1 pt.	Oysters, in their juices
2 cups	Milk, health food kind, scalded
4 tsp.	Butter, health food kind
	Salt Substitute to taste
Pinch	Coarse Ground Black Pepper

Method of Preparation
Put oysters, with their liquid, into a small soup pot. Heat on low about 5 minutes; the oysters will get plump and their edges will begin to curl. Add the milk, butter, and seasonings. Simmer until butter is melted and hot. I add a little chopped parsley, but it isn't necessary in this recipe.

Yield
Serves 4-6

Hint
Oyster crackers are absolutely the only garnish to use with oyster stew.

Cooking Method
Simmer

Nutritional Analysis

Per Serving

Energy	108 calories
Protein	6.2 gm
Fat	4 gm
Carbohydrate	11.6 gm
Fiber	0 gm
Cholesterol	45 mg
Iron	5.6 mg
Sodium	154 mg
Calcium	138 mg
Sugar	3.7 gm

Recipe Cost: $5.69

Diet Tip
Steam all your vegetables—less nutrients are lost than when you boil them.

Nutritional Analysis

Per Serving
Energy 369 calories
Protein 20.7 gm
Fat 20.1 gm
Carbohydrate 25.2 gm
Fiber 0.7 gm
Cholesterol 37 mg
Iron 0.5 mg
Sodium 183 mg
Calcium 34 mg
Sugar 0.5 gm

Recipe Cost: $9.06

Diet Tip
Include plenty of wild rice in your diet. Eliminate white rice.

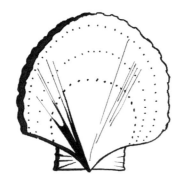

SAUTÉED SCALLOPS

In Greek mythology when Aphrodite rose from the sea, she skimmed over the Aegean waves on a scallop shell. Surely she got the shell from a chef who cooked the wonderful delicacy on the inside.

1-1/2 lbs.	Sea or Bay Scallops, fresh or frozen, washed if necessary
2 oz.	Fresh Lemon Juice
1 cup	Rice Flour
	Salt Substitute to taste
1/8 tsp.	Ground White Pepper
4-5 oz.	Olive Oil
1 Tbsp.	Chopped Garlic
1 tsp.	Chopped Shallots

Method of Preparation
Thaw the scallops if frozen. Remove any shell particles. Place the scallops in a bowl, pour on the lemon juice, and stir well for a minute or so. The scallops will turn a little white around the edges as you stir. Drain.

Combine the rice flour, salt substitute, and white pepper in a brown bag. Put the scallops in the bag and shake well.

In a large cold skillet, place the olive oil, garlic, and shallots. Turn the heat to medium. When you start to smell the garlic and shallots, turn the heat up to high.

Place the scallops in the skillet, 4 or 5 at a time, till they are all in. Cook until done (fairly firm to the touch). Take out and drain.

Place the scallops on a bed of Fried Rice (recipe in Chapter 17). Pour some Teriyaki Sauce, (see Chapter 13) or your favorite sauce, over the top. Serve with a fresh green vegetable.

Yield
Serves 4-6, depending on how much your guests enjoy scallops

Cooking Method
Sauté

308 The Executive Chef's Arthritis Cookbook and Health Guide

SHRIMP AND SCALLOP SEVICHE

Seviche makes a great summer seafood salad, or you can just eat it like it is.

1 lb.	Fresh Scallops, cut in half
1 lb.	21-25 Count Frozen Shrimp, thawed and cut in half lengthwise
6-8 oz.	Fresh Lime Juice
4 oz.	Red Onion, cut in half, then sliced thinly
4	Scallions, bias cut thinly
3 oz.	Olive Oil
1 tsp.	Garlic, mashed to a paste
1/2 cup	Fresh Chopped Cilantro

Method of Preparation
Combine all of the ingredients, mix very well, and refrigerate for 4-6 hours. Turn and mix every hour.

When serving, some people drain off the liquid while others leave it in the dish. Choose your own method.

Yield
Serves 6-8

Hint
Serve with a mixture of 2-3 lettuces for a great salad. Garnish with cucumbers, olives, etc.

Nutritional Analysis

Per Serving

Energy	*217 calories*
Protein	*21.4 gm*
Fat	*12.1 gm*
Carbohydrate	*5.1 gm*
Fiber	*0.4 gm*
Cholesterol	*105 mg*
Iron	*1.8 mg*
Sodium	*180 mg*
Calcium	*55 mg*
Sugar	*1.1 gm*

Recipe Cost: $16.18

Diet Tip
Eat more fresh green salads with plenty of fresh vegetable garnishes.

Nutritional Analysis

Per Serving
Energy	630 calories
Protein	23.3 gm
Fat	58.7 gm
Carbohydrate	2.9 gm
Fiber	0.1 gm
Cholesterol	172 mg
Iron	3.1 mg
Sodium	169 mg
Calcium	71 mg
Sugar	0 gm

Recipe Cost: $14.03

Diet Tip
Plan a good meal; it will lead to better nutrition for you.

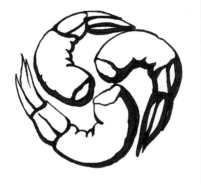

SHRIMP ON A SKEWER

Here we will bake shrimp that is so full of flavor it will make your tastebuds explode with happiness.

30	Pieces of 21-25 to a pound Shrimp, peeled and deveined

Marinade:

8 oz.	Olive Oil
4 oz.	Safflower Oil
1 Tbsp.	Chopped Garlic
1 tsp.	Chopped Shallots
1 tsp.	Chopped Parsley
1 tsp.	Chopped Chives
1 tsp.	Chopped Tarragon
1 tsp.	Chopped Basil
1 tsp.	Chopped Dill
1 tsp.	Chopped Cilantro
2 oz.	Fresh Orange or Tangerine Juice
	Salt Substitute to taste
6	Skewers, 10" long

Method of Preparation
Mix the marinade well, pour marinade over shrimp. Use a deep container (bowl, pan, etc.) so the shrimp will be practically submerged in the marinade. Refrigerate 3-4 hours; stir 3-4 times while refrigerated.

Preheat oven to 400°F. Drain shrimp from marinade (but don't put the oil down the sink!). Put 5 pieces of shrimp on each skewer. Place skewers on a sheet pan and cook 6-8 minutes, or until done.

Yield
Serves 6

Hints
Serve with Fried Rice (recipe in Chapter 17) and a nice green fresh vegetable.

Read in Chapter 10 about freeze-dried herbs.

Cooking Method
Bake

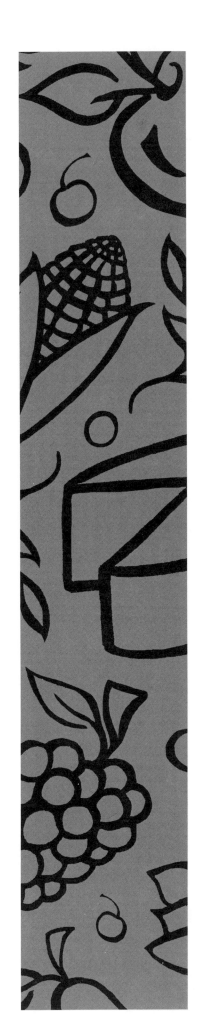
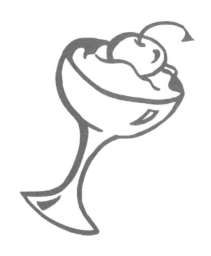
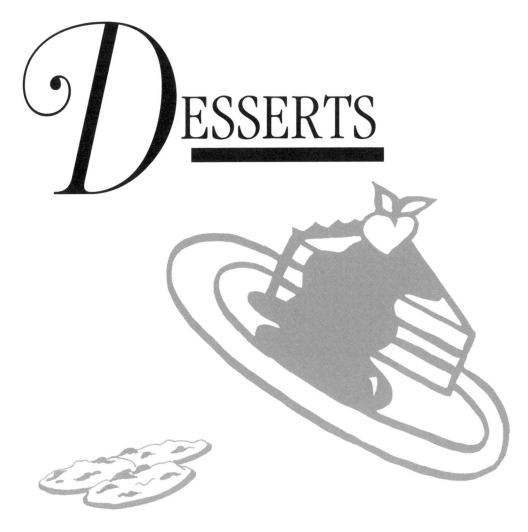

CHAPTER 22

DESSERTS

312

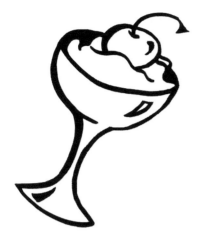

DESSERTS

Desserts, in one form or another, are enjoyed in almost all parts of the world, and have been since ancient times. Back then, eating honey alone or with other foods provided the basis for many desserts. Fruits and candied dates stuffed with nuts provided many people with simple desserts in early times. By the 14th century, desserts included cakes, rice with almonds and cinnamon, and figs prepared in a variety of ways.

When the settlers first came to America, Native Americans taught them how to make Indian pudding and many other desserts with this new product called maize or corn as we know it today.

Many countries have desserts originating within their own borders. The many types of land, population, and weather affect the different products available for cooking desserts. In many countries just fresh fruit is the dessert.

For many years desserts were served with the soup or meat course, not at the end of the meal as it is now.

Now that the world has become smaller through communication, knowledge is easily obtained about any subject, just about any time. The very same holds true for desserts. You can read the newspaper, watch cooking on TV, go to a seminar, or get on the Internet, just to name a few ways to gather dessert recipes.

Remember we want our minds to stay fit, so use it now, get up and read, research, and read some more. Make some new desserts and share them with your friends.

A chef learns many different tidbits of information. Here's a good one. My mom sent me a cartoon years ago that said, "Stressed? If you get stressed, eat desserts, because stressed is desserts spelled backwards!" I've literally told hundreds of people this throughout the years.

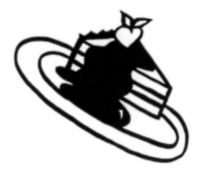

314 The Executive Chef's Arthritis Cookbook and Health Guide

A VERY SPECIAL RECIPE:
PINEAPPLE PAPAYA UPSIDE DOWN CAKE
BAKED IN A SKILLET

This is my great-grandmother's recipe. I added the papaya since we didn't have any back in Pennsylvania. When I was in junior high school I walked three blocks out of my way every day after school to sample her culinary delights with a glass of cold milk...perhaps an influence on my becoming a chef? This is the "I DON'T CARE!" great tasting, occasional treat.

1	Fresh Pineapple, skinned, cored, and sliced so you have 12 quarter-inch pieces
1	Papaya, skinned, seeds removed, sliced so you have 12 quarter-inch pieces
6 Tbsp.	Fresh Lemon Juice
1/2 cup	Butter
3/4 cup	Brown Sugar, firmly packed
1/4 cup	Oil
5/8 cup	White Sugar
2	Whole Eggs, plus 1 Egg Yolk
1-3/4 cups	All Purpose Flour
1/3 tsp.	Salt
2 tsp.	Baking Powder
5/8 cup	Pineapple Juice

Method of Preparation
Preheat oven to 350°F. Toss the pineapple and papaya in the lemon juice and drain. Arrange these alternately in the bottom of a 9" skillet. Melt half of the butter with the brown sugar, heating till all the sugar is melted. Pour this evenly over the pineapple and papaya. Set aside.

Pour the remaining butter and oil in a large mixing bowl, add the white sugar, mixing well. Add eggs and yolk and beat until light and creamy. Mix the flour, salt and baking powder together in a separate bowl. Add this alternately in 3 stages with the pineapple juice to the egg and sugar mixture, mixing well with each addition. Pour this on top of the pineapple and papaya in the skillet.

Bake in a preheated oven for 35 minutes or until done. Let rest for 15-20 minutes. Turn upside down on a cake platter, and now you have my very favorite dessert.

Yield
Serves 8-10

Cooking Method
Baked

Nutritional Analysis

Per Serving

Energy	*480 calories*
Protein	*5.4 gm*
Fat	*20.8 gm*
Carbohydrate	*70.5 gm*
Fiber	*2.1 gm*
Cholesterol	*114 mg*
Iron	*2.3 mg*
Sodium	*333 mg*
Calcium	*135 mg*
Sugar	*45.9 gm*

Recipe Cost: $6.37

Diet Tip
Use plain yogurt instead of cream and butter for low fat mashed potatoes.

Hint
You can use a boxed cake mix for this recipe. Follow the directions on the box, pour mixture over the top of the brown sugar, butter, papaya, and pineapple. Then bake according to directions on the cake mix box. This will give you about the same result as my cake mixture recipe here.

Chapter 22 Desserts 315

Nutritional Analysis

Per Serving
Energy — *357 calories*
Protein — *2.4 gm*
Fat — *13.9 gm*
Carbohydrate — *60.6 gm*
Fiber — *9.9 gm*
Cholesterol — *47 mg*
Iron — *0.9 mg*
Sodium — *31 mg*
Calcium — *71 mg*
Sugar — *42.8 gm*

Recipe Cost: $3.00 - $8.00, depending on the berries or other fruit you chose to use

Diet Tip

Remember about using too much salt. Water softeners often add a lot of sodium to your water.

Diet Tip

The USDA reports that the top sources of calories in the American diet are milk, cola, white bread, sugar, ground beef, white flour, and processed American cheese.

FRESH BERRIES WITH PURE MAPLE SYRUP

Chilled fresh berries, whatever's in season, picked fresh, with maple syrup on top, is truly one of God's exquisite culinary delights.

6 cups	Fresh Picked Berries, cleaned, washed, and chilled
6 oz.	Pure Maple Syrup
6 oz.	Whipped Cream, health food kind, whipped stiff

Method of Preparation

In a large bowl, place the berries and syrup. Mix gently so you don't damage the berries. Chill for 15 minutes.

Fill four frozen brandy snifters or small bowl with berries. Don't forget to put the whipped cream on top.

Berries: strawberries, blueberries, raspberries, boysenberries, currants, elderberries, gooseberries, mulberries

Other options: cherry varieties, apples, pears, oranges, grapes, melons of all kinds, peaches, apricots, nectarines, plums, mangoes, papaya, passion fruit, kiwi fruit. On and on and on. Just look at all the recipes from this single page.

Hint

Honey can be used instead of maple syrup, but don't use white sugar.

316 The Executive Chef's Arthritis Cookbook and Health Guide

PEACH CRISP

What is a crisp? Plain and simple, it is a pie without the bottom crust.

5 cups	Fresh Peeled Ripe Peach Slices
2 Tbsp.	Fresh Lemon Juice

Crumb mixture:

1 cup	Brown Sugar
3/4 cup	Whole Wheat Flour, sifted
3/4 tsp.	Ground Cinnamon
1/2 tsp.	Ground Nutmeg
1/4 tsp.	Ground Cloves
3/4 cup	Slivered Almonds
4 oz.	Cold Soy Margarine

Method of Preparation
Preheat oven to 300°F.

In a bowl, place peach slices and lemon juice and mix well. Now place in a well-buttered 13 x 9 x 2 inch standard baking pan.

Combine and mix well all crumb ingredients except margarine. Now mix in the margarine and crumble with your fingertips until the mixture barely clings together in lumps. Spread evenly over the peaches.

Bake in preheated oven for over 1 hour, or until lightly browned on top.

Yield
Serves 6-8

Hint
This is a basic fruit and crumb mixture. Now just think of all the different fresh fruits there are. You can use all of them in a crisp recipe. Experiment, use your imagination, and always learn, learn, learn!

Cooking Method
Bake

Nutritional Analysis

Per Serving

Energy	291 calories
Protein	4.2 gm
Fat	10.5 gm
Carbohydrate	49.2 gm
Fiber	4.2 gm
Cholesterol	0 mg
Iron	1.5 mg
Sodium	149 mg
Calcium	63 mg
Sugar	34.7 gm

Recipe Cost: $4.13

Diet Tip
Grow the fresh herbs you like in small pots on your window sill. There is nothing like the use of fresh herbs in all your favorite recipes.

Chapter 22 Desserts 317

Nutritional Analysis

Per Serving
Energy	*279 calories*
Protein	*4.4 gm*
Fat	*8.5 gm*
Carbohydrate	*49.3 gm*
Fiber	*1 gm*
Cholesterol	*74 mg*
Iron	*1.1 mg*
Sodium	*267 mg*
Calcium	*132 mg*
Sugar	*34.8 gm*

Recipe Cost: $5.83

Diet Tip
Buy some fresh ginger. Cut it into small pieces. Steep some in 10 oz. boiling water and strain into a cup: ginger tea.

WHOLE WHEAT BREAD PUDDING

Bread pudding is a very old dessert. Long ago when just about everyone was equally poor, even stale bread was put to use. That's probably why this great dessert was created.

2 cups	Soy or Rice Milk, hot
3 oz.	Soy Margarine
1/2 cup	Honey
2	Large Eggs, beaten slightly
1 tsp.	Fresh Lemon or Tangerine Juice
1/2 tsp.	Ground Cinnamon
1/2 tsp.	Ground Nutmeg
	Salt Substitute to taste
1 loaf	Whole Wheat Bread, cut into 1/2" cubes
1/2 cup	Raisins

Method of Preparation
Preheat oven to 330°F.

In a bowl, combine the milk, margarine, honey, eggs, lemon juice, and seasonings. Mix with a whisk until it's well blended.

Add the bread cubes and raisins, and mix well until the bread is completely wet.

Place the mixture in a well oiled baking pan. Bake in the preheated oven for about 1 hour, or until the mixture is puffed up and slightly brown.

Yield
Serves 6

Hint
Fresh fruit on top always tastes great!

Cooking Method
Bake

DOUBLE PEANUT BUTTER COOKIES

From *Prescription for Cooking*, p. 263.

> 2-1/2 cups Whole Wheat Flour
> 2 cups Unbleached Flour or Pastry Flour
> 1-1/2 tsp. Aluminum-Free Baking Powder
> 1 tsp. Sea Salt
> 1-1/2 cups Expeller-Pressed Vegetable Oil
> 2 cups Peanut Butter
> 1-1/2 cups Honey
> 3 Tbsp. Yogurt

Method of Preparation
Mix the dry ingredients. Cut in oil and peanut butter until resembles coarse meal. Blend in honey and yogurt. Shape into 2" roll and chill.

Slice 1/2"-1/4" thick. Place half on a cookie sheet; press, spread each with 1/2 tsp. peanut butter. Cover with remaining slices, seal edges tightly with fork.

Bake at 350°F for 12 minutes. Cool.

Yield
5 dozen cookies

Hint
Try adding a filling of carob chips and peanut butter as a filling.

Cooking Method
Bake

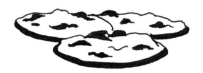

Recipe Cost: $4.84

Arthritis Tip
Never consume white distilled vinegar. Use pure apple cider vinegar.

Nutritional Analysis

Per Serving
Energy	254 calories
Protein	2.6 gm
Fat	10.3 gm
Carbohydrate	39.1 gm
Fiber	1 gm
Cholesterol	61 mg
Iron	1.3 mg
Sodium	231 mg
Calcium	11 mg
Sugar	25.6 gm

Recipe Cost: $3.06

Health Tip
Do everything in moderation. Eat, drink, exercise, and be merry—all in moderation.

Diet Tip
Red wine, red grape skin, and purple grape juice contain a polyphenol called reseveratrol, an antioxidant that appears to block tumor initiation, progression, and promotion while preventing the formation of inflammatory prostaglandins.

BANANA BREAD

This recipe is Thomas Walk's favorite. We're going against all of our own advice, but if you're able, enjoy!

2 cups	Sugar
1 cup	Butter
6	Bananas, mashed
4	Eggs, well beaten
2 tsp.	Vanilla
2-1/2 cups	Cake Flour
1/2 tsp.	Salt
2 tsp.	Baking Powder
1-1/2 tsp.	Baking Soda

Method of Preparation
Combine the sugar, butter, bananas, eggs, and vanilla. Mix well. Sift together the flour, salt, baking powder, and baking soda. Blend with banana mixture. Mix as little as possible.

Grease and flour 2 loaf pans. Pour half of the mixture in each pan.

Bake at 350°F for 55-60 minutes, or until nice and brown on top. Remove from oven, but leave in pan for 7-10 more minutes before removing to a rack to cool.

Yield
2 loaves of 10 slices each

Hint:
3/4 cup of crushed macadamia nuts are a simply marvelous addition.

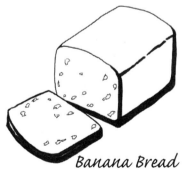
Banana Bread

320

CHAPTER

23

HEALTH FOODS

HEALTH FOODS

The use of products from health food stores is in its infancy. Yes, if you go there now they are usually pretty busy, but I believe there will be many, many more stores of this type in the near future. Healthier food, fresh from our local farms and shipped to us in a very short time is what we can all look forward to. With our ever-shrinking world of jet travel, shipping makes almost everything available to us.

You can visit your local health food store and spend an hour or so just looking at all the nice fresh fruits and vegetables, herbs, and all the other glorious products they have on hand for the betterment of your health.

Healing with food and food elimination diets is something that we have witnessed in our case studies. Food acts according to its therapeutic properties. Although it is sometimes slower to take effect, food profoundly affects all of our bodily systems.

We know that when our elimination diet is used correctly for prevention and treatment of arthritis, medicines are required less and often not at all.

Regarding health food from health food stores, we need to be knowledgeable about what we are going to eat now to replace the animal products that we have been eating for years.

Read – study – study – read – read and study!

HEALTH FOOD SUBSTITUTES

Here is a list of the major foods followed by the health food substitutes we are recommending. Research for this section was done by C. Siobhan Halstead, Manager, Down to Earth Natural Foods, and by Donnie McGean and Michele Heick, owners of Hawaiian Moons Natural Foods.

BUTTER/MARGARINE

Shedd's Willow Run Stick Margarine
lactose free, but 2.5g saturated fat per 1 Tbsp. serving
Soyco Rice Butter
no saturated fat, cholesterol, lactose, soy, or trans fats (hydrogenated oils)
Canoleo Soft Margarine
dairy free, no cholesterol or trans fats (hydrogenated oils), but l.5g saturated fat per 1 Tbsp.

324 The Executive Chef's Arthritis Cookbook and Health Guide

Canoleo 100%
canola margarine, and garlic flavored, too
The Natural Food Store
soybean soft margarine
Tryson House Buttery Delight
canola based butter flavored spray

SOUR CREAM

Tofutti Sour Supreme Soymage Low Fat Sour Cream Alternative
100% saturated fat, cholesterol, lactose, and trans fat (hydrogenated oil) free

CREAM CHEESE

Tofutti Better Than Cream Cheese
no dairy, cholesterol, butterfat, or lactose
SoyaKass Cream Cheese Style
no cholesterol, lactose, or trans fats (hydrogenated oil)
SoyCo Rice Low Fat Cream Cheese Alternative
100% saturated fat, cholesterol, soy, lactose, and trans fat (hydrogenated oil) free

SALAD OIL

Montebaldo
grape seed oil
Oils of Aloha
macadamia nut oil
Spectrum Naturals, Napa Valley, or Sadeg
cold pressed olive oil
Spectrum Naturals or Hain
pure or expeller pressed canola oil
Barlean's, Spectrum Naturals, or Flora
flax seed oil
Hempola or Spectrum Naturals
hemp oil

DRESSINGS

Follow Your Heart Dressings
available in cholesterol, dairy, and egg free flavors
NaSoya
cholesterol and saturated fat free
Annie's Naturals
available in no and low fat flavors
Paula's Dressings
no oil, no fat

Chapter 23 Health Foods

Spectrum Naturals
available in low/no fat flavors and the omega-3 line has beneficial flax seed oil
Pritikin Dressings
fat free

FRYING/COOKING OIL

Spectrum Skillet Spray
olive or canola for non-stick cooking

MILK

Rice Dream and Pacific
rice milk
Soy Dream, Better Than Milk, Edensoy, Vitasoy, Pacific, Westsoy and Silk
soy milk
Pacific
oat milk
Pacific
almond milk
Edenblend
rice and soy milk
Meyenberg
goat milk

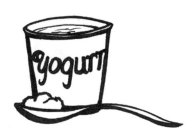

HALF AND HALF

White Wave Silk
soy milk creamer

YOGURT

Nancy's, Whole Soy, and White Wave Silk
yogurt

VINEGAR

Braggs, Spectrum Naturals, Sterling, and Natural Value
apple cider vinegar
Eden and Spectrum Naturals
red wine vinegar
Gaeta and Spectrum Naturals
balsamic vinegar

CHEESE

SoyaKaas
no cholesterol, lactose, or trans fats (hydrogenated oil). Low in saturated fat
Soymage Soy Singles and Vegan Singles
individually wrapped
Soyco
Rice Slices and Rice Parmesan
Veggy Singles and Veggy Parmesan
Rella
varieties made of tofu, almond, rice, and hemp

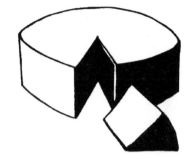

SOY SAUCE

San-J Tamari and Shoyu
Eden Tamari
Oishi Genen Shoyu
50% less salt soy sauce
Bragg Liquid Aminos

MAYONNAISE

Nasoya Nayonaise
cholesterol free, available in fat free and low fat varieties
Spectrum Naturals Lite Canola Mayonnaise
Hain Eggless Mayonnaise Dressing
Follow Your Heart Vegenaise
available in canola or grape seed varieties
Vegi Deli GourMayo
sandwich spread and dip, available in classic dijon, garlic and herb, chipotle, and pesto varieties

BREAD

Food For Life
Sprouted Breads
varieties include 7 Grain, Low Sodium, Sesame, Cinnamon Raisin, Millet Rice, and Spelt
Sprouted Hot Dog and Burger Buns
Sprouted English Style Muffins
Sprouted Bagels
French Meadow Breads and Bagels
varieties include kamut, rice, spelt, and sprouted grains
Alvarado St. Sprouted Breads
varieties include rye, barley, multigrain, and soy crunch
Alvarado St. Sprouted Bagels
varieties include granola crunch, sesame seed, onion poppy seed, and cinnamon raisin

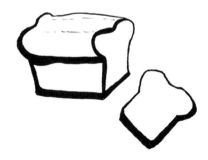

Nature's Path Manna Bread
unleavened sprouted wheat bread, varieties include whole rye, multigrain, apple and spice, cinnamon date, fruit and nut, millet rice, heritage kamut cranberry, carrot raisin, and sunseed

TORTILLA

Cedariane
blue corn, and whole wheat fat free tortillas
Alvarado St.
sprouted wheat tortillas
Rudy's Bakery
spelt tortillas
Garden of Eatin'
thin wraps

SODAS

Blue Sky, Hansen's, Knudsen Spritzer, Santa Cruz Organic, Journey, Reeds, Natural Brew, Health Valley, or Crystal Geyser Juice Squeeze
no artificial colors or flavors

ICED TEA

Tazo Tea
tea blended with juice for a natural sweetness
Honest Tea
a tiny amount of evaporated cane juice added to sweeten

JUICES

Knudsen, Santa Cruz Organic, After the Fall, Mountain Sun, L & A, or Ceres
no sugar, artificial colors, or flavors

BREAKFAST CEREAL

Barbara's
Shredded Oats, Shredded Spoonfuls, or Corn Flakes
Health Valley
Oat Bran Flakes, Amaranth Flakes, Rice Crunch-ems, or Golden Flax
Arrowhead Mills
Spelt Flakes, Kamut Flakes, Rye Flakes, Steel Cut Oats, Puffed Kamut, Puffed Millet, Puffed Rice, or Puffed Corn

328   The Executive Chef's Arthritis Cookbook and Health Guide

Golden Temple Peace Cereal
Mango Crisp with Kava and St. John's Wort, Wild Berry Crisp with Elderberry and Green Tea, Raspberry Ginger Crisp with Echinacea and Elderberry, Cinnamon Apple Crisp with Ginseng and Fo-ti, or Vanilla Almond Crisp with Ginko and Gotu Kola

Nature's Path
Millet Rice Flakes, Oaty Bites, Corn Flakes, Heritage (spelt, quinoa, and kamut)

Bob's Red Mill
5 grain, 10 grain, Scottish Oatmeal, Creamy Rice, Rolled Oats or Rolled Triticale

COOKIES
Wheat free, dairy free, no artificial colors or flavors

Health Valley
Peanut Crunch Oatmeal or Chocolate Chip Oatmeal

Pamela's
Ginger Cookies

Barbara's
Oatmeal Snackimals, Wheat Free Fat Free Fig Bars

Lotus Bakery
Peanut Butter Chocolate Chip or Peanut Butter

Newman's Own
Wheat Free Dairy Free Fig Newman's

Pride 'O the Farm
Fig Bars

The Alternative Baking Company
Choco Cherry Chunk and Mac the Chip

NUT BUTTERS
No oil, sugar, artificial colors or flavors added

Rejuvenative Foods
raw hemp seed butter, raw cashew butter, raw seed and nut spread

Maranatha
cashew, almond, peanut, or sesame tahini

Arrowhead Mills
peanut butter or sesame tahini

LM Healthy
soy nut butter

Natural Touch
soy nut butter

Health Trip
soy nut butter

JAMS AND FRUIT SPREADS

Sorrel Ridge
100% fruit black raspberry, apricot, blackberry, wild berry, strawberry, or orange marmalade
St. Dalflour
100% fruit strawberry, apricot, raspberry, or four fruits
Crofters
organic sweetened with grape juice, raspberry, apricot, blackberry, blueberry, strawberry, or black current
Eden, Knudsen, or L&A
apple butter

SOUPS

Imagine Foods
non dairy soups: creamy broccoli, creamy tomato, creamy mushroom, creamy butternut squash, creamy potato leek, vegetable broth, no-chicken broth, creamy sweet corn, or zesty gazpacho
Amy's Organic Soups
Health Valley Soups

FROZEN DESSERTS

Tofutti
pints, mini sandwiches, or popsicle style
Sweet Nothings
fat free, dairy free, and sweetened with rice syrup and fruit
Cascadian Farmer
fat free, organic, and dairy free sorbets: chocolate, strawberry, blackberry, mango, or peach
Rice Dream Ice Cream
nutty bars, cones, pies, bars or ice cream pints and quarts: vanilla, peanut butter cup, chocolate cherry chunk, pralines and dream, vanilla Swiss almond, cherry vanilla, cappuccino, cocoa marble fudge, Neapolitan, cookies and dream
Soy Delicious
the best non dairy ice cream! chocolate peanut butter, mint marble fudge, creamy vanilla, chocolate velvet, Neapolitan

MEATLESS BURGERS
Cholesterol free, low or no fat

Boca Burgers
very (97%-100%) low fat vegan original, chef Max's fave, or garlic
Garden Burger
garden vegan, roasted garlic

Amy's Organic
Texas, California, or Chicago Style
LightLife Light Burgers
BBQ or Lemon marinated grills

MEATLESS HOTDOGS
Cholesterol free, low or no fat

Yves
tofu weiners, jumbo veggie dogs, veggie wieners, veggie breakfast links
LightLife
tofu pups, smart dogs, lean Italian links

Chapter 23 Health Foods 331

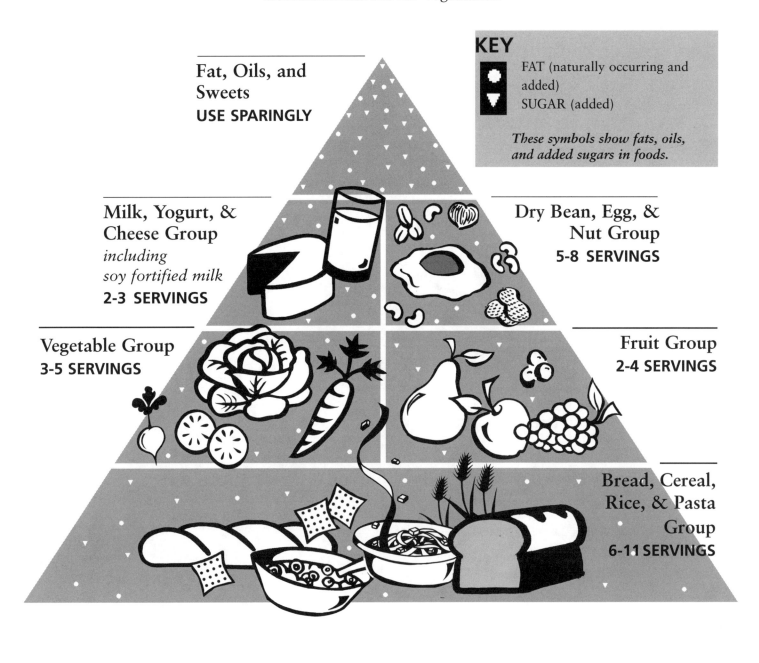

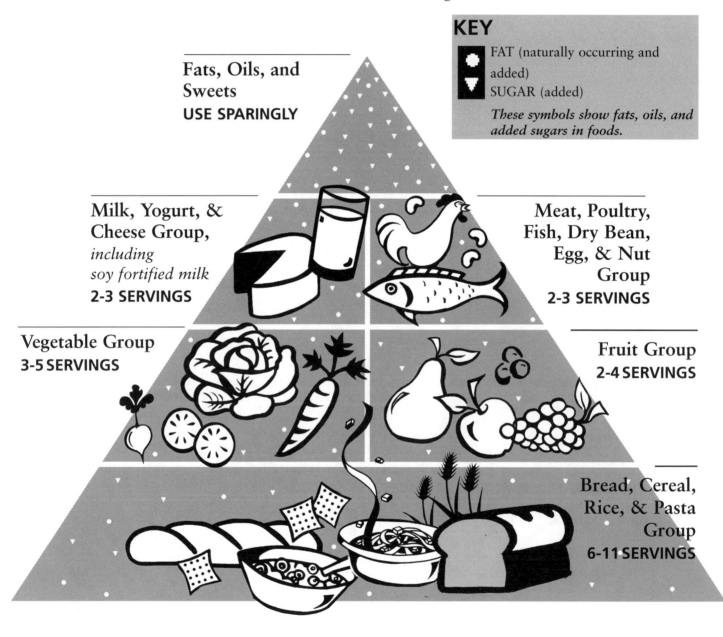

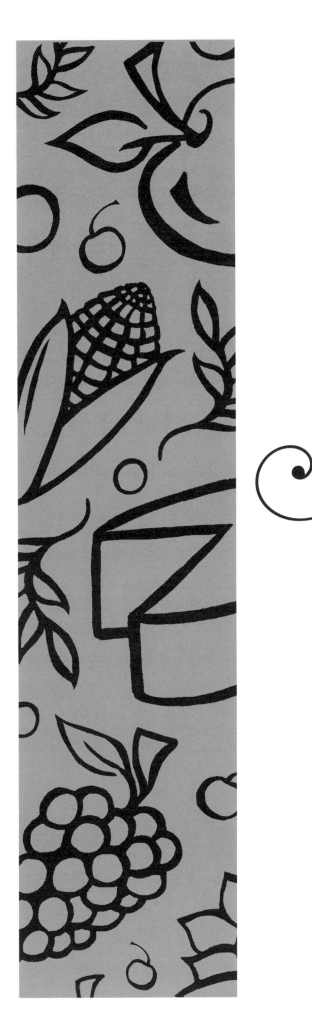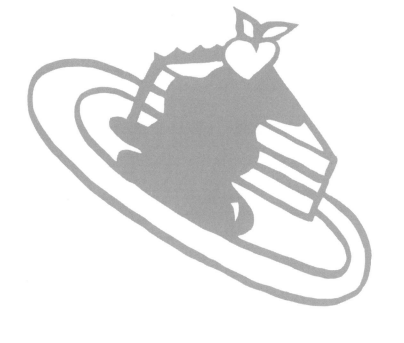

APPENDIX

Appendix

APPENDIX
TABLE OF EQUIVALENTS

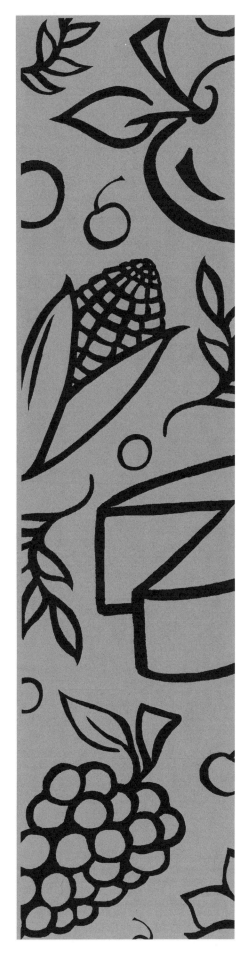

1 tsp.	=	1/6 oz.
3 tsp.	=	1 Tbsp.
2 Tbsp.	=	1 oz. (most liquids)
4 Tbsp.	=	2 oz.
8 Tbsp.	=	1/2 cup
16 Tbsp.	=	8 oz. = 1 cup = 1/2 lb.
4 oz.	=	1/2 cup
8 oz.	=	1 cup
16 oz.	=	1 lb.
1 pt.	=	16 oz.

(A pint is a pound the world around.)

2 cups	=	1 pt.
2 pts.	=	1 qt.
1 qt.	=	4 cups
1 jigger	=	3 Tbsp.

1 cup unwhipped cream	=	2 cups whipped
12-14 egg yolks	=	1 cup
8-10 egg whites	=	1 cup
1 lb. shredded cheese	=	3 - 4 cups
1/2 lb. bleu cheese, (crumbled)	=	2 cups
1 lemon	=	1-1/2 oz. juice
1 orange	=	3 - 4 oz. juice
2 cups fat	=	1 lb.
1 lb. butter or margarine	=	4 sticks
1 cup granulated sugar	=	8 oz.
1 lb. powdered sugar	=	3-1/2 - 4 cups
2-1/4 cups brown sugar	=	1 lb.
4 cups sifted flour	=	1 lb.
1/2 lb. raw macaroni	=	4-1/2 cups cooked
4 slices of bread	=	1 cup bread crumbs
15 graham crackers (crushed)	=	1 cup crumbs
22 vanilla wafers	=	1 cup crumbs
3 cups cornflakes (dry)	=	1 cup crushed
3 medium bananas	=	1 cup mashed
2 cups Oreo cookie crumbs + 2 Tbsp. melted butter	=	1 pie shell

SUGGESTED WEIGHTS FOR HEIGHTS FOR MEN AND WOMEN

Height in Inches	Weight (without clothing or shoes) Low lbs.	Med. lbs.	High lbs.
Men			
63	118	129	141
64	122	133	145
65	126	137	149
66	130	142	155
67	134	147	161
68	138	151	166
69	142	155	170
70	146	159	174
71	150	163	178
72	154	167	183
73	158	171	188
74	162	175	192
75	165	178	195
Women			
63	100	109	118
64	104	112	121
65	107	115	125
66	110	118	128
67	113	122	132
68	116	125	135
69	120	129	139
70	123	132	142
71	126	136	146
72	130	140	151
73	133	144	156
74	137	148	161
75	141	152	166

M.L. Hathaway and E.D. Foard, *Heights and Weights of Adults in the United States. Home Economics Research Report No. 10,* Table 80, p. 111. U.S. Department of Agriculture.

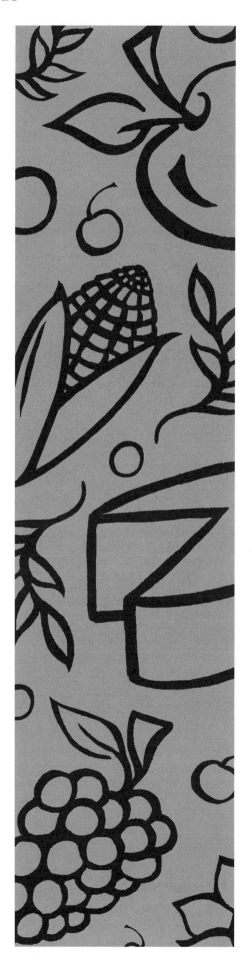

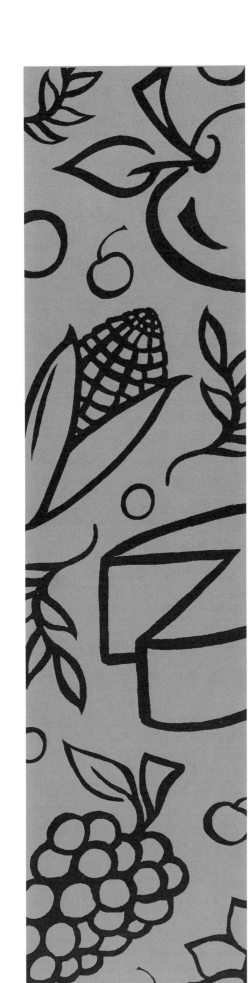

BIBLIOGRAPHY

Jethro Kloss. *Back to Eden*, 2nd ed. Loma Linda: Back to Eden Books Publishing Co., 1992.

All pamphlets from the Arthritis Foundation, especially:
Diet and Your Arthritis
Exercise and Your Arthritis

Sammons Preston™, Fred Sammons and J.A. Preston. *The Product Directory,* The Med Group, Lubbock, TX.

Phyllis A. Balch, CNC. and James F. Balch, MD., F.A.C.S. *Prescription for Cooking,* revised ed. Greenfield: PAB Books Publishing, Inc., 1987

Phyllis A. Balch, CNC, and James F. Balch, MD. *Prescription for Dietary Wellness.* Greenfield: PAB Books, Inc., 1992

James F. Balch, MD., and Phyllis A. Balch, CNC. *Prescription for Nutritional Healing,* Second Edition. Garden City park: Avery Publishing Group, 1997.

Arthritis Today Magazine. Arthritis Foundation.

Creative Brown Rice Cooking. Richvale: Lundberg Family Farms.

Publications of National Honey Board. Longmont, CO.

The Culinary Institute of America. *The Professional Chef*, 4th rev. ed. 1974

ARTHRITIS RESOURCES

The following are resources for additional educational materials and traditional treatment of arthritis that I recommend to my patients. Visit these great websites to learn more about organizations who specialize in helping people suffering from arthritis.

Organizations

1. **Arthritis Foundation**
   P.O. Box 7669
   Atlanta, GA 30357-0669
   1-800-283-7800
   www.arthritis.org

   The mission of the Arthritis Foundation is to support research to find the cure for and prevention of arthritis and to improve the quality of life for those affected by arthritis.

2. **American College of Rheumatology**
   1800 Century Place, Suite 250
   Atlanta, GA 30345
   (404) 633-3777
   www.rheumatology.org

   The American College of Rheumatology is the professional organization of rheumatologists and associated health professionals who share a dedication to healing, preventing disability, and curing the more than 100 types of arthritis and related disabling and sometimes fatal disorders of the joints, muscles, and bones.

3. **Arthritis Society**
   393 University Avenue, Suite 1700
   Toronto, Ontario M5G 1E6
   CANADA
   (416) 979-8366
   www.arthritis.ca

   Arthritis Society pursues its mission to help people with arthritis by promoting, evaluating, and funding in the area of causes, prevention, treatment, and cures of arthritis. Great website providing information, effective emotional and practical support to people with arthritis and those near them.

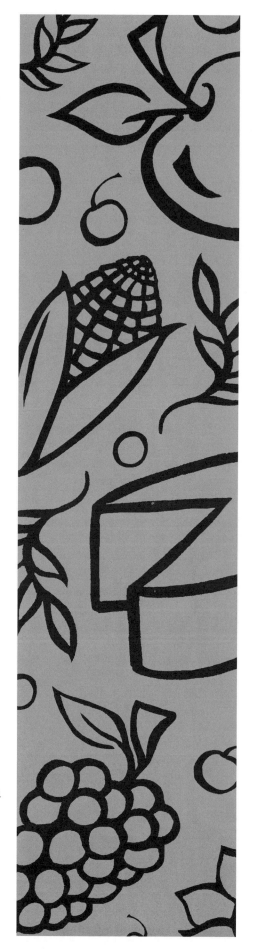

Appendix 339

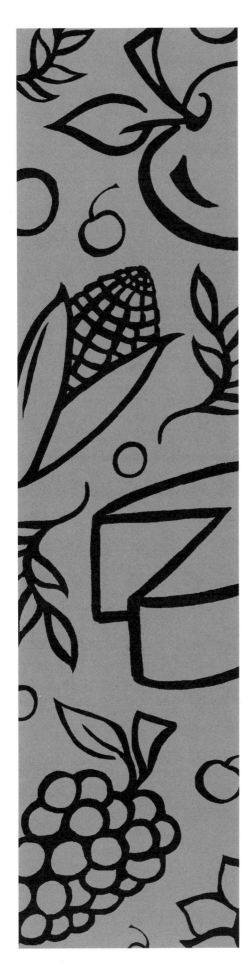

4. **National Osteoporosis Foundation (NOF)**
    1232 22nd Street N.W.
    Washington, DC 20037-1292
    (202) 223-2226
    www.nof.org

    The leading nonprofit, voluntary health organization dedicated to promoting lifelong bone health in order to reduce the widespread prevalence of osteoporosis and associated fractures, while working to find a cure for the disease through programs of research, education, and advocacy.

5. **Fibromyalgia Network**
    P.O. Box 31750
    Tucson, AZ 85751
    1-800-853-2929
    www.fmnetnews.com

    Provides educational materials on fibromyalgia syndrome and chronic fatigue syndrome such as coping techniques, research studies, medical journal listings, drug updates, non-drug treatments, disability and political issues.

Books and magazines to empower you to self-care and help you to stay current with all the latest arthritis research, new therapies, and alternative treatments

1. *Arthritis Today Magazine*
    To order call 1-800-933-0032

    Most widely read comprehensive and reliable source of information about arthritis research, care, and treatment, offering help and hope to the nearly 43 million Americans who have an arthritis-related condition.

2. *The Arthritis Foundation's Guide to Alternative Therapies*
    by Judith Horstman
    To order call 1-800-207-8633

    Get the latest, most reliable information about nearly 90 different types of alternative treatments and therapies.

3. *Celebrate Life: New Attitudes for Living with Chronic Illness*
    by Kathleen Lewis, R.N.
    To order call 1-800-207-8633

    From relationships and doctors' visits to exercise and therapy, *Celebrate Life* will guide you in rebuilding your physical, emotional, and spiritual life.

4. *Arthritis Health Monitor*
   Data Centrum Communications INC
   21 W 38th Street, Floor 4
   New York NY 10138-0981

   An ongoing information program designed to keep you up to date in arthritis news important to you.

5. *Making Sense of Fibromyalgia*
   by Daniel and Janice Wallace
   To order call 1-800-207-8633

   This unique, easy-to-understand compendium explains the history, science, and treatment of fibromyalgia.

6. *Your Personal Guide to Living Well with Fibromyalgia*
   by the Arthritis Foundation
   To order call 1-800-207-8633

   Takes you step-by-step through the fundamentals of improving your life with fibromyalgia.

Websites to assist you in your quest for optimal health. These sites are trustworthy and give valuable and reliable current information for your wellness.

1. www. drkoop.com
   This is the home page of Dr. C. Everett Koop, former U.S. Surgeon General, and others who are dedicated to improving the quality of people's lives by empowering them to improve their health

2. www.intelihealth.com
   A subsidiary of Aetna, InteliHealth provides credible information and useful tools from more than 150 top health care organizations. InteliHealth's expert editors "consumerize" health information to make it accessible to the widest possible audience.

3. www.webmd.com
   WebMD features breaking health news, live chat events, message boards, a directory of physicians, virtually anything that has to do with healthcare information and education.

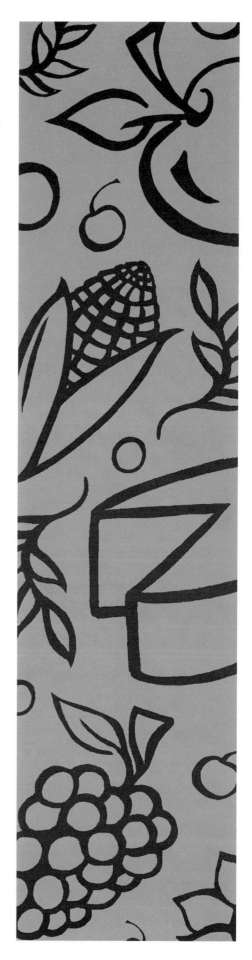

Appendix 341

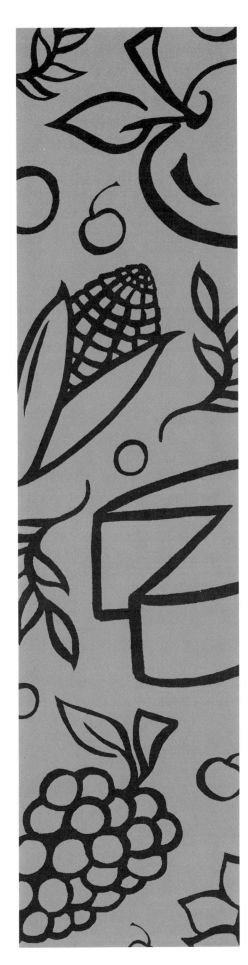

4. **www.mayohealth.org**
Mayo's website gives you access to the experience and knowledge of the more than 2,000 physicians and scientists of the Mayo Clinic.

5. **www.discoveryhealth.com**
At discoveryhealth.com, an online health service, you will learn more about the diseases, conditions, and medical breakthroughs that you've seen on Discovery Health Channel, the 24-hour television channel.

6. **www.medscape.com**
Medscape delivers products and services that provide reliable, digital clinical data and up-to-date information to healthcare professionals and consumers.

7. **www.healthcentral.com**
HealthCentral.com provides trustworthy health information and tools for consumers and healthcare institutions.

8. **www.allhealth.com**
allHealth is iVillage.com's health channel.

9. **www.jr2.ox.ac.uk/bandolier**
Bandolier is a print and Internet journal about health care, using evidence-based medicine techniques to provide advice about particular treatments or diseases for health care professionals and consumers.

10. **www.herbmed.org**
HerbMed®—an interactive, electronic herbal database—provides hyperlinked access to the scientific data underlying the use of herbs for health. It is an evidence-based information resource for professionals, researchers, and the general public. HerbMed® is a project of the Alternative Medicine Foundation, Inc., provided as a freely available, public resource.

11. **www.quackwatch.com**
Quackwatch Your Guide to Health Fraud, Quackery, and Intelligent Decisions—combats health-related frauds, myths, fads, and fallacies.

12. **www.tnp.com**
TNP.com cuts through the hype and tells you what is known and what remains to be scientifically proven regarding popular natural treatments.

342 The Executive Chef's Arthritis Cookbook and Health Guide

Resources for alternative and complementary medicine that I recommend to my patients

Organizations

1. **National Center for Complementary and Alternative Medicine**
   National Institutes of Health (NIH)
   Box 8218
   Silver Spring, MD 20907-8218
   1-888-644-6226
   www.nccam.nih.gov

2. **Center for Mind-Body Medicine**
   5225 Connecticut Avenue, NW, Suite 414
   Washington, DC 20015
   (202) 966-7338
   www.cmbm.org

3. **The Ayurvedic Institute**
   11311 Menaul NE, Suite A
   Albuquerque, NM 87112
   (505) 291-9698
   www.ayurveda.com

4. **Council for Responsible Nutrition**
   1875 Eye Street, NW, Suite 400
   Washington, DC 20006
   (202) 872-1488
   www.crnusa.org

5. **American Botanical Council**
   P.O. Box 144345
   Austin, TX 78714-4345
   (512) 926-4900
   www.herbalgram.org

6. **Herb Research Foundation**
   1007 Pearl Street, Suite 200
   Boulder, CO 80302
   (303) 449-2265
   www.herbs.org

7. **American Music Therapy Association, Inc.**
   8455 Colesville Road, Suite 1000
   Silver Spring, MD 20910
   (301) 589-3300
   www.musictherapy.org

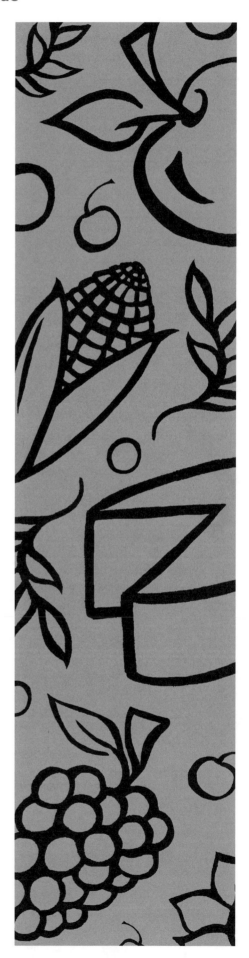

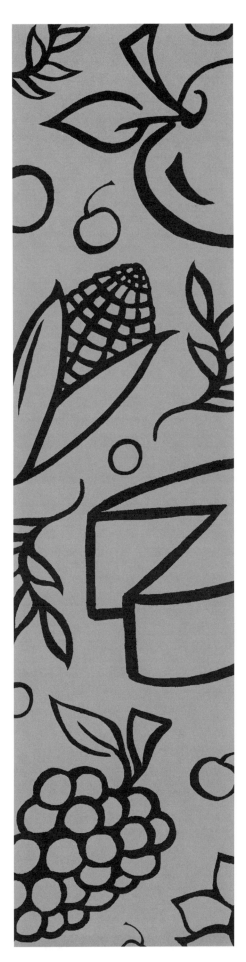

8. **American Art Therapy Association, Inc.**
   1202 Allanson Road
   Mundelein, IL 60060-3808
   1-888-290-0878 or (847) 949-6064
   www.arttherapy.org

9. **Interfaith Health Program**
   Rollins School of Public Health
   Emory University
   750 Commerce Drive, Suite 301
   Decatur, GA 30030
   (404) 592-1461
   www.ihpnet.org

10. **American Massage Therapy Association**
    820 Davis Street, Suite 100
    Evanston, IL 60201-4444
    (847) 864-0123
    www.amtamassage.org

Recommended reading about complementary and alternative approaches to wellness

1. *The Healthy Mind, Healthy Body Handbook,* by David S. Sobel, MD and Robert E. Ornstein, PhD. ISHK Book Service. 1997.

2. *Manifesto for a New Medicine: Your Guide to Healing Partnerships and the Wise Use of Alternatives Therapies,* by James S. Gordon. Perseus Pr. 1997.

3. *8 Weeks to Optimum Health: A Proven Program for Taking Full Advantage of your Body's Natural Healing Power,* by Andrew Weil, MD. Fawcett Books. 1998.

4. *Love, Medicine and Miracles: Lessons Learned About Self-Healing From A Surgeon's Experience With Exceptional Patients,* by Bernie S. Siegal, MD. Harperperennial Library. 1990.

5. *Herb Contraindications and Drug Interactions: With Appendices Addressing Specific Conditions and Medicines,* by Francis Brinker, ND. Eclectic Medical Publications. 1997.

6. *Freedom Through Health: Holistic Approach to Better Health along with Diseases and Therapies of the Twenty-First Century,* by Terry Shepherd Friedmann, MD. Harvest Publishing. 1998.

Websites recommended that are trustworthy and of interest for a complementary/alternative approach to wellness

1. **www.compmed.ummc.umaryland.edu**
   Great source for research in complementary/alternative therapies and pain, from the University of Maryland Complementary Medicine Program.

2. **www.consumerlab.com**
   Find out whether your herb or supplement contains exactly the ingredients it claims to have. ConsumerLab.com's site provides results of independent tests of products that affect health and well-being.

3. **www.herbs.org**
   Herb Research Foundation's website focuses on medicinal plants. Site features news, scientific research, regulatory updates, photo gallery, and extensive herb links.

4. **chili.rt66.com/hrbmoore/homepage/homepage.html**
   Michael Moore's Home Page features more than 1,400 botanical photographs and illustrations, as well as various herb manuals.

5. **www.drweil.com**
   Ask Dr. Weil offers a large database of commonly asked questions by patients about various complementary/alternative treatments for various diseases. Great links to lots of useful information.

6. **www.drkarenwolfe.com**
   Dr. Karen Wolfe is an international speaker, author of six books and Principal of Healing Quest. She is a licensed physician in Australia and worked in the administration of national health care.

Here are the addresses for two sources of arthritis-friendly tools:

C.R. Newton
1575 S. Beretania Street, Suite 101
Honolulu, HI 96826
Phone (808) 949-8389
Fax (808) 955-4721

Sammons Preston
P.O. Box 5071
Bolingbrook, IL 60440-5071
Phone 1-800-323-5547
Fax 1-800-547-4333

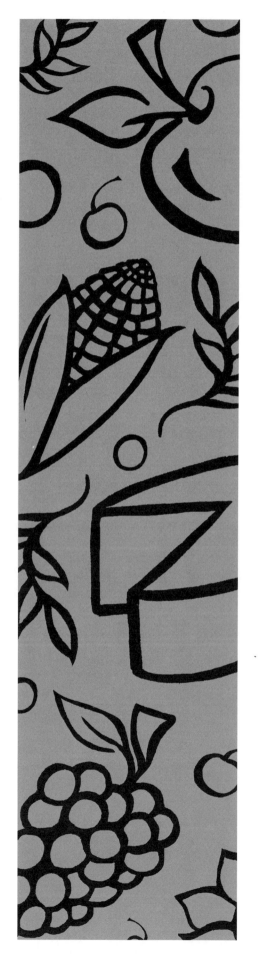

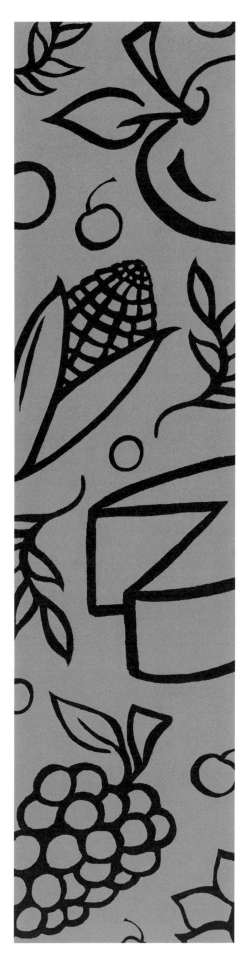

GLOSSARY

Here are definitions of commonly used terms in arthritis care:

American College of Rheumatology (ACR)
The American College of Rheumatology is the professional organization of rheumatologists and associated health professionals who share a dedication to healing, preventing disability, and curing the more than 100 types of arthritis and related disabling and sometimes fatal disorders of the joints, muscles, and bones. Members include practicing physicians, research scientists, nurses, physical and occupational therapists, psychologists, and social workers.

Arthralgia
Arthralgia is aching of the joint.

Arthritis
Arthritis is the most prevalent of chronic diseases. The word *arthritis* means 'inflammation' or 'damage to joints.' Warning signs of arthritis are pain, stiffness, swelling in or around a joint, associated with loss of motion. There are more than 100 different forms of arthritis.

Arthritis Foundation
The Arthritis Foundation is a national, nonprofit health organization that works for all people affected by any of the 100-plus forms of arthritis or related diseases. The vision of the Arthritis Foundation is to support research to find the cure for and prevention of arthritis and to improve the quality of life for those affected by arthritis.

Bursitis/Tendonitis
Inflammation of a bursa or tendon that occurs most commonly in the shoulder, elbow, hip, and knee. This usually occurs after the joint has been overused or when the joint has become deformed by arthritis. Bursitis/tendonitis makes it painful to move or put pressure on the affected joint.

DMARD (disease modifying anti-inflammatory rheumatic drug)
Drug used for rheumatoid arthritis and other chronic inflammatory arthritis diseases. DMARDs reduce inflammation and may slow progression of the disease.

Gelling
Stiffness and tightness of a joint after a period of inactivity, which improves after a few minutes of moving the joints.

Impingement
Impingement generally refers to inflammation of the tendons and bursae of the shoulder that causes a painful elevation of the shoulder past a certain point (anywhere between 65 degrees and 105 degrees).

Myalgia/Myositis
Myalgia is aching of the muscles, which differs from myositis that is inflammation of the muscles with associated weakness.

Myofascial Pain
Diffuse muscle aching that localizes to one anatomical location association with trigger/painful points of the muscle (i.e., upper neck and across shoulder).

NSAID (nonsteroidal anti-inflammatory drug)
A type of drug that does not contain steroids, but is used to help relieve pain by reducing inflammation.

Occupational Therapist
One who has completed an approved educational program to help improve a person's ability to perform daily tasks, facilitate successful adaptation to disruptions in lifestyle, and prevent loss of function. Patients are trained in alternate methods and the use of adaptive equipment for performing daily self-care, work/school, or leisure/play tasks.

Physical Therapist
One who has completed an approved educational program to help others work toward the achievement of optimal function and the relief of pain. The ultimate goal is to assist the patient's physical recovery and re-entry into the home, community, and work environment at the highest level of independence and self-sufficiency. The therapist uses therapeutic exercise to improve a patient's muscle strength and joint mobility. Therapists also use numerous modalities (heat, cold, electrical therapy, hydrotherapy, etc.) to help relieve pain.

Rheumatologist
A rheumatologist is an internist or pediatrician who is qualified by additional training and experience in the diagnosis and treatment of arthritis and other diseases of the joints, muscles, and bones. Many rheumatologists conduct research to determine the cause and better treatment for these disabling and sometimes fatal diseases.

Rheumatology
Field of study that specializes in research, diagnosis, treatment, and prevention of arthritis and related disorders.

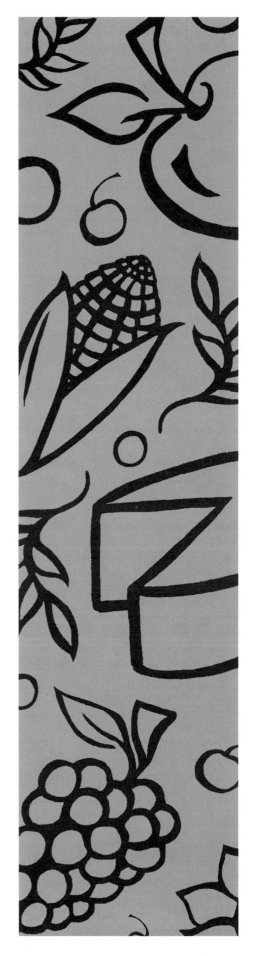

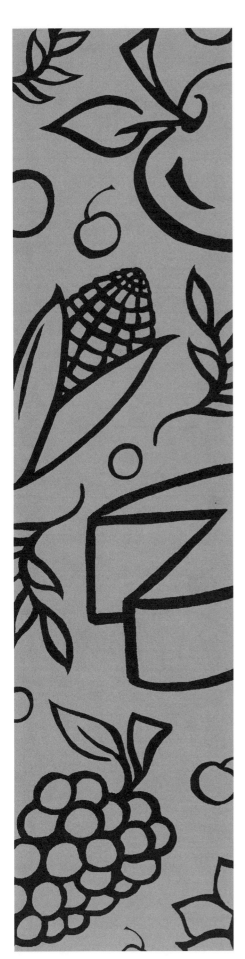

Syndrome
A collection of symptoms and/or physical findings that characterize a particular abnormal condition or illness (e.g., fibromyalgia pain syndrome, chronic fatigue syndrome)

Tenderpoints
Areas in the body that are abnormally sensitive, causing pain when pressed. People with fibromyalgia have tender points in certain areas of the body. Presence of these tender points helps in the diagnosis of fibromyalgia. Has been used interchangeably in the past with *trigger point*.

NUTRITIONAL ANALYSIS

The nutritional analyses that accompany the recipes were created with Computrition, Inc.'s Nutritional Software Library. Given the ingredients, their quantities and number of servings, the program automatically calculates serving size and nutritional content. The program uses a database of nutritional values for foods ranging from raw ingredients to pre-packaged foods, including spices and organic products. These values were primarily obtained from the U.S. Department of Agriculture's Nutrient Database. In addition, new foods or whole recipes can be added to the database and used as ingredients in subsequent recipes. Some 24 nutrients are available for each food item.

CONTACT PAGE

Arthritis Cookbook Corporation
P. O. Box 880130
Pukalani, HI 96768
E-Mail: arthritiscookbook@maui.net
Fax: (808) 572-6746

Heavenly Hawaiian Recipes

In 1986, Executive Chef Carl Haupt published his first cookbook, *Heavenly Hawaiian Recipes*. We have a few signed, first edition copies available. If you would like a copy, please use the order form in the back of the book. Here's what Chef Carl wrote about the book in his introduction.

"Heavenly Hawaiian Recipes has been an idea of mine for some years. I finally found the time to complete the project. This booklet contains many Hawaiian recipes that were tested and made better for today's world and for the cooking methods of today. This booklet was designed for the housewife and the homestyle cook. You don't have to be a chef to make these dishes. I wrote the recipes as if I were there telling you how to do them.

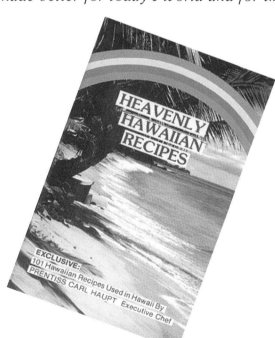

This is a simple book to understand if you have a small understanding about cooking. It should also be a lot of fun. You will also be able to impress your friends and relatives. Some of these recipes are not Hawaiian but are used here in the Hawaiian world of cooking. They are still very nice. I hope you enjoy these recipes which include many of my favorites." ALOHA!

Prentiss Carl Haupt
Certified Executive Chef

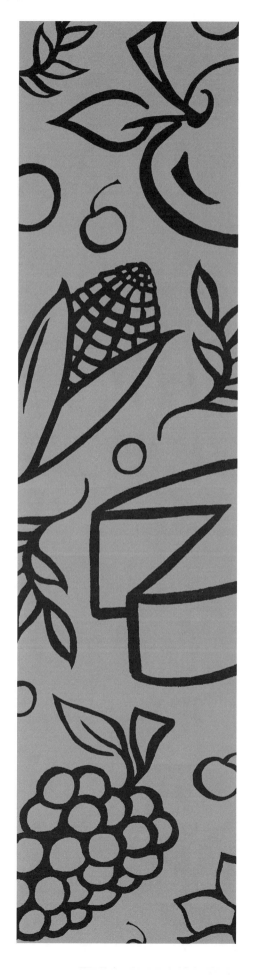

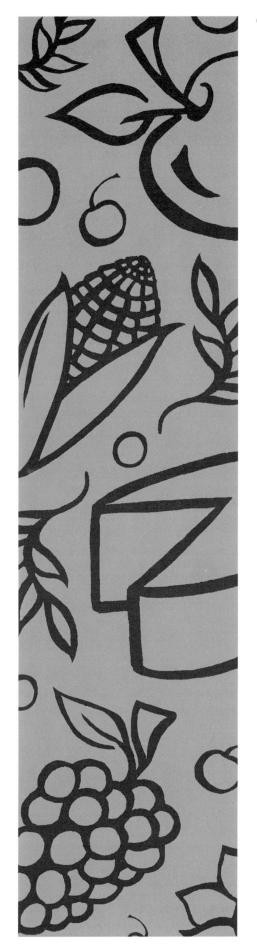

Carl's little brother...

KURT'S KANDLES
The Kandle with a Kandle in the Lid™
- **Handkrafted**
- **Superior Fragrance**
- **Extended Burn Time**

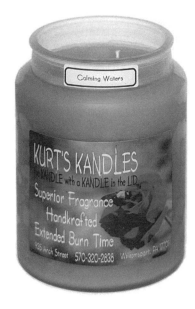
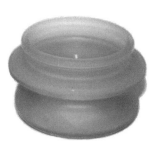

Kurt's Kandles are handcrafted with TWO wicks to give you an even burn. Kurt's special wax makes the kandle burn longer than most candles of the same size. You'll love the superior fragrance in Kurt's Kandles. Best of all, you get two kandles in one. The lid of each kandle is a separate 3 oz. kandle in itself that you can burn somewhere else or when the main kandle is finished.

Kurt's Kandles come in three size jars:

	10 oz.	16 oz.	24 oz.
Burns up to:	65 hours	105 hours	160 hours

Aromatherapy uses essences of plants to promote the well-being of our mind and emotions through our sense of smell. You can create different moods such as Calming, Revitalizing, Restful, Passion, and more. Some of these essences are bergamot, cedarwood, sandalwood, patchouli, lavender, jasmine, rose, rosemary, peppermint, and ylang ylang.

Request a catalog or order from:
Kurt's Kandles
935 Arch Street
Williamsport, PA 17701
(570) 320-2838
Website: www.kurtskandles.com
E-Mail: chaupt@blazenet.net

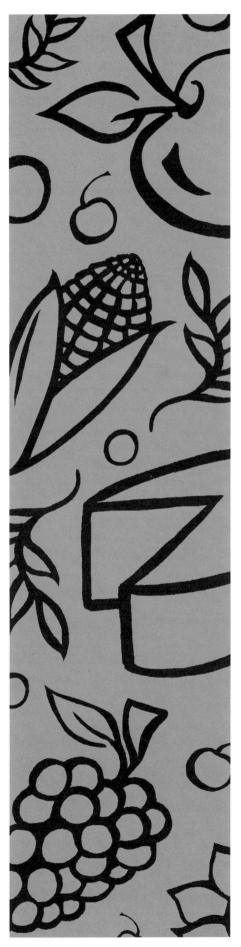

ORDER FORM

You can order extra copies of this book from our website at www.arthritiscookbook.com or fill out and fax this form to (808) 572-6746 or mail this form to the address below.

#	Title	Price	Total
__	Executive Chef's Arthritis Cookbook (hard cover)	$32.95	$ _____
__	Executive Chef's Arthritis Cookbook (paperback)	$24.95	$ _____
__	Heavenly Hawaii Cookbook (paperback)	$ 9.95	$ _____

Subtotal _____

Shipping and Handling: U.S. $4.95 per book   Shipping _____

4% Tax (HI only) _____

TOTAL _____

Name: _____
Company: _____
Address: _____
City: _____ State: _____ ZIP: _____
Phone: _____ Fax: _____
E-Mail Address: _____

❏ Check enclosed   ❏ Visa   ❏ Mastercard
Card Number: _____
Name on card: _____ Exp. Date: _____
Signature: _____

Arthritis Cookbook Corporation
P. O. Box 880130
Pukalani, HI 96768
E-Mail: arthritiscookbook@maui.net
Fax: (808) 572-6746

Your satisfaction is guaranteed or your money will be cheerfully refunded!

352

Appendix 353

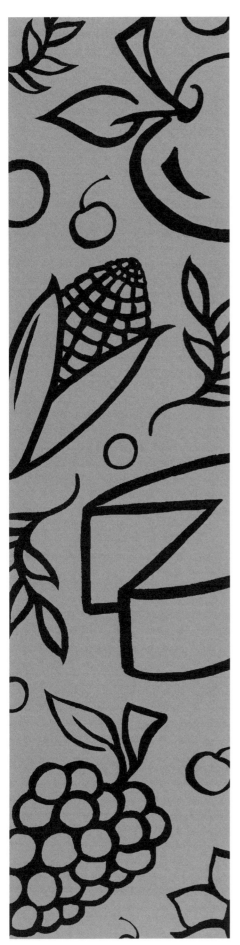

ORDER FORM
You can order extra copies of this book from our website at www.arthritiscookbook.com or fill out and fax this form to (808) 572-6746 or mail this form to the address below.

#	Title	Price	Total
___	Executive Chef's Arthritis Cookbook (hard cover)	$32.95	$ _____
___	Executive Chef's Arthritis Cookbook (paperback)	$24.95	$ _____
___	Heavenly Hawaii Cookbook (paperback)	$ 9.95	$ _____

Subtotal _____
Shipping and Handling: U.S. $4.95 per book   Shipping _____
4% Tax (HI only) _____

TOTAL _____

Name: _____
Company: _____
Address: _____
City: _____ State: _____ ZIP: _____
Phone: _____ Fax: _____
E-Mail Address: _____

❏ Check enclosed   ❏ Visa   ❏ Mastercard
Card Number: _____
Name on card: _____ Exp. Date: _____
Signature: _____

Arthritis Cookbook Corporation
P. O. Box 880130
Pukalani, HI 96768
E-Mail: arthritiscookbook@maui.net
Fax: (808) 572-6746

Your satisfaction is guaranteed or your money will be cheerfully refunded!

354

INDEX

A

Advice for Those Seeking an Herbal Cure 51
Alternative Treatments 51
Appendix 335
    Arthritis Resources 338
    Bibliography 337
    Contact Page 348
    Glossary 345
    Heavenly Hawaiian Recipes 348
    Kurt's Kandles 349
    Nutritional Analysis 347
    Order Form 351
    Suggested Weights for Height 336
    Table of Equivalents 335
Appetizers 181-186
    Citrus Salsa 184
    Fruit Salsa with Red Onion 185
    Garlic Bread 183
    Guacamole 186
    Mushrooms Stuffed With Crabmeat 182
Apples 99
Arava (leflunomide) 43
Arthritis 21-38
    Osteoarthritis 21
    Rheumatoid Arthritis 23
Arthritis and Nutrition 69
Arthritis Treatment 74
Artificial Sweeteners 78
Asparagus 252
    Steamed Asparagus 253
    Stir Fried Asparagus with Chicken and Nuts 252

B

Beans 254
    Green Bean Salad with Mushrooms and Sprouts 255
    Green Beans in Olive Oil with Garlic and Nuts 256
    Green Beans Sauteed with Sliced Almonds 254
    Yellow Beans with Nuts and Garlic Chives 257
Beets 258
    Sauteed Beet Greens 258
Bread 79
Broccoli 259
    Steamed Broccoli 259

Broth 153-158
    Vegetable broth 153
Brussels Sprouts 260
    Brussels Sprout Salad 260

C

Cabbage 262
    Sauteed Red Cabbage 262
Carbohydrates 75
Carrots 261
Case Studies 70
Chicken 283
    Chicken Breast Teriyaki Style 286
    Orange Chicken Salad 283
    Papaya Surprise Filled with Chicken Salad 285
Chronic Fatigue Syndrome 32
Complementary Treatments 51
    Chronic Fatigue Syndrome 56
    Fibromyalgia 56
    Osteoarthritis 54
    Rheumatoid Arthritis 55
Cooking Fish and Seafood 295
Cooking Methods 147-150
    Dry Heat 148
    Dry Heat Using Fat 147
    Moist Heat 147
COX-2 Inhibitors 41
Croutons 210

D

Desserts 313
    Banana Bread 319
    Double Peanut Butter Cookies 318
    Fresh Berries with Pure Maple Syrup 315
    Peach Crisp 316
    Pineapple Papaya Upside Down Cake 314
    Whole Wheat Bread Pudding 317

E

Exercise and Arthritis 28

F

Fats 119
    Monounsaturated Fats 121
    Polyunsaturated Fats 120
Fibromyalgia Syndrome 30

Fish 291
Fish Flavors 292
Poached Cold Fish with Oil, Lemon
Juice, and Fresh Herb Dressing 297
Food Pyramid - Non-Vegetarian 332
Food Pyramid - Vegetarian 331

G
Game Hens 284
Apricot and Tangerine Glazed Game
Hens 284
Garlic 263
Cream of Roasted Garlic Soup with
Chicken 265
Garlic Oil 266
Gene Therapy 45
Grains 230
Green and Leafy Vegetables 251

H
Health Food Substitutes 323
Health Foods 323
Herbs 137-144
Basil 137
Bay Leaf 138
Cilantro 137
Dill 138
Mint 140
Oregano 140
Parsley 138
Rosemary 139
Sage 139
Tarragon 139
Thyme 139
Watercress 138
Herbs And Spices, How To Select 142
Herbs And Spices, How To Store 142
Homemade Yogurt 220
Honey 100-104
Buying and Storage 101
Forms and Flavors 102
Honey Nutrition Facts 101
Honey Tip Sheet 100
Honey Glazed Carrots 261

I
Innovative Treatments 41
Arava (leflunomide) 43
COX-2 Inhibitors 41

Gene Therapy 45
Prosorba Column 44
Remicade (infliximab) 44
TNF-Blocking Agents 44
Viscosupplementation 41
Instant Non-Fat Dry Milk 222

K
Kitchen Tools 127-134

L
Leeks 267
Lettuce 207

M
Marinades and Bastes for Fish 174-178
Basting Mixture for Boiled or Barbecued Fish
176
Fish Marinade for Baking 176
Ginger Soy Marinade 175
Lemon Butter with Garlic Baste 174
Tangerine Basil Parmesan Marinade 175
Mind/Body Medicine 59-66
Aromatherapy 60
Guided Imagery 60
Meditation 60
Music Therapy 61
Spirituality 60
Support Groups 61
Yoga 61
Miracle Spread, Low-Fat 222
Mushrooms 267
Sauteed Mushrooms with Orange Mustard
Sauce 268

N
NO Foods 87-96
Foods High in Purines 91
Nightshades 87
Other Foods 92
Nutrition and Arthritis 27

O
Onions 269
Maui Onions and Mushrooms 270
Osteoarthritis 21

Osteoporosis 34
   Drug Treatment 37
   Monitoring, Prevention, and Treatment 36
   Risk Factors 36

P
Pea Pods 271
   Stir Fried Pea Pods with Shrimp and Water
      Chestnuts 271
Potatoes 239-248
   Baked Stuffed Potatoes 243
   Candied Sweet Potatoes 245
   German Potato Salad 246
   Mashed Potatoes 244
   Oven Roasted Potatoes 247
   Parsley Buttered Potatoes 242
   Perfect Baked Potato 241
   Potatoes Fried in Garlic Oil 241
Poultry 277
   Buying, Storing and Handling 278
   Classification and Pointers 279
Prosorba Column 44

R
Refined Flour 79
Remicade (infliximab) 44
Rheumatoid Arthritis 23
   Diagnosis 25
   Evaluation 24
   Management 25
   Nonpharmacologic Therapy 26
   Symptoms 23
Rice 229
   Brown Rice 232
   Electric Rice Cooker 231
   Fried Rice 233
   Lundberg Wild Blend 234
   White Rice 235
   Wild Rice 231
Roux 122
   Brown Roux 123
   White Roux 122

S
Salad Dressings 207-226
   Bleu Cheese Dressing with Fresh Basil 210
   Chutney Dressing 216
   Creamy Coconut Dressing 226

Creamy Horseradish Dressing 212
   Fruit Salad Dressing with Honey 226
   Mustard Vinaigrette 209
   Orange Cream Dressing 218
   Pineapple Lemon Dressing 216
   Tangerine Mayonnaise 209
   Toasted Coconut Chips 218
Salads 207-226
   Ambrosia Salad Hawaiian Style 217
   Carrot and Raisin Salad with Pineapple
      224
   Chicken and Fruit Salad 215
   Coleslaw 211
   Coleslaw and Pineapple Salad 225
   Marinated Broccoli Salad 219
   Six Fruit Salad Maui Style 213
   Spinach and Romaine Salad 212
   Spinach, Turkey, Bacon, and Mushroom
      Salad 208
   Stuffed Papayas or Avocados 214
Salt 80
Salt Substitute 84
Sauces 161-178
   Barbecue Sauce 171
   Basic Sauce Veloute 168
   Bechamel 166
   Brown Sauce 165
   Categories of Sauces 162
   Cheese Sauce 170
   Hollandaise Sauce 169
   Mushroom Sauce 170
   Orange Mustard Sauce 173
   Pesto 177
   Sauce Poulette 172
   Sweet and Sour Sauce 171
   Tartar Sauce with Capers 173
   Teriyaki Sauce and Marinade 172
   Tomato Sauce 168
   White Sauce No. 1 (Light) 166
   White Sauce No. 2 (Medium) 166
   White Sauce No. 3 (Heavy) 167
Seafood 291
   Artichoke Bottoms with Kula Style
      Crabmeat 299
   Baked Stuffed Shrimp 304
   Broiled Seafood Brochettes with Lemon
      and Herbs 298
   Crab Dip 305
   Crab Louis 303

Seafood (Continued)
Crab Salad Kula Style 296
How to Select Seafood 294
Oyster Stew 306
Sauteed Scallops 307
Scampi Olowalu 301
Shrimp and Scallop Seviche 308
Shrimp Cocktail on a Plate with Basil
  Mayonnaise 300
Shrimp on a Skewer 309
Shrimp Salad with Basil Mayonnaise 302
Shallots 272
Roasted Shallots and New Potatoes 272
Shallot Oil 273
Sodium Compounds 83
Soups 189-204
Avocado Soup 193
Broccoli Soup with Diced Chicken 194
Chicken Barley Soup 198
Chicken Corn Soup with Noodles 195
Chicken Noodle Soup 196
Chilled Yogurt Soup with Fruits 190
Cream of Broccoli Soup 191
Cream of Crab Curry Soup 192
Cream of Mushroom Soup 201
Hawaiian Style Seafood Chowder 197
Onion Soup with Cheese and Croutons 199
Split Pea Soup with Chicken 200
Sweet Potato Soup 203
Vegetable Soup with Chicken Broth 202
Sour Cream, Low-Fat 222
Soy Milk 223
Spices 140-144
Allspice 141
Celery Seed 141
Chili Powder 141
Cinnamon 142
Cloves 141
Fennel 141
Ginger 141
Nutmeg 141
Paprika 140
Pepper 140
Sprouts 273
Stocks 153-158
Chicken Stock 154
Court Bouillon 155
Fish Stock 156
Turkey Stock 157

Stress and Arthritis 28
Top 10 Stressors 29
Sugar 77

T
TNF-Blocking Agents 44
Tofu 223
Turkey 280
Carl's Perfect Way to Roast a Turkey 287
Turkey Noodle Soup 280
Turkey Rice Soup 280
Turkey Salad Sandwich 282
Watercress Soup with Turkey 281

V
Viscosupplementation 41

W
Water 107-116
How Safe Is Your Water? 109
Major Contaminants 112
Six Ways To Get Safe Water 113
Sources Of Drinking Water 110
Testing Your Tap Water 114
Whipping Cream, Low Fat 221

Z
Zucchini 274
Grilled Zucchini 274